FOUNDATIONS OF AURAL REHABILITATION

Children, Adults, and Their Family Members

A Singular Audiology Textbook
Jeffrey L. Danhauer, Ph.D.
Audiology Editor

FOUNDATIONS
OF
AURAL REHABILITATION

Children, Adults, and Their Family Members

Nancy Tye-Murray, Ph.D.

Central Institute for the Deaf
St. Louis, Missouri

With a Chapter by

William Clark, Ph.D.

Central Institute for the Deaf
St. Louis Missouri

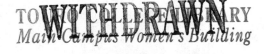
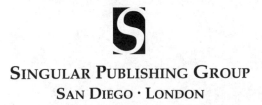

SINGULAR PUBLISHING GROUP
SAN DIEGO · LONDON

WB

COPYRIGHT © 1998
Singular Publishing Group is a division of Thomson Learning. The Thomson Learning logo is a registered trademark used herein under license.

Printed in the United States of America
5 6 7 8 9 10 XXX 05 04 03 02 01

For more information, contact Singular Publishing Group, 401 West "A" Street, Suite 325 San Diego, CA 92101-7904; or find us on the World Wide Web at http://www.singpub.com

Library of Congress Cataloging-in-Publication Data:
ISBN: 1-5659-3701-5

11/21/02

Contents

Preface

What exactly is aural rehabilitation? The answer to this question can conceivably include almost every aspect of audiology and deaf education. Under the rubric of aural rehabilitation may fall any of the following topics: identification and diagnosis of hearing loss and other hearing-related communication difficulties, patient and family counseling, selection and fitting of listening devices, follow-up services for the prescribed listening devices, communication training, noise protection, tinnitus, speech and language therapy, literacy promotion, classroom management, parent instruction, and speech perception training.

If a survey of recent textbooks for aural rehabilitation is any indication, increasingly, a primary component (if not the essence) of what we define as aural rehabilitation has come to mean the provision and maintenance of appropriate listening devices.

This indeed is an important activity in any aural rehabilitation service delivery model. However, this textbook represents a bit of a departure from many current texts and, to some extent, a return to the roots of aural rehabilitation. Although it includes chapters and sections on identification and quantification of hearing loss, and on hearing aids and other listening devices, these topics are not the book's primary focus. Instead, the emphasis is placed on three other topics: (1) understanding the patients who are served by speech and hearing professionals, (2) providing them with appropriate professional support and counseling, and (3) maximizing their communication success in their everyday environments, once they have received appropriate amplification.

In the spirit of this orientation, this book presents in-depth considerations of different patient populations, provides a review of research that is pertinent to furnishing aural rehabilitation to patients, and offers nuts-and-bolts procedures for providing services. It is hoped that students will gain an understanding of why we do what we do as speech and hearing professionals. Also, it is anticipated that readers will return to this book once they have finished their professional training for reference and practical how-to ideas.

The book is divided into four parts. Part I deals with conversation and communication-strategies training. Communication strategies and conversational styles are considered, and data from both speech and hearing and sociolinguistics literature are reviewed. This information provides a firm foundation for a consideration of assessment procedures for conversational fluency and communication handicap and for developing specific training protocols for both adults and children.

Part II concerns speech recognition: How to assess speech recognition, how to maximize speech listening through the use of technology, and how to develop speech perception skills. The chapters on speech perception training do not take us back to the days when speechreading training was the sole component of aural rehabilitation. However, it is recognized that speech perception training still has an important place in the arsenal of speech and hearing professionals, particularly when they provide intervention for young children. Although adults may not receive as much benefit from speech perception training per se, it is important that they and their families understand the difficulty of the speech recognition task in the presence of reduced auditory capabilities.

The third part of the book concerns the adult population with hearing loss. Part III begins with individuals who are under the age of 65 years, and then discusses adults who are older. Comprehensive descriptions of the patient groups are provided, as are specific tactics for developing aural rehabilitation plans. The guiding theme in this section is that aural rehabilitation services must be tailored to meet the needs of the individual. A strength of Part III is William Clark's chapter regarding noise protection and the role of the aural rehabilitation specialist (Chapter 13). With the aging of our population and with ever-increasing noise levels in our everyday world, this topic will grow in importance for the professions who are involved with aural rehabilitation.

Part IV deals with children. Topics include hearing loss and assessment, the design of an intervention plan, and speech, language, and literacy achievement. A chapter is devoted to each of two especially timely topics. Chapter 17 pertains to parent-centered conversation and language instruction whereas Chapter 18 deals with patient management and cochlear implants in children.

The structure of the text has three notable features. First, supplemental or tangential information to the main text is provided in shaded inserts. These inserts are meant to provide an added dimension to the text and/or add interest for the student. In addition, final remarks appear at the end of every chapter, and important concepts are summarized. Key terms are defined in the margins.

This book was designed to be used by both undergraduate and beginning graduate students in audiology and speech-language pathology. In addition, it may serve as a text for training programs in deaf education, special education, medicine, nursing, occupational therapy, and vocational rehabilitation counseling.

This is an exciting time to be involved with aural rehabilitation. We know more about hearing loss and how to manage its consequences than ever before in history. Advances in hearing measurement and hearing-related technology and increased understanding in the areas of sociolinguistics, psychology, speech acquisition, and speech perception have created a climate in which providing aural rehabilitation is both rewarding and wonderfully challenging to the speech and hearing professional. The goal of writing this book was to create a valuable resource for those who will be involved with aural rehabilitation in the coming years.

Acknowledgments

I thank Pam Conley for creating the figures in this book. Much hard work and imagination went into their preparation. Thanks also to Kim Readmond at Central Institute for the Deaf for contributing the photographs, and to Kathleen Campbell for contributing suggestions for Chapter 1.

Dedication

For Ellen Thornber Murray and Aubrey Fox Murray.

Introduction

Topics

- Definitions of Aural Rehabilitation: Step-by-Step
- Hearing Loss and Prevalence
- Relevance of Aural Rehabilitation

- Final Remarks
- Key Chapter Points
- Key Resources

Hearing loss often has been called the "invisible condition," yet its impact may be anything but invisible. The consequences of hearing loss may be manifested in a broad spectrum of an individual's life. For example, everyday communication may be difficult and, for some persons, impossible without a great deal of effort. The adult may feel the ramifications of hearing loss at home, in the workplace, and in the community. The young child may share similar difficulties in everyday communication, and may also experience delays in speech, language, educational achievement and social development.

In this introductory chapter, we will consider prevalence of hearing loss in today's world and define what we mean by the term *aural rehabilitation*. We will do so in the context of considering relevance. That is, why is aural rehabilitation so necessary in the service delivery models provided by speech and hearing professionals?

Aural rehabilitation is intervention aimed at minimizing and alleviating the communication difficulties associated with hearing loss.

The answer to the question of the relevance of aural rehabilitation is two-pronged. First, the ranks of persons who have hearing loss continue to swell, and they include individuals who are both old and young. The demand for aural rehabilitation is likely to demonstrate a concomitant growth. Second, aural rehabilitation can improve the quality of life for individuals who have hearing loss, and can minimize the negative consequences of this invisible disability, in a manner that is cost-effective.

DEFINITIONS OF AURAL REHABILITATION: STEP-BY-STEP

Rehabilitation services are designed to help individuals overcome the challenges posed by a disability. The logic behind rehabilitation is to provide an individual with the most appropriate technological support, and then to help the person build skill levels in functioning. Skill levels are developed in small increments, and in a way that is not overwhelming. For instance, a patient who has a knee injury may first receive a knee brace. A physical therapist may then help the patient perform simple leg extensions early on in a rehabilitation program. Much later, the patient may progress to one-legged hopping.

Similarly, much of what we do in aural rehabilitation is designed to provide appropriate technical support, and then develop the individual's skill levels step-by-step. For example, a child with a profound hearing loss may receive a cochlear implant. Initially, a speech and hearing professional may help the child learn to detect the presence or absence of sound. Only later will the child learn to identify words. Mastering this, the child may then progress to an even more advanced skill level, and learn to comprehend ongoing discourse.

What are the Goals of Aural Rehabilitation?

The goals of aural rehabilitation are to

■ Alleviate the difficulties related to hearing loss and
■ Minimize its consequences.

Aural rehabilitation may include diagnosis and quantification of the hearing loss and the provision of appropriate listening devices. In addition, for the adult, aural rehabilitation may include communication strategies training, counseling related to hearing loss, vocational counseling, noise protection, and counseling and instruction for family members. Less commonly, an aural rehabilitation program for an adult also may include speech perception training, such as speechreading training. For the child, aural rehabilitation may include diagnostics, provision of appropriate amplification, and speech perception and communication strategies training, as well as intervention related to speech, language, and academic achievement. Children's family members also often receive services under the umbrella of an aural rehabilitation plan.

Other Terms Related to "Aural Rehabilitation"

Sometimes the terms aural habilitation or audiologic rehabilitation are used when discussing the provision of services related to alleviating the problems associated with hearing loss. The term *aural habilitation* instead of aural rehabilitation is used when the person receiving the services is a child rather than an adult. This is because in the strict sense, *rehabilitation* means to restore something that was lost. When we provide speech perception training or speech and language therapy to children who have hearing loss, we are not aiming to restore lost func-

continued

Aural habilitation is intervention for persons who have not developed listening, speech, and language skills.

Audiologic rehabilitation is a term often used synonymously with aural rehabilitation or aural habilitation; may entail greater emphasis on the provision and follow-up of listening devices and less emphasis on communication stategy and speech perception training.

tion, but rather, to develop (that is, to habilitate or furnish) skills that were not present beforehand. Although this is a cogent distinction between the terms rehabilitation and habilitation, in this text, we shall use the two synomonously for simplicity's sake.

The term audiologic rehabilitation closely parallels the term *aural rehabilitation*, but usually encompasses a narrower breadth of services. The term *audiologic rehabilitation* implies an emphasis on the diagnosis of hearing loss and the provision of listening devices, and a lesser emphasis on follow-up support services, such as communication strategies training.

Where Does Aural Rehabilitation Occur?

Now that we have defined what aural rehabilitation may encompass, let us consider where it might be provided. Aural rehabilitation may occur in a variety of locales. For example it may be provided in any of the following settings:

■ A university speech and hearing clinic
■ An audiology private practice
■ A hearing-aid dealer private practice
■ A hospital speech and hearing clinic
■ A community center or nursing home
■ A school (Figure 1–1)
■ An otolaryngologist's office
■ A speech-language pathologist's office
■ Consumer organization meetings

Who Provides Aural Rehabilitation?

Aural rehabilitation might be provided by an audiologist, a speech-language pathologist, or a teacher for the hard-of-hearing and deaf. Typically, an audiologist takes a lead role in developing an individual's aural rehabilitation plan, and coordinates the services provided by other professionals. Particularly with adults, the audiologist is the primary health-care professional in the management of the hearing loss.

In some cases, however, the speech-language pathologist may play the lead role for a child, especially in a school environment. For instance, the speech-language pathologist is most likely to provide speech and language therapy, and often is the professional who provides auditory and speechreading train-

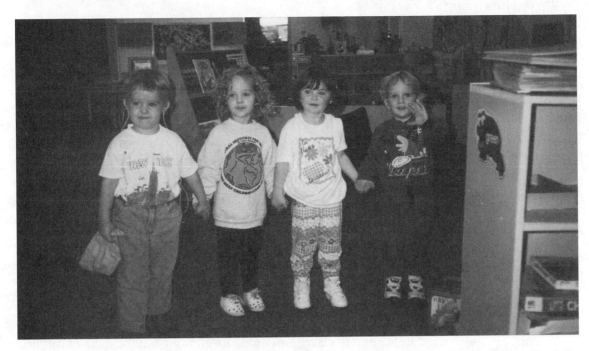

Figure 1-1. Aural rehabilitation for young children often occurs in educational settings. By Julia Rottjakob, courtesy of Central Institute for the Deaf.

ing. Whereas the audiologist may fit and maintain a child's hearing aids and/or equip the classroom with appropriate assistive listening devices, the speech-language pathologist may be the person who has extended one-on-one contact with a child, and the one who knows the child well. We will revisit the issue of "who" in Chapter 14, when we address hearing loss and children.

HEARING LOSS AND PREVALENCE

Individuals who have hearing loss represent a heterogeneous group. They vary in the nature of their hearing loss and in their aural rehabilitation needs. In this section, we will briefly consider how hearing loss may be parameterized (Figure 1–2).

Hearing loss may be categorized along three dimensions: degree, onset, and time course. In terms of degree, hearing loss may be characterized as mild, moderate, moderate-to-severe, severe, or profound (Chapter 5). A person who has a mild, moderate, or moderate-to-severe hearing loss (i.e., a hearing loss between 26 and 70 dB) is often called *hard-of-hearing*. A person who has a severe or profound hearing loss (i.e., hearing loss greater than 70 dB) may sometimes be called *deaf*.

Hard of hearing means having a hearing loss; usually not used to refer to a profound hearing loss.

Deaf: having minimal or no hearing.

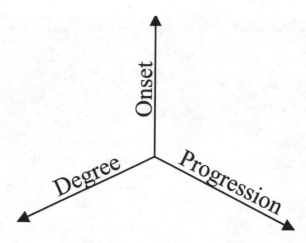

Figure 1–2. Hearing loss can be parameterized on three dimensions: onset, degree, and time course.

Prelingual refers to a hearing loss acquired before the acquisition of spoken language.

Perilingual refers to a hearing loss acquired during the stage of acquiring spoken language.

Postlingual refers to a hearing loss incurred after the acquisition of spoken language.

A **progressive hearing loss** is a hearing loss that increases over time.

A **sudden hearing loss** is a hearing loss that has an acute and rapid onset.

In terms of onset, a hearing loss may be described as prelingual, perilingual, or postlingual. A person who has a *prelingual* hearing loss incurred the loss before the acquisition of spoken language skills. Although there is no universally agreed cut-off time as to when the prelingual phase ends, generally, when a child incurs a hearing loss before the age of 2 years, he or she is said to have a prelingual loss. A child who lost the hearing after acquiring some spoken language but before acquisition was complete is said to have a *perilingual* hearing loss. Finally, a *postlingual* loss is one that occurred after the acquisition of speech and language. Again, there is no agreed-on age at which the perilingual stage ends and the postlingual stage begins, but it may be around the age of 5 years.

Finally, a hearing loss may be categorized as progressive or sudden. An individual who has a hearing loss that occurs over the course of several months or years has a *progressive hearing loss*. An individual who lost hearing suddenly, say as a result of head trauma, has a *sudden hearing loss*.

We will consider in more detail levels of hearing loss and onset in Chapters 5 and 14, respectively. As we shall see, an aural rehabilitation plan for an individual patient may vary as a function of the degree, age of onset, and progression of the hearing loss.

RELEVANCE OF AURAL REHABILITATION

Now let us tackle the issue of relevance. Aural rehabilitation is an important component of the speech and hearing professionals' service delivery program for at least two reasons. These reasons relate to demographics and cost-effectiveness.

Demographics and Service Needs

The Importance of Aural Rehabilitation Training for Speech-Language Pathologists

Because aural rehabilitation is provided to persons who have a hearing loss, we sometimes think that only audiologists provide it. As the following except from a letter to *ASHA Leader* indicates, this is not true. Speech-language pathologists often play a major role:

> The changes taking place in the profession and populations served will require speech-language pathologists who are prepared to deal with issues in aural rehabilitation. Universal neonatal hearing screening is rapidly becoming a reality in many states and will result in a dramatic increase of hearing impaired babies and their families entering early intervention programs. Because the hearing loss will be identified so early, the children will be staying in the system for nearly three years—longer than if they had been identified at a later age. Babies with milder degrees of hearing loss will be identified, as well as those who are deaf. Cochlear implants are also becoming a reality for many young hearing impaired children with implantation occurring at an earlier age. These children are the "hard of hearing deaf" who, once destined for schools for the deaf, will most likely be mainstreamed into regular classrooms. In both these settings, early intervention programs and the public schools, the only professional on hand who is expected to have any training in hearing impairment is the speech-language pathologist.
>
> At the end of the age spectrum, the fastest growing segment in our society is the over 80 year olds, a population
>
> *continued*

> with a high percentage of hearing loss. Again, the speech-language pathologist in the nursing home or rehabilitation facility will be the only one with any credible training in hearing disorders and appropriate intervention.
>
> The demand for skilled clinicians who are competent to plan and implement appropriate and effective aural (re)habilitation programs across the life span will become greater in the near future. (Letter to the editor, David Luterman and Ellen Kurtzer-White, *ASHA Leader*, February 17, 1998)

Many different segments of our society require aural rehabilitation:

Older Persons

With the aging of the "baby boom" population, age-related hearing loss (which is called presbycusis, Chapter 13) is affecting an increasing percentage of our citizens. These individuals often are unwilling to, nor should they be expected to, sit on the sidelines of life because they are unable to communicate with those around them. They have a demand for services that will enhance their ability to communicate with their families and friends, to participate in community activities and volunteer work, and to stay in touch with their world via multimedia technology. Some desire to continue in their professional careers and postpone retirement. With increased awareness of preventative medicine routines and a growing sophistication in medical practice, an ever-growing number of older persons are living longer, and many have few health problems other than hearing loss that restrict their day-to-day functioning.

Infants and Children

On the other end of the life cycle, advances in neonatology and critical-care medicine have led to better survival rates of high-risk babies. Infants who might have died in earlier times now survive, often with a myriad of medical conditions that might include hearing loss. Families of babies who have hearing loss desire and expect assistance and support that will enable their children to grow up and achieve their full potential. Public policy reflects these trends. There is now a greater emphasis on earlier identification and service provision for young children who have hearing loss, under the auspices of Public Law 94-142 (Chapter 14).

Adults

In addition to the youngest and oldest members of our society, individuals in the center of the life cycle also may desire aural rehabilitation services. They have learned that, with appropriate support, they can make meaningful contributions in both the work place and in their communities. Indeed, this realization helped lead to the passage of the American with Disabilities Act, which is landmark legislation that calls for equal access for all persons with disabilities (Chapter 10).

Unserved and Underserved

There is evidence from the Institute on Rehabilitation Issues that individuals who have hearing loss are currently unserved or underserved (Robards-Armstrong & Stone, 1994). *Unserved* means this population is a group that is not served as a result of policy, practice, and/or environmental barriers. *Underserved* denotes a population that is inadequately served, in part because of:

An **unserved** population refers to a group of patients in need of but not receiving services.

An **underserved** population is a group of patients receiving less than ideal services.

- A dearth of outreach and immediate or extended support services.
- The attitudes of service delivery personnel.
- The lack of reimbursement policies for aural rehabilitation.
- Communication and/or environmental barriers.

Increasingly, persons with hearing loss and their families are exerting pressure on lawmakers and policy makers to ensure that more services are provided to individuals who have hearing loss and deafness. There will be a need for aural rehabilitation specialists to provide these services.

Incidence

Statistics underscore the fact that a significant number of persons have hearing loss. About 28 million people in the United States have some degree of reduced hearing sensitivity. Of this number, about 80% have an irreversible hearing loss. Hearing loss occurs in young and old persons. For example, data suggest that one of every 22 infants born in this country has some kind of hearing problem. One in every 1,000 infants have a severe or profound hearing loss, which means hearing thresholds that are poorer than 70 dB HL. One in three persons over the age of 65 years has decreased hearing. In fact, hearing is the third most prevalent chronic condition in the older population (NIDCD, 1989).

Cost-Effectiveness and Costs

Cost-effectiveness also relates to the relevance of aural rehabilitation, whereas the costs of providing services relate to the reality of providing services in an environment where health-care expenses are spiraling, and services are being cut for economic purposes.

Cost-Effectiveness

In recent years, there has been a growing awareness of the importance of rehabilitation services for individuals who have acute or chronic disabilities. We have learned that rehabilitation can promote an individual's quality of life and increase his or her productivity in the home, work place, and community. In the case of children, appropriate rehabilitation can promote success in school as well.

In areas other than aural rehabilitation, such as occupational therapy and physical therapy, we have documented that rehabilitation is very cost-effective. By providing appropriate support services, we can reduce dramatically medical and education costs, as well as other costs related to supporting individuals who are not as productive and independent as they might be.

We are realizing gradually that this also is true with aural rehabilitation. For instance, children who receive cochlear implants and abundant aural rehabilitation, particularly auditory speech stimulation are more likely to demonstrate benefit than those who do not receive such follow-up support (Osberger, Robbins, Todd, & Riley, 1994). Spitzer (1997) reviewed evidence that demonstrates the cost effectiveness of providing a cochlear implant and related support services to adult patients.

Costs and Reimbursements

Perhaps the primary obstacle to providing aural rehabilitation pertains to the short-term costs of service provision. Aural rehabilitation can be expensive for two reasons: Listening device technology is often costly, and providing services such as communication strategies training is labor-intensive. Often these kinds of costs are not covered by insurance companies, and must be borne by the private individual.

Insurance policies can be classified as private (e.g., Health Maintenance Organizations [HMOs]), state (e.g., Blue Cross and Blue Shield), and/or as federal plans (e.g., Medicare). Sometimes when insurance plans provide coverage for services following receipt of a listening device, they do so only when the services are provided by a speech-language pathologist rather than an audiologist. If coverage is provided for a hearing aid or cochlear implant, follow-up services may not be included. In these instances, it is not unusual for an audiologist to bundle aural rehabilitation costs into the price of the listening device.

FINAL REMARKS

In the following chapters, we will review both traditional and cutting-edge practices in aural rehabilitation. In the first half of the text (Parts One and Two), we will consider some of the components of an aural rehabilitation service delivery model, including communication strategies training, diagnostics and assessment, provision of listening devices, and speech perception training. In the second half (Parts Three and Four), we will consider specific populations and how an aural rehabilitation plan can be customized to meet the needs of individual patients.

A number of professional journals deal with aural rehabilitation. These journals are listed in Key Resources at the end of each chapter. They can provide interested readers with additional and timely information about the topics covered in this text.

KEY CHAPTER POINTS

✔ Hearing loss can affect several aspects of an individual's daily life at home, at work, in school, and in social situations.
✔ Aural rehabilitation for the adult may include diagnosis and quantification of hearing loss, provision of appropriate listening devices, training in communication strategies, counseling related to hearing loss, vocational counseling, noise protection, and counseling and instruction for family members. It may or may not include speech perception training.

✔ Aural rehabilitation for the child may include diagnostics, provision of appropriate amplification, speech perception training, communication strategies training, family training, and intervention related to speech, language, and educational development.

✔ Aural rehabilitation may occur in a variety of locales, including university speech and hearing clinics and audiology private practices.

✔ Aural rehabilitation may be provided by an audiologist, speech-language pathologist, or educator.

✔ Hearing loss may be categorized by degree, onset, and time course.

✔ Aural rehabilitation is relevant for two general reasons: demographics and cost-effectiveness.

KEY RESOURCES

Professional Journals

American Annals of the Deaf

American Journal of Audiology: A Journal of Clinical Practice

American Journal of Speech-Language Pathology: A Journal of Clinical Practice

Asha (American Speech-Language Hearing Association)

Audiology

British Journal of Audiology

Contact

Deafness and Education

Ear and Hearing

Educational Audiology

Hearing Journal

Journal of the American Academy of Audiology

Journal of the Academy of Rehabilitative Audiology

Journal of Child Language

Journal of Communication Disorders

Journal of Speech, Language and Hearing Research

Language and Speech

Language, Speech, and Hearing Services in the School

Noise Regulation Report

Scandinavian Audiology

Seminars in Hearing

Seminars in Speech and Language

Speech Communication

Topics in Language Disorders

Trends in Amplification

Volta Review

Volta Voices

PART I

Conversation and Communication Strategies

2

Communication Strategies and Conversational Styles[1]

Topics

- Conversation
- Classes of Communication Strategies
- Factors That Influence Reception of Spoken Messages
- Facilitative Communication Strategies
- Repair Strategies

- Stages in Repairing a Communication Breakdown
- Research Related to Community Strategy Use
- Conversational Styles and Behaviors
- Final Remarks
- Key Chapter Points

[1]The transcripts of conversation in this chapter are based on actual interchanges. Some have been edited for the sake of brevity or clarity.

Communication training is instruction provided to a person with a hearing loss to maximize his or her communication potential.

With this chapter, we begin our consideration of communication training in the aural rehabilitation setting. *Communication training* is a catchall term used to denote communication strategies, auditory, and speechreading training collectively. Ideally, all speech and hearing-related professionals offer communication training to their patients. In reality, however, communication training is not proffered universally, and when it is, it is often provided in a cursory fashion.

Successful everyday communication for individuals with hearing loss is influenced by many variables, including the effectiveness of their listening device, their lipreading skills, and the amount of residual hearing. In addition, success in communication is affected greatly by how well people use communication strategies. A *communication strategy* is a course of action taken to facilitate a conversational interaction or to rectify a problem that arises during conversation. During communication strategies training, patients receive instruction about how to manage their conversational interactions effectively. In recent years, many hearing professionals have recognized that communication strategies training is a powerful way to enhance individuals' abilities to manage everyday listening problems.

A **communication strategy** is a course of action taken to enhance communication.

In this chapter, the foundation will be laid for subsequent chapters about communication assessment and communication training. We will consider briefly general issues related to conversation, and then we will focus on communication strategies and conversational styles.

CONVERSATION

Much of the fabric of human relationships is woven by our conversations—by what we say, how we say it, and how we listen. We engage in conversation for several reasons (Figure 2–1):

- ■ To share ideas
- ■ To relate experiences
- ■ To tell stories
- ■ To express needs
- ■ To effect a result
- ■ To instruct
- ■ To influence
- ■ To establish intimacy

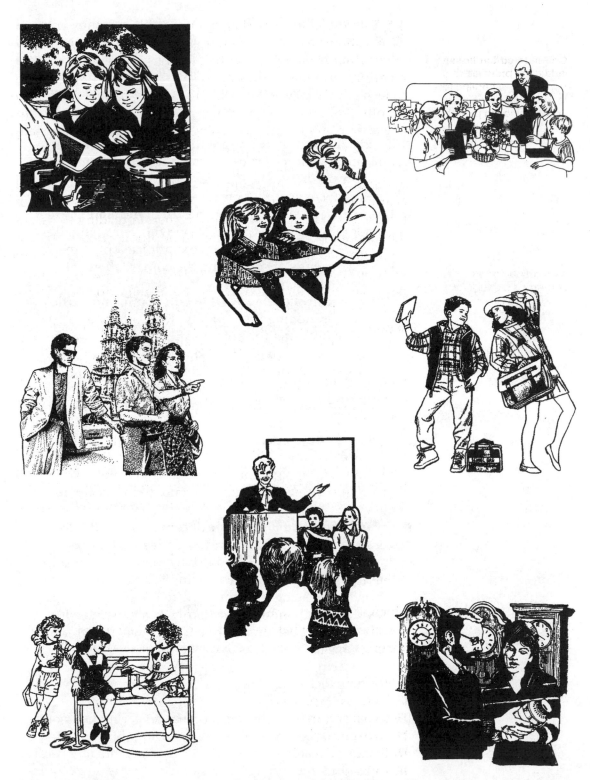

Figure 2-1. We engage in conversation for a variety of reasons, for example, to share, to inform, or to instruct.

Conversational rules are
implicit rules that guide the
conduct of participants in a
conversation.

The way we talk with others is guided by our knowledge of implicit *rules of conversation*. If you reflect in a metaphysical fashion about the way we converse, you may realize that most of us typically adhere to culturally established conventions. For example, when two or more people begin a conversation, they each:

■ **Tacitly agree to share one another's interests.** We commit our mental resources to attending to our communication partner's message, and respond to the messages in a way that furthers the discussion.

■ **Ensure that no single person does all of the talking.** We do not dominate the conversation with our own talking, and we do not expect our communication partners to bear the onus of continuing the conversation alone. We share speaking turns.

■ **Participate in choosing what to talk about, and participate in developing the topic.** Typically, there is not a "chief" who leads the conversation, and who alone decides what is talked about and how that subject is developed. Rather, all participants play a role, at some point or other, in deciding what is talked about and in shaping the direction in which the discussion progresses.

■ **Take turns in an orderly fashion.** Everyone should have a chance to contribute to the conversation, and to end a contribution before someone else begins their speaking turn. This means that interruptions do not occur too often.

■ **Try to be relevant to the topic of conversation.** If a conversation is centered on automobiles and someone abruptly begins to talk about a recipe for cornbread, that individual has violated an implicit rule of conversation by not being relevant to the discussion.

■ **Provide enough information to convey a message without being verbose.** In a conversation, we expect our communication partners to deliver their messages in a fairly succinct way, and in a manner that maintains our interest in listening.

If one participant in a conversation has a hearing loss, some of the rules of conversation may have to be modified or adapted. For instance, interruptions may occur more frequently because the individual must frequently ask for clarification of a misperceived message. Other participants may have to exert a greater effort to ensure that the person has an opportunity to contribute to a topic's development. If he or she did not understand or misunderstood something that has been said, the hard-of-hearing person may sometimes contribute remarks that are not relevant to the ongoing discussion. The person with hearing loss may also have to use communication strategies, ideally in a way that does not violate the more universally established rules of conversation.

Erber (1996, p. 20) suggests that conversations involving someone who has a hearing loss may have any of the following characteristics:

■ **Disrupted taking of turns.** When we come to an end of speaking turn, we often begin to speak slower and our intonation contour begins to fall. The person with hearing loss may not hear these signals and, thus, inappropriate silences may occur because he or she does not initiate a conversational turn on cue.
■ **Modified speaking style.** A communication partner may speak slowly with precise articulation in order to facilitate speech recognition for the hard-of-hearing person.
■ **Inappropriate topic shifts.** The hard-of-hearing person may not recognize previous remarks, and may inadvertently (and inappropriately) change the subject.
■ **Superficial content.** Because speech recognition is difficult for the hard-of-hearing individual, the participants in a conversation may avoid certain topics for discussion, and avoid topics that might evoke unusual vocabulary or complex syntax.
■ **Frequent clarification.** Misunderstandings are commonplace in conversations, even when all participants have normal hearing. When someone has a hearing loss, misunderstandings may become even more frequent. Both the hard-of-hearing person and communication partner may need to engage in clarification more often, and diversions from the topic may occur regularly.

CLASSES OF COMMUNICATION STRATEGIES

Now that we have considered how conversations may unfold when one of the participants has a hearing loss, let us review strategies that can be used to modify conversational interactions. Persons with hearing loss may use two kinds of commu-

Facilitative strategies include instructing the talker and structuring the listening environment, to enhance the listener's performance.

A **receptive repair strategy** is a tactic used by an individual when he or she has not understood a message.

A **communicaton breakdown** occurs when one communication partner does not recognize another's message.

nication strategies during the course of a conversation to minimize or prevent communication difficulties, facilitative and repair. Individuals use *facilitative strategies* to influence the talker, the structure of the message, the environment, or themselves. *Repair strategies* provide explicit instruction to the communication partner about what to do immediately following a communication breakdown. A *communication breakdown* is an instance in which one person says something and another person does not recognize the message.

FACTORS THAT INFLUENCE RECEPTION OF SPOKEN MESSAGES

Before we consider communication strategies in depth, it is important to analyze the factors that influence how successfully a hard-of-hearing person participates in conversation. Four such factors are the talker, the message, the environment, and the listener. As we will learn in the next section, facilitative strategies are used to influence these four factors.

The Talker

How a communication partner delivers the message, and whether the partner uses appropriate speaking behaviors effect message reception. For instance, the sentence, "Geeze, yashouldaseendagameFridee, it'dovblownyaway!" would be difficult for a hard-of-hearing individual to understand for at least three reasons: The talker spoke quickly, blurred together word boundaries and omitted some of the words' component sounds. If the talker had been chewing gum, or had covered his face with his hand (Figure 2–2), recognition would have been even more difficult.

The Message

The second factor that influences someone's ability to recognize a message is the message itself. For example, the sentence above spoken slowly is, "Geeze, you should have seen the game Friday, it would have blown you away." This sentence could be revised to make it even easier to recognize. The talker might say instead, "I saw the baseball game Friday. The game was great." This alternative version is easier for a hard-of-hearing person to recognize because this version has the following characteristics:

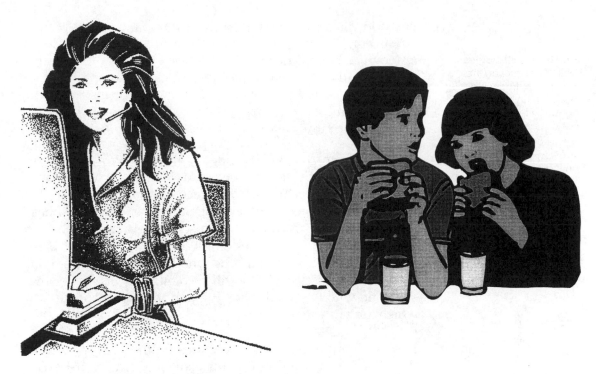

Figure 2–2. Chewing or obstructions in front of a talker's mouth can decrease a hard-of-hearing person's ability to recognize a spoken message.

Simple syntax.
Repetition of an important keyword, *game.*
Two sentences rather than a single, long one.
No ambiguous references, such as *it*.
No colloquialisms, such as *blown you away.*

Environment

The third factor that influences an individual's speech recognition performance is the environment. It is not hard to imagine that a person with hearing loss will experience difficulty when attempting to communicate in a dimly lit room with loud music playing in the background. Most hard-of-hearing persons have an especially difficult time recognizing speech in the presence of background noise, particularly when they cannot see the talker's mouth and face clearly to speechread. Environments that have the following characteristics are much more suitable:

Quiet, without background noise.
Well-lit, without light shining into the hard-of-hearing person's eyes.

■ Good distance (i.e., 4–6 ft) from the communication partner.
■ No visual distractions.
■ Good viewing angle of the talker.

The Patient

The final factor we will consider that influences message reception is the patients themselves. An individual who is inherently a good speechreader will recognize more of a spoken message than someone who is not. Someone with a mild hearing loss will recognize more than someone who has a severe loss, unless that person uses amplification and receives excellent benefit. Of course, someone who has appropriate amplification and corrected vision will recognize speech better than someone who has similar hearing and visual capabilities, but which are untreated.

How well an individual concentrates on the message also influences message reception. For example, a hard-of-hearing person may feel anxious, stressed, or fatigued while engaging in conversation. "Oh no," he or she may think, "I'm not getting any of this, they are going to think I'm stupid or not interested." These kinds of emotional states are self-defeating. One's ability to recognize speech decreases when he or she allocates mental resources to considerations other than comprehending the message being spoken at the moment.

FACILITATIVE COMMUNICATION STRATEGIES

Table 2–1 summarizes four types of facilitative communications strategies. Each type is designed to influence each of the four factors we have just considered, factors that impinge on message recognition success.

Strategies that Influence the Talker

In an **instructional strategy**, the listener asks the talker to change the delivery of the message.

Hard-of-hearing persons use *instructional strategies* to influence communication partners' speaking behaviors. A person asks the talker to change the delivery of the message, as in these examples:

■ "Slow down."
■ "When you cover your mouth with your hand, I have a hard time speechreading you."

Table 2–1. Facilitative and repair strategies.

Facilitative strategies may be used to influence:

■ **Patient's speech recognition skills**
Adaptive strategies: the individual with hearing loss implements relaxation techniques.

Attending strategies: the individual pays attention to situational, linguistic, and facial cues for the purpose of inferring partially recognized messages.

Anticipatory strategies: the individual prepares for conversational interactions in advance by anticipating conversational content and potential listening difficulties.

■ **Communication Environment**
Constructive strategies: a person structures the environment to optimize communication by minimizing background noise and ensuring a favorable view of the talker.

■ **Communication partner**
Instructional strategies: a person influences the communication partner's speaking behaviors by asking the partner to speak clearly, facing forward.

■ **Message**
Message-tailoring strategies: individuals encourage communication partners to use short sentences or they control the topic of conversation.

Source: Adapted from Tye-Murray, N., Knutson, J. F., and Lemke, J. (1993). Assessment of communication strategies use: Questionnaires and daily diaries, *Seminars in Hearing, 14,* 338–353.

■ "Could you face me please?"
■ "Please slow down your talking. I understand more that way."

To use instructional strategies, hard-of-hearing persons must identify behaviors that impede their speech recognition efforts. Then they may instruct the communication partner about how to change the behavior.

Strategies that Influence the Message

Message-tailoring strategies, the second kind of facilitative strategy, influence the way someone constructs a message. A person might ask, "Did you go swimming or biking last night?" This question sets the stage for one of two responses, *swimming* or *biking*. Alternatively the individual may not use a message-tailoring strategy, and instead ask, "What did you do last night?" which opens the floodgate for a multitude of answers and a greater likelihood of communication breakdown.

Using a message-tailoring strategy requires some meta-communication skills. That is, persons must be able to think about

Message-tailoring strategy: phrasing one's remarks to constrain the respones of a communication partner.

not only what they want to say, but also, how best to say it in order to effect the desired result.

Strategies That Influence the Environment

Constructive strategy: a tactic designed to optimize the listening environment for communication.

John Dooling, a father who has a significant hearing loss, is talking to his daughter in the kitchen. His son is running water in the sink, the refrigerator is humming, the dishwasher is gurgling, and their dog is barking. John motions toward the living room and says to his daughter, "Let's go into the living room and finish talking about your plans for the weekend." In this instance, John employed a *constructive strategy* to enhance the communication environment. Constructive strategies are a third kind of facilitative strategy, and are used to effect a modification in environmental listening conditions.

The success of constructive strategies hinges on the ability of the person to analyze the communication environment and identify those elements that can be modified or exploited to optimize communication. Table 2–2 presents a list of other constructive strategies that patients may use to optimize communication.

Maladaptive Strategies

Maladaptive strategy: an inappropriate behavioral mechanism for coping with the difficulties caused by hearing loss in a conversation.

Sometimes people who are hard of hearing adopt *maladaptive strategies* to cope with their communication difficulties. These strategies include bluffing and pretending to understand, social withdrawal to avoid communication difficulties, dominating conversations so to be ever aware of what is being talked about, and succumbing to feelings of anger, hostility, or self-pity. Some individuals become unduly anxious and tense, either as they anticipate an upcoming communication interaction (such as a meeting with their boss), or during the interaction itself, as problems in understanding begin to arise. It is well within the purview of a communication strategies training program to encourage alternative behaviors in lieu of maladaptive strategies.

Strategies That Influence the Patient's Reception of the Message

Adaptive, attending, and anticipatory strategies are ways in which persons can adapt to their hearing losses and minimize

Table 2–2. Examples of constructive strategies that can be used to optimize the listening and speechreading task. This list might be provided to the person who has hearing loss.

- If possible, ensure that the talker is well-lit so that you watch the talker's face.
- If the talker is far away, move closer.
- If background noise is present, try to either reduce the noise or move to a quieter setting.
- Try to avoid rooms or auditoriums that have sound reverberation. You might request that a meeting be held in a room with good acoustics; typically, a room that has carpet, draperies, and minimal noise from air conditioners and radiators.
- Arrive early so that you can get favorable seating, near the talker.
- Eliminate visual distracters, such as a curtain flapping in an open window.

communication difficulties. These strategies influence a person's reception of a message.

Adaptive and *attending strategies* serve to counteract maladaptive behaviors, and include relaxation techniques and other means of dealing with emotions and negative behaviors that stem from hearing loss. For example, some hard-of-hearing persons feel anxious during a conversation with someone who is unfamiliar to them, and they worry about what they might miss and/or what their communication partners think of them. In these instances, they might have to take a deep breath, consciously relax, purposefully redirect their thoughts toward the present conversation, and attend to the talker's lip movements. This adaptive behavior not only can decrease anxiety, but also, enhance message recognition.

Adaptive and attending strategies: methods of counteracting maladaptive behaviors that stem from hearing loss.

An individual uses an *anticipatory strategy* to prepare for a communication interaction. These strategies include anticipating potential vocabulary and conversational content. For example, before a job interview, a person with hearing loss might study related information about the company, such as employee handbooks or news clippings. The individual might buy books about recruitment procedures, and learn what kinds of questions are standard during interviews. Should the interviewer mention names of key employees, the person may thus recognize the names because they are already familiar. When the interviewer asks routine questions, they also may be easier to recognize because the person has the appropriate framework in which to listen. Erber (1996) suggested that patients can anticipate spoken remarks by attending to situational cues (e.g., talking with a ticket seller at a movie theater). They can make predictions on the basis of "knowledge of a partner's typical conversational style (e.g., use of colloquialisms or ges-

Anticipatory strategies are methods of preparing for a communication interaction.

tures); common conversational sequences (e.g., as in greeting rituals); and expected responses to utterances of particular types (e.g., to choice questions)" (p. 42).

Resolving Difficulties in Speech Recognition by Using Facilitative Strategies

Figure 2–3 summarizes the process that hard-of-hearing persons might engage in when they experience difficulty in recog-

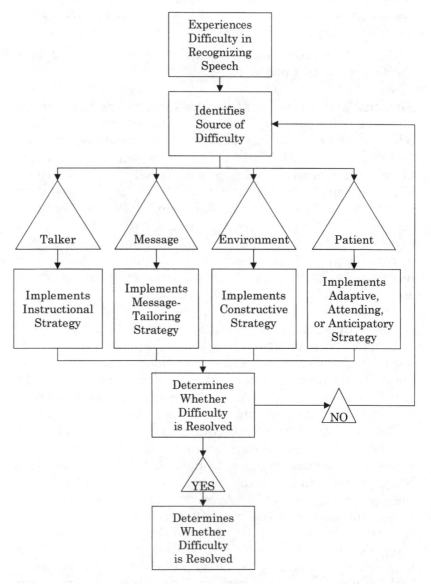

Figure 2–3. Process someone may follow when encountering a communication difficulty.

nizing speech during conversation. The individual identifies the source of difficulty, implements a facilitative strategy, and determines whether the difficulty is resolved. If it is, then the conversation can continue. If it is not, the person might implement another strategy.

REPAIR STRATEGIES

Now that we have reviewed the various facilitative communication strategies, we will now consider repair strategies. As we have noted, a *communication breakdown* occurs when one communication partner speaks a message and another does not recognize it. After signaling the occurrence of a communication breakdown, people can request information by using one of many possible *receptive repair strategies* (Table 2–3). The word *receptive* indicates that the repair strategy is used to rectify a communication breakdown when the recipient of a message (in this case, a hard-of-hearing person) does not recognize the sender's (talker's) message. Examples include: "Could you say that again?" (the *repeat repair strategy*), "Who is going to give you a ride?" (the *request for information repair strategy*) and, "I missed that completely, what are you talking about?" (the *key word repair strategy*). An individual also might ask for more information (the *elaborate repair strategy*): "Tell me more, I didn't catch that."

Receptive repair strategy: a tactic used by a listener when the message presented by a communication partner is not understood.

Table 2–3. Repair strategies that can be used by hard-of-hearing individuals to repair breakdowns in communication.

Specific repair strategies request the communication partner to:

Repeat all or part of message

Rephrase message

Elaborate message

Simplify the message

Indicate the topic of conversation

Confirm the message

Write

Fingerspell

Nonspecific repair strategies ask:

What

Huh

Pardon

Depending on how well individuals know their communication partners, they might feel comfortable in asking them to write, use gestures and hand signals, or to spell important topic words. Selection of a particular repair strategy may hinge on a variety of factors, including how useful a particular strategy has been in the past, how much of the message was understood, and an assessment of how well a communication partner might follow the instructions.

STAGES IN REPAIRING A COMMUNICATION BREAKDOWN

Figure 2–4 indicates that there are at least three stages involved in repairing a communication breakdown. First, the breakdown must be detected by either the hard-of-hearing person or the communication partner. The person may have missed all of the message, missed only a part of the message, or perceived it incorrectly.

Once the communication breakdown has been detected, one of the communication partners must initiate a repair of the breakdown (Stage 2). If the hard-of-hearing person initiates repair, he or she first chooses a course of action and then implements it. The individual might choose to attempt repair, decide that

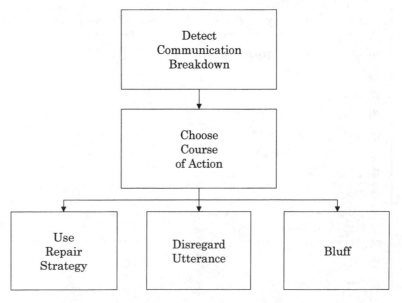

Figure 2–4. Stages associated with communication repair.

the message was not important enough to pursue understanding, or bluff and pretend to understand. The action is then implemented (Stage 3). If the individual chooses to implement a repair strategy, and the strategy leads to successful repair, the conversation carries on. If the hard-of-hearing person still does not understand, the repair process must continue.

Detection of a Communication Breakdown (Stage 1)

Stage 1 of the model depicted in Figure 2–4 is detection of a communication breakdown. When communication breakdowns occur, hard-of-hearing persons might detect immediately that they did not recognize the message. In such cases, an individual might alert the partner, and seek repair. "Hold on," the person might say, "I missed that."

Sometimes, a person might recognize that his or her response to a remark was inappropriate, perhaps by his or her communication partner's facial expression or by attempts at clarification. For example, a communication partner may ask, "What are you reading?" If the hard-of-hearing person responds, "Chicken salad," the communication partner might then say, "Not 'eating,' I said 'reading.'"

It sometimes happens that an individual does not realize a breakdown has occurred until much later in the conversation, as in the following example:

Professor (who has hearing loss):	"What was your last assignment?"
Film student:	"I did a 10-minute educational film on Arctic moss."
Professor:	(thinking the film student said Arctic *moths*) "Oh, you must have had to do that over the summer then."
Film student:	"Believe it or not, some species live embedded in ice crystals, so we did some shots in early November."
Professor:	"What do they do, live in caverns?"
Film student:	"Huh?"
Professor:	(beginning to wonder whether he has missed something) "Live in caverns?"

Film student:	"Well, I guess there's some moss in caverns up there, but I've never seen any caves."
Professor:	"*Moss*?" (blushing) "Oh, I thought we were talking about *moths*!"

As the professor sensed an incongruence between the film student's and his own remarks, he gradually realized that he misunderstood an utterance earlier on in the conversation. This is a prime example of not realizing that a breakdown has occurred at its onset.

Dealing With a Breakdown in Communication (Stages 2 and 3)

The second and third stages of the model depicted in Figure 2–4, which shows the stages associated with communication breakdown and repair, are choosing a course of action and then implementing it. We will consider what may happen when someone uses a repair strategy and what may happen when someone bluffs.

Using a Repair Strategy

Once a misunderstanding becomes apparent, an individual might alert the communication partner and provide instruction about how to repair it. For instance, he or she may ask about the topic of conversation (e.g., "What are you talking about?").

Usually, breakdowns are repaired with the use of one or two repair strategies. There are occasions, however, especially when one of the participants has a severe or profound hearing loss, when several exchanges are required to repair a communication breakdown. In the worst of circumstances, these interchanges can be awkward for all parties involved in the conversation, as in the following example in which a husband and wife (who recently received a cochlear implant) talked while seated in a speech and hearing test room:

Husband:	"Laura is going to catch the train on Tuesday."
Wife:	"What? I didn't catch any of that."
Husband:	"I said, Laura is going to catch the train on Tuesday."
Wife:	"No, none of it."

Husband:	"Laura . . ."
Wife:	"Something about more?"
Husband:	"No, watch me. Laura is going to get the train."
Wife:	"Oh, yeah. I got 'train'."
Husband:	"Yes, a train. Laura is . . ."
Wife:	(shaking her head) "Nope, nope, none of it. Spell it."
Husband:	"L-A-U-R-A"
Wife:	"Oh Laura! What about Laura and the train?"

At this point, several repair strategies have been implemented and the message is still not conveyed. This is an example of an *extended repair*, because many repair strategies are needed before the breakdown is resolved. It would be very easy for both participants in the conversation to abandon repair, and say, "Never mind, it's not that important." And indeed, in situations such as this, that is often exactly what happens.

Extended repair: when many repair strategies are needed to mend a communication breakdown.

It is important that use of a repair strategy does not create a concomitant disruption of conversation. Sometimes when someone uses a repair strategy to repair a breakdown in communication, the topic of conversation can shift, as indicated in Figure 2–5. Ideally, people use repair strategies in such a way that they do not cause the conversation to stagnate or veer off into a different direction. For example, a student with a hearing loss, Janet, did not use a repair strategy very effectively in the following exchange:

Cynthia:	"I got my grades in the mail last Saturday."
Janet:	"Grapes? Why are you getting grapes in the mail?"
Cynthia:	"No, I said *grades*, not *grapes*."
Janet:	"Oh, I know you make wine, so I thought you had joined some kind of mail-order program. By the way, when am I going to get my bottle?"

The problem with this interchange is that the topic of conversation changed inappropriately (from grades to a promised bottle of wine) as a result of the repair strategy used. A seemingly more cooperative and congenial way to repair this communication breakdown is as follows:

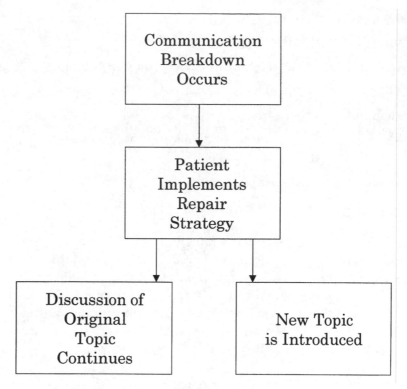

Figure 2–5. Possible effects of using a repair strategy.

Cynthia:	"I got my grades in the mail last Saturday."
Janet:	"Grapes?"
Cynthia:	"No, I said *grades*."
Janet:	"Oh, you got your grades in the mail. How did you do?"

In this latter version, Janet asked for confirmation, and then steered the conversation back on track.

Bluffing

Sometimes patients bluff and pretend to understand following a communication breakdown, nodding and smiling in agreement with what they do not know. The consequences of bluffing can be unpleasant. The person may appear insensitive, uninterested, dull, or inattentive. He or she may begin to feel powerless to manage communication difficulties. When bluffing is used excessively, conversation may leave the person feeling like a failure or angry at him or herself.

The following conversation, which occurred between two women who had just met, presents an instance in which bluffing led to the appearance of insensitivity. Woman 2 has just said that she is about to take a trip. Woman 1 has a hearing loss:

Woman 1: "Where are you going?"

Woman 2: "To Portland to see my daughter. She is having a baby."

Woman 1: (nodding; she understood the word *baby*, but not much else) "I see."

Woman 2: "She has been bedridden for several weeks because she has diabetes and high blood pressure, and now the doctor says they are going to have to induce or the baby you know might be in trouble if it goes much longer than it's been going, even though it will be 4 weeks premature which we are pretty worried about especially since it's her first."

Woman 1: (lost by the length and convoluted syntax of her partner's utterance, and still not understanding much) "Oh, how nice."

Woman 2: "No, not really, this is pretty serious."

Inadvertently, Woman 1 has created an unfavorable impression because she bluffed and pretended to understand instead of repairing the communication breakdown. There are at least two reasons why people bluff extensively as in the above conversation: (1) reluctance to acknowledge a hearing loss, and (2) spirit of cooperation.

Many people are reluctant to admit a hearing loss. The first reason that someone may bluff is because use of a repair strategy may require a person to acknowledge a hearing loss. For instance, an individual might say, "Can you say that again please?" and the communication partner might respond, "What's-a matter?" For some people, it is difficult to acknowledge, "I have hearing loss, and I can't always catch all that is said to me."

We could devote an entire chapter to issues regarding the difficulty of acknowledging hearing loss. Many persons are reluctant to admit a hearing loss, in part because of personal vanity and perceived social stigmata (Blood, Blood, & Danhauer,

1978; Danhauer, Johnson, Kasten, & Brimacombe, 1985; Hétu, Riverin, Getty, Lalande, & St-Cyr, 1990). Unfortunately, many people have stereotypical views of hard-of-hearing persons. Some see them as difficult to communicate with, or as deserving pity. With respect to our present discussion, suffice it to say that, for many people, revealing a hearing loss to someone who does not know they have one can be a daunting challenge and, hence, they may be reluctant to use repair strategies.

A second reason why people may bluff relates to a desire to be cooperative and agreeable. Some people are unwilling to use repair strategies, and so bluff because they feel guilty and embarrassed about introducing difficulties into a conversation. Typically, when we converse, we try to ensure that a conversation is as pleasant and rewarding an experience for our communication partner(s) as it is for ourselves. If someone frequently halts the conversation for clarification, it may become less pleasant and rewarding (Figure 2–6).

If you were a participant in the following conversation, you probably would conclude that Richard, who, unknown to you, has a hearing loss, is both uncooperative and troublesome, and not a lot of fun to talk with:

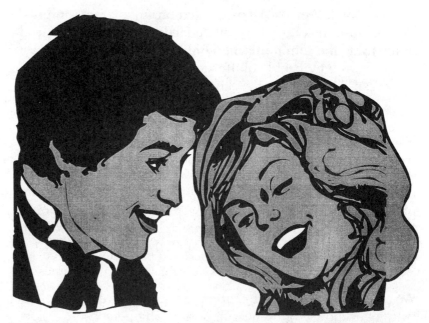

Figure 2–6. When we engage in conversation, we usually try to be cooperative and help make the conversation a pleasurable or meaningful experience for all participants.

Patrick:	"I am going on spring break next week."
Richard:	"Huh?"
Patrick:	"I said *spring break.*"
Richard:	"Oh."
Patrick:	"We are driving to Florida in Jason's parents' car."
Richard:	"Huh?"
Patrick:	"We are driving to Florida in Jason's parents' car."
Richard:	"Oh."
Mary:	"I wish I was going somewhere."
Richard:	"Huh?"
Mary:	"I wish I was going somewhere."
Richard:	"Yeah, me too."

As the interchange unfolds, the spontaneity of the conversation becomes stifled by Richard's continual requests for clarification. Maintaining continued conversation will prove laborious and effortful for all involved. It is for such reasons that many hard-of-hearing people opt to bluff, particularly when talking to people they do not know well.

Interruptions

Research has shown that frequent requests for clarifications may lead a communication partner to view a hard-of-hearing person unfavorably. Robinson and Reis (1989) found that people who interrupted their communication partners were perceived as less sociable than those who did not. Gagné, Stelmacovich, and Yovetich (1991) and Tye-Murray, Witt, Schum, and Sobaski (1995) found that a hard-of-hearing person was perceived more favorably when few communication breakdowns occurred during the course of a conversation. More research is needed about communication breakdowns and repair strategies. We need to explore how the hard-of-hearing person might gracefully indicate that a communication breakdown has occurred, when it is important for the individual to alert the communication partner (which might not be necessary in every instance of communication breakdown), and how long a hard-of-hearing person should attempt to repair the breakdown before giving up or moving on.

Expressive Repair Strategies

Heretofore, discussion has centered around receptive repair strategies, that is, a course of action someone may take when he or she does not recognize (receive) a spoken message. In addition to using receptive repair strategies, many children who have hearing loss need to use expressive repair strategies. *Expressive repair strategies* are used to rectify a communication breakdown that occurs because the hard-of-hearing person (the sender) produces an unintelligible utterance, and the conversational partner (the receiver) is unable to recognize it.

Many children who have hearing impairments have limited language skills or poor articulation. As a result, their conversational partners often may not recognize their spoken messages. Thus, it is important for them to learn how to cope with these kinds of communication breakdowns by using expressive repair strategies. Expressive repair strategies include repeating their original message using their best speech (e.g., they might slow down their speaking rate and emphasize important key words), breaking their longer sentences into shorter sentences, using another communication modality such as writing or mime, and using hand gestures, such as pointing. For instance, a child may say, "Hu mah meh mah," and her communication partner might respond, "Huh?" The child then may repeat the message using her best speech, "He make me *mad*." In this example, the child has implemented an expressive repair strategy. She has articulated her words more precisely and emphasized the keyword *mad*.

Expressive repair strategies are used when the sender produces an unintelligble utterance and the conversational partner cannot understand it.

RESEARCH RELATED TO COMMUNICATION STRATEGY USE

Several investigators have studied how hard-of-hearing individuals use repair strategies, and have converged on interesting conclusions. This research provides an important theoretical substratum for the content of a communication strategies training program.

The Repeat Repair Strategy and Nonspecific Repair Strategies

One issue investigators have addressed pertains to which repair strategies are used most commonly. The findings reveal that most individuals are more likely to ask their communication partners to repeat a message following a communication breakdown than to simplify it, restructure it, or elaborate (Tye-Murray, Knutson, & Lemke, 1993; Tye-Murray, Purdy, Woodworth, & Tyler, 1990; Tye-Murray & Witt, 1996). Moreover, their most common repair tactic is to say, "What?" "Huh," or "Pardon?" This kind of repair strategy (i.e., what-huh-pardon) is called a *nonspecific*, as opposed to a specific, *repair strategy*. When using a *specific repair strategy*, the hard-of-hearing person provides explicit instruction to the communication partner about how to repair the breakdown.

Specific and nonspecific repairs: Providing explicit instructions to the communication partner about how to repair the breakdown, as opposed to simply indicating lack of understanding.

Another issue that researchers have examined is what happens after particular repair strategies are used. For instance, when a person says, "Pardon?" how is a communication partner likely to respond? One of the most noteworthy findings pertains to the use of the repeat repair strategy and nonspecific repair strategies. When these are used following a communication breakdown, the communication partners typically repeat the original message verbatim (Tye-Murray, Witt, Schum, & Sobaski, 1995). Thus, if someone says "Huh?" to you, there is a high probability that you will repeat exactly what you have just said.

Interestingly, additional research suggests that someone is more likely to understand a message following a communication breakdown if the communication partner restructures it rather than simply repeating it (Gagné & Wyllie, 1989), especially if the talker already has repeated the message one time and the hard-of-hearing person still has not recognized it. Suppose someone says, "I bought a new car," and your patient responds "Huh?" Then the person repeats, "I bought a new car." This verbatim repetition may be less helpful to the patient than if the person had rephrased the message as, "I bought a Buick." New words, especially the more visible word *Buick* as opposed to *car*, may be easier for the patient to recognize audiovisually.

These findings suggest that many persons with hearing impairment typically use repair strategies that are apt to elicit the least effective response from their communication partners. That is, they often say "Huh?" and, in turn, receive a verbatim repetition of the very message they did not understand the first time around.

The results of another set of investigations suggest there may be another drawback to using nonspecific repair strategies. When persons often say "What?" or "Huh?" during a conversation to rectify communication breakdowns, their communication partners are more likely to perceive them unfavorably and to enjoy the interaction less (Gagné, Stelmacovich, & Yovetich, 1991; Tye-Murray, Witt, Schum, & Sobaski, 1995). Some laboratory studies have found that individuals who asked "What?" or "Huh?" following a breakdown in communication are more likely to be perceived unfavorably. In the experimental paradigm that was used in these experiments, audiovisual recordings were made of spontaneous conversations between two people, one of whom had a real or simulated hearing loss. The recordings were then shown to a team of judges, who were asked to view the recordings and rate the person with hearing loss on a personality 6-point rating scale (e.g., *this person is competent-incompetent*). The judges also rated the hard-of-hearing persons on a scale of emotional responses, using a second 6-point rating scale (e.g., *this person makes me feel composed-irritated*). The results revealed that, when individuals used nonspecific instead of specific repair strategies, they were rated unfavorably and they elicited unfavorable reactions from the judges. Thus it appears that some hard-of-hearing persons often tend to use the very repair strategies (nonspecific) that are most likely to elicit an unfavorable response from their communication partners.

Before we conclude our review of this area of research, two caveats must be appended. First, communication breakdowns that occur during spontaneous conversation between adults in which one partner has a hearing loss often are resolved after the use of a single repair strategy, even if it is a nonspecific strategy (Tye-Murray, Witt, Schum, & Sobaski, 1995). These data suggest that nonspecific repair strategies can be effective. Secondly, a nonspecific repair strategy is minimally disruptive to the flow of ongoing conversation. For instance, when an individual asks, "huh?" he or she assumes the speaking floor briefly, and the communication partner can easily continue a speaking turn. However, when someone uses other repair strategies, such as, "I missed that, can you tell me what you are talking about?" and uses them frequently, a conversation can become stilted and less fluent. By using a nonspecific repair strategy, the individual takes a phantom speaking turn, and may appear more cooperative in the conversational interchange.

Who Uses Repair Strategies, When, and What Are the Benefits?

Some research has focused on how the use of communication strategies relates to attitudinal variables and social-interaction indices, how repair strategy use varies as a function of whether the communication partner is familiar or unfamiliar, and the characteristics of hard-of-hearing adults who are most likely to use repair strategies. Hard-of-hearing persons have been surveyed about their use of communication strategies, and their responses have then been related to attitudinal variables, social-interaction indices, audiograms, or demographic variables.

These kinds of studies have yielded the following results. People are generally more likely to use communication strategies if their communication partner is familiar rather than unfamiliar. For instance, if they know the person, they might ask, "Can you tell me what you are talking about?" If they do not know the person, they may pretend to understand.

Some individuals are more likely than others to use a repair strategy than to say nothing following a communication breakdown. Individuals who use repair strategies also are less likely to feel frustrated with their speechreading skills and less likely to avoid social interactions than individuals who say nothing.

Persons who are least likely to use communication strategies tend to share certain characteristics (Tye-Murray, Purdy, & Woodworth, 1992; Tye-Murray, Knutson, & Lemke, 1993):

■ They have attained lower levels of education.
■ They have experienced a sudden hearing loss.
■ They receive minimal benefit from their listening devices.

In summary, research data suggest that an important component of an aural rehabilitation program might be provision of practice in using types of repair strategies other than nonspecific strategies. Nonspecific repair strategies comprise one of the most commonly used class of repair strategies but are the least effective. Moreover, patients should practice communication strategies with both familiar and unfamiliar communication partners, because some persons use strategies differently depending on who they are talking with. Finally, some persons may have a greater need for communication strategies training than others; for example, people who have experienced sudden hearing loss.

Informing a Communication Partner About a Hearing Loss

As noted earlier, some people are reluctant to use repair strategies because they do not want their communication partners to know they have hearing losses. One investigation examined what happened when adults who use cochlear implants talked with someone they did not know, and who did not know about the hearing loss (Tye-Murray & Witt, 1996). In this investigation, one patient was seated at a table with someone who had normal hearing. The normally hearing person was told that he or she was participating in a study about conversation, but did not know that his or her communication partner had a hearing loss. Each dyad tested in the experiment talked for 10 minutes. The conversations were videotaped and later analyzed.

Analyses showed that only 44% of the patients revealed their hearing losses, even though most experienced many communication breakdowns during the course of the 10-minute conversation. What is perhaps most interesting is what happened when a patient did reveal a loss. Once the patient did so, the conversation began to center around the topic of hearing loss and difficulties associated with hearing loss, rather than other shared topics of interest. This may be yet another reason why people are reluctant to reveal a hearing loss—they do not want the loss to become the focus of discussion.

Adjacency pairs: linked speaking turns.

You Say, I Say

When hard-of-hearing persons implement a repair strategy, they invite a response from their communication partners, thereby establishing a linked speaking turn. Schegloff and Sacks (1973) call linked speaking turns *adjacency pairs*. Examples of adjacency pairs include question-answer (e.g., "Who asked?"—"Bob asked.") and greeting-greeting combinations (e.g., "Hey there"—"Hi"). Particular repair strategy-response adjacency pairs often emerge when a hard-of-hearing person interacts with a normally hearing person. These include:

1. *Nonspecific repair strategy-message repetition response.* When a hard-of-hearing individual implements a nonspecific repair strategy following a communication breakdown, the communication partner typically repeats the original message.
2. *Request for information repair strategy-provide information response.* When a hard-of-hearing person requests specific information, the communication partner typically provides it.
3. *Confirmation repair strategy-feedback response.* When a hard-of-hearing person restates the message content, the communication partner usually either confirms or corrects the statement (see Tye-Murray and Witt, 1996, p. 467).

CONVERSATIONAL STYLES AND BEHAVIORS

Many communication training curricula include materials that are aimed at developing desirable conversational styles and conversational behaviors. Although there are no right and wrong ways per se of engaging in conversation, and what is appropriate will vary with the situation, some conversational styles and behaviors are nonetheless more effective when communication is hampered by the presence of hearing loss than are other styles and behaviors.

Conversational Styles

Kaplan, Bally, and Garretson (1985, pp. 19–20) described three kinds of conversational styles that adults with significant hearing impairment may exhibit: (1) passive, (2) aggressive, and (3) assertive. A person with a *passive conversational style* is someone who often does the following:

■ Withdraws from conversation
■ Frequently bluffs and pretends to recognize utterances
■ Avoids social interactions and group gatherings in order to avoid communication difficulties

A person with a **passive conversational style** tends to withdraw from conversations and social interactions rather than attempt to repair conversations.

Someone who sits at the bridge table, smiling and quietly nodding, is probably someone who can be characterized as having a passive conversational style. The person gains little by being in the game, and may begin to feel frustration and helplessness.

A person with an *aggressive conversational style* is the opposite extreme of the person with a passive conversational style. He or she may exhibit some of the following characteristics during conversation:

A person with an **aggressive conversational style** may blame others for misunderstanding.

■ Hostility
■ Belligerence
■ Bad attitude

The person may inadvertently embarrass, hurt, or anger his or her communication partners and often blame others for their communication difficulties. "Quit mumbling, and try to help me out!" someone may demand, or "I may as well not be here, you're talking to everyone but me." The first utterance is a tacit insult (i.e., it implies, "You could help me out but you have chosen not to"), whereas the second is demanding ("I have hearing loss and no one else does, so you should accommodate me "). These kinds of utterances have the potential to alienate communication partners, and may result in the hard-of-hearing person being ineffective and even avoided.

During communication training, patients often are encouraged to minimize their use of a passive or aggressive conversational style, and instead implement an assertive style. Persons who adopt an *assertive conversational style* usually follow these guidelines during conversation. They:

A person who adopts an **assertive conversational style** takes responsibility for managing communication difficulties in a way that is considerate of communication partners.

■ Respect the rights of their communication partners, while honestly and openly expressing their own needs and emotions.
■ Take responsibility for managing communication difficulties, but do so in a way that is considerate of their communication partners.

"Let's get a seat away from the stereo speaker," an assertive person may suggest, "and then you won't have to repeat everything you say." This remark is courteous and provides direct explanation of how to remedy a communication problem.

These three types of conversational styles (passive, aggressive, and assertive) are often reviewed in a communication training program. Hard-of-hearing persons can learn to develop assertive ways of dealing with communication problems, and minimize their passive or aggressive responses.

Communication Behaviors

Figure 2–7 presents three constellations of behaviors that complement the model of conversational styles described by Kaplan et al. (1985) (Tye-Murray & Witt, 1996). The model consists of three circles that are labeled interactive, noninteractive, and dominating.

Interactive behavior is the use of cooperative conversational tactics, consistent with an assertive conversational style.

Persons who fall within the *interactive* circle use cooperative conversational tactics (Grice, 1975; Wardhaugh, 1985), which are consistent with an assertive conversational style. These individuals share responsibility with their conversational partners for advancing a topic of conversation and selecting topics of conversation. They do not dominate discussion, and they show interest in what their communication partners say and attempt to respond appropriately to their remarks.

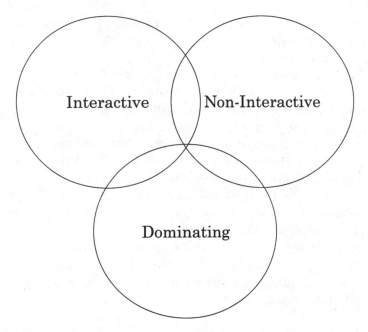

Figure 2-7. Constellations of behaviors that characterize some hard-of-hearing persons.

Persons who fit the *noninteractive* constellation of behaviors often can be characterized as having a passive conversational style. They may bluff following a communication breakdown. They may not contribute much to the development of a conversation topic, and they may not participate in selecting a topic to talk about. They also may not respond to turn-taking signals. For instance, a communication partner may say, "So . . . you know . . . hmmm," hoping that the person with hearing impairment will contribute a remark. The following interchange illustrates a noninteractive conversational style (exhibited by Rose, who has a hearing loss):

Noninteractive behavior is characteristic of a passive behavioral style.

Marie:	"I saw a great movie last night."
Rose:	"Oh."
Marie:	"It was on the old movies channel on cable."
Rose:	"Hmmm."
Marie:	"It had Fred Astaire and Ginger Rogers, lots of dancing and, you know, that kind of old movie stuff . . ."
Rose:	(nods)
Marie:	"I just love that . . ."
Rose:	(nods)

| Marie: | "I guess it takes me back to when I was going to the movies as a kid." |

In this interchange, Rose does not express interest in Marie's remarks and does not share in advancing the topic. Marie begins to talk more in order to fill in the silences.

A noninteractive conversational style often yields unfavorable consequences. In a series of interviews with hard-of-hearing adults, Cowie and Douglas-Cowie (1992) were told by one participant, "There are many occasions when I would like to ask questions, but in case I don't hear the answer I just don't do it. I think that probably gives the impression that I'm not interested which isn't the case, it's just to save embarrassment" (p. 269). An individual's withdrawal can elicit negative reactions from communication partners and create an internal source of stress for oneself.

Dominating behaviors are characteristic of an aggressive conversational style.

The final constellation in Figure 2–7 denotes a constellation of *dominating conversational behaviors*, which are characteristic of an aggressive conversational style. Persons who fall into this circle may take extended speaking turns, interrupt, and use abrupt topic changes. They may try to dominate the conversation, in order to always be aware of what is being talked about. Sometimes they will avoid asking questions so that they do not have to give up the speaking floor to hear the answers. Here is an excerpt from one conversation in which Deidre, an older woman with hearing loss, was conversing with her friend's daughter, Carrie:

Deidre:	"Sharon says you are going on vacation."
Carrie:	"Yes, I am flying with my brother to . . ."
Deidre:	(interrupting) "Oh, I went on a plane once, to see my brother in South Carolina. He has a house down there, one he built himself on a lake."

With one remark, the two are suddenly talking about Deidre's plane trip and her brother rather than Carrie's upcoming travels.

As is the case with a passive conversational style, a dominating conversational style also may have undesired effects. One participant in the interviews conducted by Cowie and Douglas-Cowie (1992) reported, "I have to dominate the meeting, I make myself the artificial center of attention so that people will just speak to me . . . instead of speaking to the chairman they would be speaking to me" (p. 269). One can surmise that colleagues (or at least the chairman) might react unfavorably to such a dominating conversational style.

In the model illustrated in Figure 2–7, the three circles overlap because an individual usually demonstrates behaviors that are characteristic of more than one constellation. An individual's use of conversational behaviors may vary during a conversation, as the person becomes more comfortable or the dynamics of the interchange are established. Behavior may vary as a function of the familiarity of the communication partner too, as well as the circumstances in which the conversation is occurring.

FINAL REMARKS

In this chapter, we have considered communication strategies and conversational styles and behaviors. Patients have a myriad of means for managing their communication difficulties. Although many of the strategies we considered in this chapter seem like common sense, it is surprising that many people either have not explicitly thought about them or do not use them effectively. Moreover, many people are not aware that they may be using a conversational style or conversational behaviors that alienate their communication partners. Although these may have been adopted as a means of coping with hearing-related difficulties, they may create problems in and of themselves.

KEY CHAPTER POINTS

✔ The accepted rules of conversation often must bend when one of the conversational partners has a hearing loss. The overall quality of conversation also may be diminished. For instance, there may only be superficial content.
✔ There are two classes of communication strategies, facilitative and repair. Within each of these classes are several kinds of strategies that hard-of-hearing individuals can use to facilitate conversational interchanges.
✔ There are at least three stages involved in repairing a communication breakdown: detection, selection of a course of action, and implementation.

✔ Hard-of-hearing persons often bluff and pretend to understand. They may do this because they are reluctant to admit a hearing loss, or because they do not want to appear uncooperative.

✔ Much research has centered on the use of repair strategies. One conclusion that emerges is that the most commonly used repair strategy is the repeat strategy.

✔ Hard-of-hearing persons may be passive, assertive, or aggressive, during conversation.

Assessment of Conversational Fluency and Communication Handicap

Topics

- Conversational Fluency
- Communication Handicap and Disability
- General Considerations for Assessing Conversational Fluency and Communication Handicap
- Interviews
- Questionnaires

- Daily Logs
- Group Discussions
- Structured Communication Interactions
- Final Remarks
- Key Chapter Points
- Key Resources

Typically, a communication strategies training program begins and ends with an assessment of individuals' conversational fluency and communication handicap, two terms that will be defined shortly. The goals of the initial assessment are to:

■ Determine the communication demands placed upon individuals in their everyday life.
■ Evaluate the impact of hearing loss on daily activities.
■ Identify the settings in which communication problems arise.
■ Document the kinds of social activities in which a person is likely to engage.
■ Assess how effectively they use communication strategies in a variety of settings.
■ Chronicle their employment responsibilities.

The goals of assessment will guide your selection of which measures you administer. For example, if the goal of assessment is to identify communication problems that are especially troublesome, you might interview the patient or administer a questionnaire. On the other hand, if the goal is to document conversational fluency, you might determine how well information can be exchanged between two communication partners, while maintaining a give-and-take dialogue. Assessment techniques for this purpose may include structured communication interactions or informal conversations.

The final assessment indicates whether a person's actual or perceived conversational fluency and communication handicap have improved as a result of training. Some of the original measures might be repeated to determine whether performance has changed. One-time-only measures also might be administered, such as a questionnaire, in which participants can critique the success of an aural rehabilitation plan.

You will want to know what the patient's audiogram looks like, both aided and unaided. In addition, you will assess his or her ability to recognize words in an audition-only condition and in an audition-plus-vision condition. In Chapter 5, we will consider the audiogram and assessment of word recognition. In this chapter, we will consider those assessment instruments that pertain to communication difficulties in everyday situations and conversational fluency.

CONVERSATIONAL FLUENCY

Now we will consider the definition of conversational fluency. *Conversational fluency* relates to how smoothly conversation unfolds. The following factors help to define conversational fluency (Erber, 1996, pp. 204–205):

■ **Time spent in repairing communication breakdowns**. If during a course of a conversation, numerous communication breakdowns occur and they require many interchanges between the hard-of-hearing person and communication partner before they are resolved, then conversational fluency is low. On the other hand, if need for clarification is minimal, conversational fluency is high.

■ **Exchange of information and ideas**. If the participants in a conversation successfully and easily share information and ideas, and the conversation seems to them to be spontaneous and not stilted, then conversational fluency is high.

■ **Speaking time is shared**. When conversation is smooth-flowing, participants have ample opportunity to speak, and no one person dominates with protracted speaking times. Prolonged silences or frequent interruptions are not characteristic of fluent conversations.

Sociolinguists (scientists who study conversational interactions and how they are influenced by social and cultural factors) often index the sharing of speaking time with a measure called *mean length turn ratio (MLT ratio)*. To determine this ratio, *mean length of speaking turn (MLT)* is first computed for each participant in a conversation by determining the average number of words each person speaks, for some set number of conversational turns (often, 50 turns). A *conversational turn* begins when one communication partner starts to speak. The turn ends when the person stops talking, and someone else responds to the remark. The MLT ratio is computed by taking a ratio between the MLTs of the two communication partners. Table 3–1 illustrates how MLT and MLT ratio are determined.

The dialogues in Table 3–1 also illustrate two different levels of conversational fluency. In the first example, conversational fluency is high. The two communication partners exchange information with ease, and they share responsibility in ad-

Conversational fluency relates to how smoothly conversation unfolds.

Sociolinguistics is a branch of linguistics that studies the effects of social and cultural differences within a community on its use of language and conversational patterns.

Mean length (speaking) turn (MLT) is computed by determining the average number of words spoken during a set number of conversational turns.

Mean length turn ratio (MLT ratio) is the ratio of the MLTs of two speakers in a conversation.

A conversational turn is the period during which a participant delivers a contribution to the conversation.

Table 3–1. Dialogues that illustrate two levels of conversational fluency. Example 1 presents a sample with high conversational fluency, whereas Example 2 presents a sample with low conversational fluency.

Example 1

Joan: "Has your new furniture arrived yet?"

Ann: "Yes, and I'm thrilled with it."

Joan: "You said that it was going to be French regency."

Ann: "No, I didn't go with that. My husband wanted a deco look."

Analysis: Joan's MLT = 8.0 words (16 words divided by 2 utterances)

Ann's MLT = 9.0 words (18 words divided by 2 utterances)

MLT ratio: 0.9, where 1.0 = equal length speaking turns

Example 2

Martha: "Has your new furniture arrived yet?"

Tom: "Huh?"

Martha: "Your furniture?"

Tom: (looks around, shakes head)

Martha: "How are you doing? How is your wife?. . . . Mary?"

Tom: "Fine."

Analysis: Martha's MLT = 5.6 words (17 words divided by 3 utterances)

Tom's MLT = 0.7 (2 words divided by 3 utterances)

MLT ratio: 6.2, where 1.0 = equal length speaking turns

MLT = mean length turn

vancing the topic of discussion. They talk about a content-dense subject, period furniture. The MLT ratio for this conversation is approximately equal, which is often characteristic of fluent interchanges.

The second conversational excerpt in Table 3–1 presents a sample of low conversational fluency. The topic of discussion quickly becomes superficial, as communication breakdowns occur. In this conversation, Martha bears the onus of responsibility for advancing the conversation. She must fill in the awkward silences, and develop the topic. Conversational fluency like this is not uncommon when one of the conversational partners has a significant hearing loss.

Traditional Audiologic Tests Versus Measures of Conversational Fluency

There are at least three reasons why traditional tests of word recognition sometimes do not index how well patients perform in real-world conversational interactions (e.g., Binnie, 1991; Cox, Alexander, & Gilmore, 1987; Erber, 1992; Tye-Murray & Tyler, 1988). "First, most audiologic test lists present unrelated speech stimuli. In typical conversations, utterances are related by linguistic, and often situational, context. Second, clients usually must repeat what they hear verbatim. In everyday conversation, they listen more often for the gist of the message and not for the purpose of repeating every word (Tye-Murray, Purdy, & Woodworth, 1992; see also Bransford & Frank, 1971, and Sachs, 1967, for related research). Finally, clients usually interact with their conversational partners during the give and take of an ongoing conversation. If a client does not recognize an utterance, the individual can ask the partner to repeat or modify the message. Clients who repair communication breakdowns effectively might experience fewer difficulties in conversations than standard audiologic test results would predict; clients who do not repair breakdowns very well might experience more difficulties" (Tye-Murray, Witt, & Castelloe, 1996, p. 396).

COMMUNICATION HANDICAP AND DISABILITY

An issue closely related to conversational fluency is that of communication handicap. *Communication handicap* refers to the psychosocial disadvantages that result from hearing loss. These disadvantages include limitations that occur in performing activities of daily life. When we discuss how well a patient can talk to a business associate on the telephone, we are considering that person's communication handicap.

A **communication handicap** consists of the psychosocial disadvantages that result from hearing loss.

The term *communication handicap* contrasts with the term *communication disability*, which is any restriction resulting from hearing impairment to perform an activity in the range that is considered normal (World Health Organization, 1980). When we say that a person cannot detect the /s/ sound in the word *soup*, we are talking about that person's disability.

A **disability** is a loss of function.

GENERAL CONSIDERATIONS FOR EVALUATING CONVERSATIONAL FLUENCY AND COMMUNICATION HANDICAP

Conversational fluency and communication handicap can be challenging for a speech and hearing professional to assess for a number of reasons. First, conversational fluency and success in managing communication difficulties vary as a function of the conversational setting and situation, and as a function of the communication partner. For instance, conversational fluency may be high when an individual talks with a seasoned speech and hearing professional but poor when the person converses with an unfamiliar store clerk. The speech and hearing professional is likely to be accustomed to talking to persons with hearing loss, and probably speaks slowly and clearly and checks for comprehension. The store clerk may not know how to facilitate speech recognition for the person with hearing loss, may turn away when talking (and hence, limit the hard-of-hearing person's ability to speechread), and may speak quickly. A measure of conversational fluency taken from the same hard-of-hearing individual probably would be high for the first communication partner but low for the second.

A second reason that assessment of conversational fluency may be problematic is because measures vary with the topic of discussion. For instance, conversational fluency may be high for a superficial topic such as the weather but low for a topic centering on local politics. Thus, depending on what you talked about, you might rate conversational fluency with a particular patient as either high or low.

A third reason conversational fluency and communication handicap are difficult to assess is because communication difficulties do not always arise during a conversation. A person may experience numerous difficulties in conversing in the workplace, but none while talking to a family member in a speech and hearing clinic test room. If communication breakdowns do not occur during the course of an assessment, a speech and hearing professional may not gain an appreciation of how an individual manages communication difficulties.

Finally, conversational fluency and communication handicap are difficult to index because no one measure can capture adequately the "construct" of conversational fluency or communication handicap, because both are defined by several dimensions. That is, both are abstractions that reflect a multitude of factors, such as those we considered above for conversational fluency (i.e., the occurrence of breakdowns and pauses, the fluidity of conversation, MLT ratio, and the superficiality of discussion). A number of measures must be performed, and the results aggregated and then interpreted.

For all of these reasons, assessment can be challenging. In the next sections, we consider specific assessment procedures that may be used. These procedures are listed in Table 3–2, along with some of their advantages and disadvantages.

INTERVIEWS

The most straightforward assessment procedure is the *interview*. Individuals talk about their conversational problems, and they consider possible reasons as to why communication breakdowns happen (Figure 3–1). They comment on their subjective impressions of conversational fluency in a variety of settings (e.g., the workplace, the home). "Are you able to use the telephone?" a clinician might ask, or the clinician might ask a more open-ended question, such as, "Tell me about your listening difficulties." People's answers will indicate their particular concerns, and their perceptions of their situation and problems.

Interviews are a basic assessment procedure used to elicit specific information about each individual's hearing problem.

Table 3–2. Some general procedures for measuring conversational fluency and communication needs, and one advantage and disadvantage of each.

Procedure	Advantage	Disadvantage
Interview	Yields patient-specific information	Difficult to quantify information
Questionnaire	Quick and easy to administer	May miss patient-specific information
Daily log	Provides quantitative information about an extended time period	Can be a reactive procedure
Group discussion	Stimulates patients to introspect and reflect	Some patients may be reluctant to participate
Structured communication interaction	Has good face validity because assessment is based on actual conversational interactions	Can be time-consuming to score

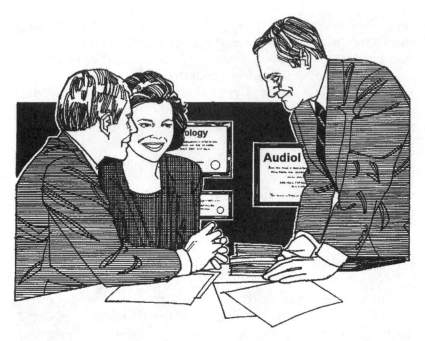

Figure 3–1. A clinician may interview the patient or the patient and a family member to learn about communication difficulties that are being experienced.

Interviews are effective because they elicit information that is specific to an individual. For instance, you may learn that one individual has difficulty communicating during office conferences whereas another experiences problems while watching television. An open-ended discussion about the workplace may trigger a patient to reflect about particular instances in which communication was difficult in his or her recent past and may provide direction for the aural rehabilitation plan.

The disadvantage of interviews is that remarks cannot be quantified. This is problematic when changes in communication behaviors that result from intervention must be documented (Stephens & Hétu, 1991). Documentation is essential when you seek reimbursement for providing training to patients from third party health care providers.

QUESTIONNAIRES

Questionnaires are procedures used to gain subjective information about conversational fluency and communication handicap from respondents.

Another assessment instrument that is used to assess conversational fluency and communication handicap is the questionnaire. *Questionnaires* might query respondents about how often communication breakdowns occur, and whether they typically attempt to repair communication breakdowns and how. Questionnaires are a means of gathering general information easily and quickly (Figure 3–2).

One drawback in using questionnaires is that it is possible to miss important information about communication difficulties that are specific to an individual simply because they are not covered by items in the questionnaire (Stephens & Hétu, 1991). For instance, a true/false statement such as, *I always verify what I understood during a meeting with a co-worker afterwards*, is irrelevant to the respondent who does not work or does not attend meetings. Moreover, responses to questionnaires may not reflect the importance of each communication difficulty or communication situation to the individual. For example, an inability to talk on the telephone may be devastating to the lifestyle of one person but only a minor annoyance to another.

A number of self-assessment questionnaires have been developed. Several are summarized in the Key Resources section at the end of the chapter. The recent popularity of these instruments relate in part to the fact that subjective impressions of communication difficulties often do not correspond to patients' audiograms (Brainerd & Frankel, 1985; Demorest & Walden, 1984; Speaks, Jerger, & Trammel, 1970; Weinstein &

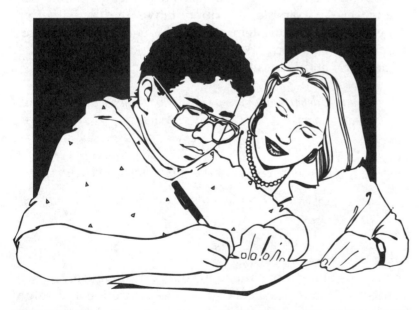

Figure 3–2. Questionnaires are an effective means of obtaining information about communication and conversation in an easy and fast way.

Ventry, 1983). For example, an audiogram may indicate that a person has a significant hearing loss. However, the individual, when completing a questionnaire, may describe the loss as a minor nuisance, but not overly problematic. In considering the discrepancy that sometimes exists between audiological and questionnaire information, Erdman (1994) notes:

> Self-reports simply constitute different measures; the method of measurement differs as does the content of the measurement. Audiometric tests assess maximum potential or best performance of the central or peripheral hearing mechanism. Self-report instruments, on the other hand, assess typical performance in behavioral utilization of hearing ability (p. 69).

Questionnaires may yield either quantitative or qualitative information, depending on the design of the questionnaire items. *Open-ended questions* typically elicit qualitative data. Examples of open-set items include the following:

Open-ended questions elicit qualitative information.

■ *Describe the situations wherein you typically have problems communicating.*
■ *What do you usually do when you do not understand someone?*

Closed-ended questions are used to gather quantitative information.

Closed-ended questions may be used to gather quantitative information. An example of a quantitative questionnaire item appears below. On this item, the respondent's task is to write a number between one and ten on each response blank, where *1* means *never* and *10* means *always*:

> *I am at a department store. The clerk asks me a question, but I do not understand her. I am most likely to:*
>
> _____ *ask the clerk to repeat the question*
>
> _____ *ask the clerk to say the question in a different way*
>
> _____ *shake my head to indicate that I missed what the clerk said*
>
> _____ *say and do nothing*

Both kinds of questionnaire items offer advantages and disadvantages. Open-ended items are less restrictive and might yield information from a patient that could not have been anticipated. However, sometimes answers to open-ended items are rambling or off-topic, and they may be difficult to quantify, which may be important if a clinician desires to compare pre- and postintervention performance. Closed-ended items allow for a quantitative analysis of responses. However, important information may be missed if the questionnaire does not include items that tap information relevant to a patient's communication difficulties.

DAILY LOGS

In completing a *daily log* (Figure 3–3) , respondents perform a self-monitoring procedure regarding behaviors of interest, and provide self-reports. For example, they may log how many times a day they experience communication difficulties, and in which communication settings (e.g., the home, the workplace). In completing logs, patients may answer a series of questions about their communication difficulties and/or behaviors every day for a set number of days. Example items from a daily log appear in Table 3–3.

Daily logs are self-reports of behavior used by respondents for self-monitoring.

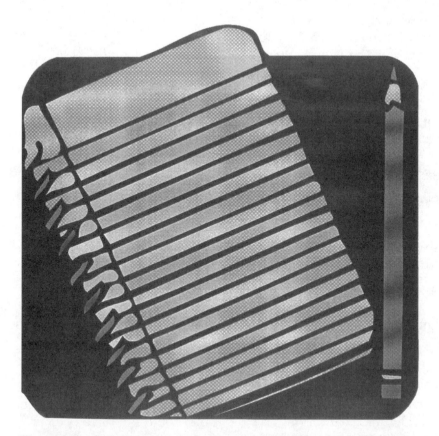

Figure 3–3. Daily logs usually are completed every day for a set period of time, often a week.

Table 3-3. Example items from a daily log, designed to monitor someone's communication behaviors.

1. **Think about your communication interactions today. For the following situations, circle the term (*never, a few times, many times*) that best describes how much time you spent talking today (beyond a greeting). Circle one response for each condition:**

In a quiet place	Never	a few times	many times
In a noisy place	Never	a few times	many times
On the telephone	Never	a few times	many times
From another room	Never	a few times	many times
In a group of people	Never	a few times	many times

2. **For the following two situations, write down a number between 0 to 100 (0 = nothing and 100 = everything) that indicates how much of what was said to you today you believe you understood.**

    ___ while watching the talker and listening

    ___ while listening only

3. **Did you ever indicate that you did not understand a spoken message today (Yes or No)?**

    _____

4. **What did you do when you did not understand a message (Check all that apply.)**

    ___ I asked the talker to repeat the message.

    ___ I said, "Huh" or "Pardon."

    ___ I asked the talker to rephrase the message.

    ___ I asked the talker to indicate what he or she was talking about.

    ___ I decided the message was not important enough to keep trying.

    ___ I asked the talker to spell or write the message.

    ___ Other (describe)_____

5. **Consider the conversations that you had with relatives today. Check all of the statements below that apply.**

    ___ I felt anxious when I tried to talk with my relative today.

    ___ I was able to understand my relative's spoken messages.

    ___ I felt satisfied with the success of our communication interactions.

    ___ I avoided talking about unimportant topics.

When patients complete a log for several consecutive days, their responses provide a general index of their daily use of communication strategies, their conversational fluency, and their communication handicap. Responses also may provide information about their aural rehabilitation needs. For example, if an individual reports that he never spoke on the telephone during six consecutive days, it might be inferred that this person may be unable to use the telephone successfully, and therefore avoids telephone conversations. The aural rehabilitation plan may thus be designed to provide telephone training and a telephone receiver amplifier.

Individuals can perform a daily log activity before and after participating in a communication strategies training program, and trends in responses can be compared before and after training. For example, if after completing a communication strategies training program and after receiving a telephone receiver amplifier, the man above reported he used the telephone an average of two times every day (as compared to never), then it might be concluded that intervention provided some benefit to this individual.

Guidelines for Constructing a Daily Log

Few examples of daily logs for aural rehabilitation applications are available in the literature. Therefore, you may have to design your own, and tailor them to track the pertinent activities and behaviors of each patient. Below are five guidelines you might consider when developing a daily log:

1. Include detailed instructions at the beginning of the daily log and at the start of each section that initiates a new format. Make the instructions clear and concise.
2. Use active sentences rather than passive sentences when writing daily log items.
3. Log items should have a minimum of prepositional phrases.
4. Avoid professional jargon or terms often used within the speech and hearing communication field but not by the general public.
5. Limit the number of items in a daily log to a maximum of seven. Otherwise, it may be too taxing for your client to complete, or too much of an imposition in the daily routine.

Self-monitoring can provide **reactive** procedure as it may influence how a person uses communication behaviors and strategies.

Self-monitoring can be a *reactive* procedure because it may influence a person's communication behaviors and how he or she uses communication strategies. For example, researchers have shown that when individuals complete self-monitoring diaries, they often improve their academic performance, reduce their consumption of alcohol, or decrease the number of cigarettes smoked (e.g., Johnson & Wilhite, 1971; McFall, 1970). Similarly, by monitoring use of communication strategies, patients may actually improve their use of them. As such, the use of daily logs can be used as a training procedure as well as an assessment procedure. However, for this very reason, it can be problematic when one is trying to assess the effects of an intervention program.

GROUP DISCUSSION

Group discussion provides a forum for class members to discuss communication issues.

In a *group discussion* (Figure 3–4), usually convened on the first meeting of a communication strategies training program,

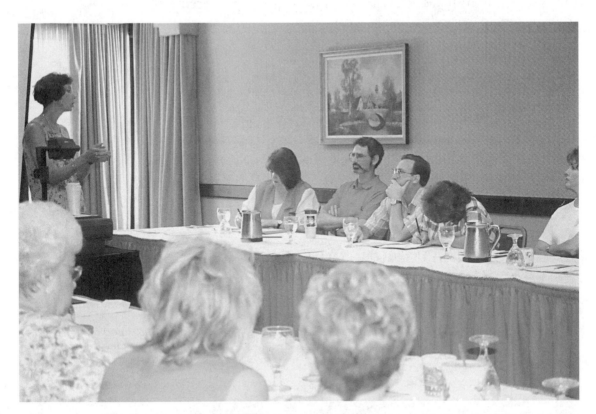

Figure 3–4. The success of a group discussion may well hinge on the skill of the group leader. In this session, the clinician is using an overhead projector to record the group participants' comments. By Kim Readmond, courtesy CID.

members of the class construct a list of their communication problems and the topics they would like included in the syllabus. The remainder of the program then focuses on these issues. This procedure is excellent, and can be used any time that instruction occurs in a group setting as opposed to one-on-one. Table 3–4 lists some concerns that have emerged during this kind of group session.

Tips on Conducting a Group Discussion

The success (or failure) of a group discussion often hinges on the skill of the speech and hearing professional who conducts the session. Below are a list of suggestions that might be followed when conducting a group discussion (Trychin, 1994):

■ Encourage everyone to participate in the discussion, perhaps by asking group members to take turns one at a time around the table.

■ Record remarks on a chalkboard, on an overhead projector slide, or an oversized hanging notebook, even if they seem off-topic or minor.

■ Make sure that no one is made to feel embarrassed or foolish for making a contribution.

■ Ask some questions that guide the discussion and engage the students in the discussion. For example, you might say, "Mrs. Smith, you work in a pharmacy. What kinds of listening difficulties do you experience when you are behind the counter?"

■ Come to the class prepared to draw specific material from the participants.

STRUCTURED COMMUNICATION INTERACTIONS

Structured communication interactions also can be used during both assessment and training. *Structured communication interactions* are simulated conversations, and reflect some of the difficulties that actually occur in a patient's typical day. *TOPICON* (Erber, 1988) is an example of a structured communication interaction activity that may be used for both assessment and training purposes. In this procedure, the patient carries on a conversation with the clinician. The clinician monitors and evaluates conversational difficulties that occur. Afterwards, the

Structured communication interactions are simulated conversations used to reflect a patient's communication difficulties.

TOPICON is an example of a structured communication interaction activity.

Table 3-4. Common concerns that might by identified during a group discussion.

Difficulty talking on the telephone

Impatience on the part of a spouse

Inability to manage communication breakdowns effectively

Avoidance by old friends

People talk to my spouse instead of me

Feelings of isolation and loneliness

Feelings of incompetence and anger

Difficulty conversing in noisy settings

Difficulty in communicating with my co-workers

Anxiety about not being able to hear warning signals

Frustration that family does not understand my hearing loss

Frustration that most people do not know what it is like to have a hearing loss

Feelings of being "left out"

Source: Adapted from Trychin, S. (1994). Helping people cope with hearing loss. In J. G. Clark and F. N. Martin (Eds.), *Effective counseling in audiology: Perspectives and practice* (pp. 247–277). Englewood Cliffs, NJ: Simon and Schuster Co.

clinician and student discuss the fluency of the interaction. They talk about the problems that arose, and alternative ways of handling them. They consider who spoke more during the interaction and why. They discuss the direction of information flow, and identify which communication strategies were applied and whether or not they were effective. Conversation fluency can be evaluated with a consideration of the following: (1) number of prolonged pauses, (2) number of restarts, (3) number of topic shifts, (4) interruptions of turn-taking, (5) level of abstraction and superficiality, (6) presence of self-consciousness, and (7) the degree of understanding (Erber, 1988, p. 79).

Question-Answer Sessions (Quest?AR)

Quest?AR is a structured communication procedure that can be used to assess communication difficulties.

Quest?AR is a structured communication procedure that can be used to assess communication difficulties. In the procedure, the clinician asks a series of scripted questions, and the patient responds. Occasionally, listening difficulties are added to induce communication breakdowns. Performance is then evaluated in terms of the frequency of communication breakdowns, and the patient's facility in repairing them. An example of the procedure is presented below (quoted from Erber and Lind, 1994, p. 280).

	Difficulty Added	Difficulty Identified?
1. Why did you go there?		
2. When did you go?	fast	no
3. How many people went with you?		
4. Who were they (relations/ names)?	soft	yes
5. What did you take with you?	long	yes
6. Where is (the place where you went)?		
7. How did you get there?		
8. What did you see on the way?	fast	yes
9. What time did you get there		

FINAL REMARKS

In this chapter, we have considered a variety of ways to assess conversational fluency and communication handicap. Each procedure has advantages and disadvantages, and a major challenge for a speech and hearing professional may lie in the optimum selection and use of the measurement procedures. It is not uncommon for clinicians to use a test-battery approach and employ more than one type of assessment procedure. This approach can provide a more well-rounded portrait of communication difficulties than the use of a single measure. However, you need to be careful not to overwhelm patients with assessment procedures. For example, if they spend their entire first class of communication training with assessment, and do not perceive they have benefitted by attending, they are not likely to show up for a second class.

KEY CHAPTER POINTS

✔ Most communication strategies training programs begin and end with an assessment of conversational fluency and communication handicap. Conversational fluency relates to how smoothly conversation unfolds. Communication handicap pertains to the psychosocial disadvantages related to the hearing loss.

✔ Conversational fluency and communication handicap are difficult to assess for many reasons. For example, conversational fluency may vary as a function of the communication partner (Is the person familiar? Is the person experienced with talking to hard-of-hearing people?) and with the topic of conversation.

✔ A variety of assessment procedures are available. These procedures include interviews and questionnaires. Each offers both advantages and disadvantages. Often, clinicians opt to use a test-battery approach.

KEY RESOURCES

Self-Assessment Questionnaires for Assessing Hearing Handicap and Disability

Communication Assessment Profile
Schow, R. & Nerbonne, M. (1982). Communication screening profile: Use with elderly clients. *Ear and Hearing, 3,* 135–147.

Communication Profile for the Hearing Impaired
Demorest, M., & Erdman, S. (1987). Scale composition and item analysis of the communication profile for the hearing impaired. *Journal of Speech and Hearing Disorders, 52,* 515–535.

Denver Scale of Communication Function
Alpiner, J. G., Cheverette, W., Clascoe, G., Metz, M., & Olsen, B. (1974). Printed in J. Alpiner and P. McCarthy (Eds.). (1993). *Rehabilitative audiology: Children and adults.* Baltimore, MD: Williams and Wilkins.

Hearing Handicap Inventory for the Elderly
Ventry, I., & Weinstein, B. (1982). The hearing handicap inventory for the elderly: A new tool. *Ear and Hearing, 12,* 355–357.

Hearing Handicap Scale
Fairbanks, G., & Glorig, A. (1964). Scale for self-assessment of hearing handicap. *Journal of Speech and Hearing Disorders, 29,* 215–230.

Hearing Measurement Scale
Noble, W., & Atherley, G. (1970). The hearing measurement scale: A questionnaire for the assessment of auditory disability. *Journal of Auditory Research, 10,* 229–250.

Hearing Performance Inventory (Revised)
Lamb, S., Owens, E., & Schubert, E. (1983). The revised form of the hearing performance inventory. *Ear and Hearing, 4,* 152–157.

Nursing Home Hearing Handicap Index (NHH)
Schow, R., & Nerbonee, M. (1977). Assessment of hearing handicap by nursing home residents and staff. *Journal of the Academy of Rehabilitative Audiology, 10,* 2–12.

Profile Questionnaire for Rating Communicative Performance in a Home Envrionment
Sanders, D. (1988). Hearing and orientation and counseling. In M. Pollack (Ed.), *Amplification for the hearing impaired.* New York, NY: Grune and Stratton.

Communication Strategies Training

Topics

- General Program Content
- Issues to Consider When Developing a Training Program
- Model for Training
- Short-Term Training
- Communication Strategies Training for Frequent Communication Partners
- Communication Strategies Training for Children
- Efficacy of Training
- Final Remarks
- Key Chapter Points

There are many ways to provide training in the use of communication strategies. Current practices range from simply making printed materials available in the clinic waiting room to presenting a weekly program that may extend several weeks or even months. Training activities may include paper and pencil tasks, role-playing, group discussions, and workbook exercises. When possible, the training program should be designed to meet the participants' expectations, age, socioeconomic background, lifestyle, and particular communication problems.

In the following sections, we will consider the stages of a communication strategies training program, and training activities for each stage. Because it is not always feasible to implement this model, we also will consider alternative models.

Sensitivity to People's Self-Perceptions

"[Speech and hearing professionals] may find it particularly helpful when working with hard-of-hearing adults and their families to remember that how people perceive communication problems (i.e., their meaning or significance to the people involved) is a very important factor to consider. For example, some hard-of-hearing people believe that, due to their hearing loss, they are a burden on other people, and this belief leads them to withdraw from social contact and also probably leads to depression. As another example, many people believe that hearing aids correct hearing problems to the same degree that glasses correct visual problems. It is difficult for people holding this belief to understand why a person wearing hearing aids does not understand what is being said, and it does not occur to them to think about doing anything else to remedy the situation. So, included in the [communication strategies training] programs I conduct are some ways to help people separate fact from fiction pertaining to hearing loss, and methods for helping hearing-impaired people develop a more realistic appraisal of themselves and their hearing problem" (Trychin, 1994, p. 248).

GENERAL PROGRAM CONTENT

The content of a communication strategies training program typically concerns problems specifically related to hearing loss and how these problems can be minimized. Excessive sympathy for individuals is not expressed, and personal problems unrelated to hearing loss are not considered. Content may include training for the two types of communication strategies, facilitative and repair (see Chapter 2). During this training, people learn to modify the four factors that affect communication success (the talker, the message, the environment, themselves), and learn to rectify breakdowns in communication. They typically learn about assertive versus nonassertive behaviors too, and work on developing their skills to deal assertively with communication difficulties.

ISSUES TO CONSIDER WHEN DEVELOPING A TRAINING PROGRAM

In developing a training program, several nuts-and-bolts issues must be considered. One issue is the optimum program length. Some persons will have minimal time to devote to a communication strategies training program, and 1 hour may be all that is available. Standard programs usually require 12 to 40 hours, and are presented in one of two formats. The course may provide intensive instruction during a week-long period, meeting 4 to 7 hours per day or may be spread over an 8 to 15 week period, with each session lasting several hours each week.

Another issue to consider is the class format. Communication strategies training may be provided during a one-on-one class, a couple's session, or in a group. Common wisdom suggests that the most effective means is the group setting, where people interact with other persons who have hearing loss, and also interact with their family members. Defenses and recriminations between a hard-of-hearing person and a family member may subside when they recognize that other families share common experiences, and when they share solutions with individuals who are in similar situations.

When you work with a group, it is important to develop a group spirit and *esprit de corps*. Table 4–1 presents attributes of a class group where participants receive optimal benefit from participation.

Other issues to consider include the participants' gender, age, life stage, culture, motivation to participate in training, and specific communication difficulties. The program material and the teaching activities may need to be modified to meet these variables.

Table 4–1. Attributes of an optimal class spirit.

1. Every class member accepts every other class member with an appreciation of the individual's strengths and a tolerance of the individual's quirks and weaknesses.

2. There is a familiarity of approach among the members of the class, with an awareness of each person's hearing difficulties and backgrounds.

3. Contributions from each class member are encouraged and recognized.

4. Class members can communicate easily with one another, possibly with the use of assistive listening devices.

5. There is acceptance of and conformity to a code of behavior (e.g., "only one person may speak at a time"), usually involving courtesy, mutual respect, and empathy.

6. There is an ability to recognize and use wisely the experiences of individual class members to educate other participants in the class.

7. There is a clear definition of the class agenda and format so each individual knows what to expect.

8. Discussion remains focused, and comments are not made to distract the class.

9. Class members are encouraged to be specific and use examples.

Source: Adapted from Houle, C. O., (1997). *Governing boards.* San Francisco, CA: Jossey-Bass Publishers.

MODEL FOR TRAINING

The model presented in Figure 4–1 provides a useful framework for conceptualizing the stages of communication strategies training (Tye-Murray, 1992a; modified by Witt, 1997). The first stage entails formal instruction. The second stage centers around guided learning, and the third stage involves real-world practice. In the ideal program, students move through the three stages sequentially, with one stage providing the foundation for the next. Sometimes a student may revisit a previous stage before advancing to the next one, perhaps to review or refresh important concepts.

Formal instruction provides individuals with information about various types of communication strategies and appropriate listening and speaking behaviors; the first stage in a communication strategies training program.

Formal Instruction

During *formal instruction*, the first stage in the model presented in Figure 4–1, individuals are introduced to the various types of communication strategies and other appropriate listening and speaking behaviors, and they receive examples of each. In a group setting, you might ask people to talk about

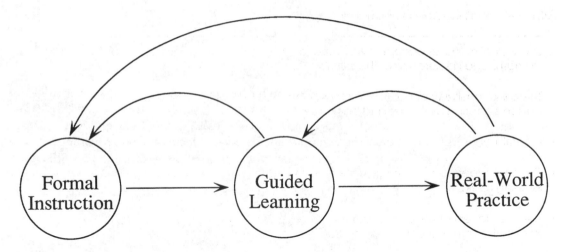

Figure 4-1. A framework for conceptualizing the stages of communication strategies training. (From: Witt, S. (1997). *Effectiveness of an intensive aural rehabilitation program for adult cochlear implant users: A demonstration project.* Unpublished master's thesis, Iowa City: University of Iowa. Reprinted with permission.)

ways they manage their communication difficulties. You may find it valuable to write participants' ideas and responses on a chalkboard or an oversized hanging notebook to stimulate contributions to an ongoing discussion. Formal instruction usually is most effective when the clinician engages everyone in a dialogue as opposed to making a formal presentation as might occur in a typical university classroom. You will quickly discover that a long-winded lecture and advice-giving alienate (and anesthetize) students (Trychin, 1994).

Example of a Formal Instruction Training Activity

When sections on passive, aggressive, and assertive behaviors are included in the content of a communication strategies training program, participants must reflect on their own styles of handling communication difficulties and consider alternative, perhaps more effective, styles. Below is a paper-and-pencil exercise from Kaplan, Bally, and Garretson, (1985) that asks respondents to identify communication styles exhibited in each situation. Answers and discussion are provided afterwards.

A. "Penny entered the office of her boss, the dean. She noticed it was dark and probably it would be hard to speechread. She pushed past the dean's desk (he was sitting at it!) and

(continued)

opened the blinds. Then she sat down and said, 'Let's get this meeting over with.'"

B. "Wilma replaced the battery in her hearing aid and entered the classroom for the course she signed up for, Feminism in the Deaf Community. She immediately noticed that the room was arranged with desk-chairs in a circle. She was relieved to think that this would facilitate speechreading. However, when the rapid-fire discussions began, she had difficulty identifying which of the 22 participants was speaking. Although she was really interested in the topic, she dropped the course the next week."

C. "Harry stopped at his instructor's office after the first day of his geometry class. He was feeling really frustrated because he was unable to understand the questions being asked of the instructor by class members in front of him; he couldn't see their lips. The instructor suggested he move to the front row and look back at the questioners. The next day he was back again. 'I still have a problem,' he admitted. 'I can't identify the speaker quickly enough to speechread. Could we ask the questioners to identify themselves by holding up their hands a little bit longer?' Harry was able to follow class discussions after that."

ANSWERS

A. "Aggressive. Penny's behavior was both rude and demanding.

B. Passive. Wilma didn't try to solve her problem; she gave up on it.

C. Assertive. Harry recognized his problem and worked it out with his instructor" (pp. 37–38).

Guided Learning

In **guided learning**, the second stage in a communication strategies training program, students use conversational strategies in a structured setting.

The purpose of *guided learning*, the next stage in the model depicted in Figure 4–1, is to encourage people to use conversational strategies in a structured setting. Activities for guided learning include role-playing, analysis of videotaped scenarios, continuous discourse tracking, and drill activities. Any number or combination of these activities can be included.

In **role-playing**, individuals participate in hypothetical real-world situations and interactions.

A hypothetical conversational interaction is staged during *role-playing*. Participants practice using communication strategies and other assertive listening behaviors. If possible, the situation parallels one that is relevant to the participants' everyday experiences.

Videotaped scenarios help patients identify and talk about their communication problems by providing concrete examples. Individuals view videotaped scenarios that contrast inappropriate with appropriate use of communication strategies (Trychin, 1987a, 1987b). For instance, one scenario might show a couple in the living room. One person has a hearing loss, the other one does not. The person with normal hearing talks behind a newspaper to the other one. The hard-of-hearing person accuses the talker of mumbling, and leaves the room in anger. The videotape is stopped at this point so that the class can discuss how the hard-of-hearing person might have effectively implemented an instructional strategy in this context. After the discussion, the class views a second videotape scenario, where the hard-of-hearing person demonstrates how to use an instructional facilitative strategy appropriately.

Videotaped scenarios provide examples of communication interactions that can be used to discuss communication strategies and stimulation techniques.

Continuous discourse tracking is another means to provide guided learning. In *continuous discourse tracking* (DeFillipo & Scott, 1978) the clinician plays the role of *sender* and the patient plays the role of *receiver*. The sender reads a selection from a book, phrase by phrase. After each phrase, the receiver attempts to repeat it verbatim. If the receiver cannot recognize it, then he or she must bear the onus of repair, and be responsible for using a repair strategy. For instance, the receiver may say, "Can you tell me in a different way?" The instructor provides coaching and suggestions in how to select and implement particular repair strategies effectively.

Continuous discourse tracking is an aural rehabilitation technique in which the listener attempts to repeat verbatim text presented by a reader.
Sender: an individual who presents a message.
Receiver: an individual who receives a message from a sender.

Example of a Guided Learning Training Activity

After the patient views the picture in Figure 4–2, a clinician will ask him or her to perform a continuous discourse tracking procedure, with the clinician assuming the role of sender and the patient assuming the role of receiver. The following passage corresponds to the picture (Tye-Murray, 1997). The sender reads it sentence by sentence, and the receiver attempts to repeat it verbatim. When unable to do so, the sender encourages the receiver to use a repair strategy, and request an alteration of the passage so that it can be tracked correctly.

(continued)

PASSAGE: "This young man's name is Bill. Bill likes to back-pack in the mountains of Montana. He usually likes to start in the early morning. Along the way he usually spots many different animals and objects. Bill often sees moose and bears. Butterflies land on blooming wild flowers along the trail. (p. 35).

This is what might happen during a continuous discourse tracking exercise:

Sender: "This young man's name is Bill."

Receiver: "Something about a man."

Sender: "Yes. A man named Bill."

Receiver: "A man named Bill. What was the first part?"

Sender: (nodding head) "This young man's name is Bill."

Receiver: "This young man's name is Bill."

Sender: (presents next sentence in the paragraph)

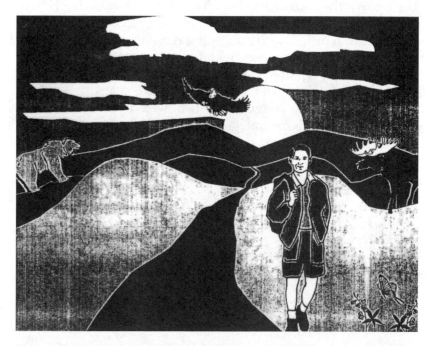

Figure 4–2. A picture that provides a context for a continuous discourse tracking task. (From: Tye-Murray, N. (1997). *Communication strategies training for older adults and teenagers* (p. 34), Austin, TX: Pro-Ed. Reprinted with permission.)

Exercise drills also can provide guided learning. An example of a ***drill activity*** is a sentence identification task (Tye-Murray, 1997), which proceeds as follows. The clinician reads a sentence from a printed text (Table 4–2). A four- or nine-split picture page (Figure 4–3) is laid before the client. The patient's task is to choose the picture that illustrates the sentence. The pictures in a picture-split share similar actors or actions, there-

Drill activity: repeated exercises and rote activities.

Table 4-2. For a drill activity, the clinician presents the sentences below. The sentences correspond to the picture set shown in Figure 4–2.

___

Upper Left Corner

■ I bought a magazine and a newspaper at the newsstand.

> I only picked up a magazine and newspaper at the store. (Rephrase)
> I bought a magazine and a newspaper. (Simplify)

■ A magazine and a newspaper are examples of print media.

> Print media include magazines and newspapers. (Rephrase)
> A magazine and newspaper are media materials. (Simplify)

Upper Right Corner

■ News can be conveyed by printed materials such as magazines and newspapers and by voices from television and radio.

> We can get our news from printed sources such as magazines and newspapers and from the spoken word by television and radio. (Rephrase)
> News can be conveyed by magazines, newspapers, television, and radio. (Simplify)

Lower Left Corner

■ The newspaper man wants to catch the next bus.

> The boy is running to catch the bus. (Rephrase)
> The boy runs to the bus. (Simplify)

■ The newspaper man hurries by the media display.

> The newspaper man runs past the magazine, newspaper, television, and radio. (Rephrase)
> The man hurries by. (Simplify)

Lower Right Corner

■ We have only a television and radio to entertain my nephew.

> We can listen to either the television or the radio. (Rephrase)
> We only have a television or a radio. (Simplify)

___

Source: From Tye-Murray, N. (1997). *Communication training for older teenagers and adults* (pp. 186–187). Austin, TX: Pro-Ed. Reprinted with permission.

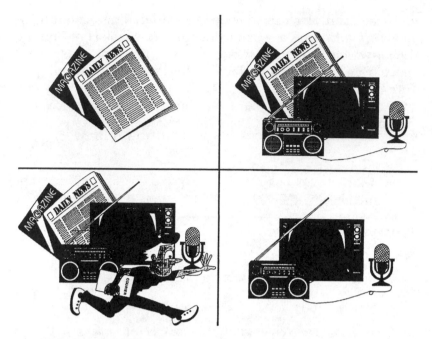

Figure 4–3. A four-split picture set that can be used during a guided-learning training exercise. (From Tye-Murray, N. (1997). *Communication strategies training for older adults and teenagers* (p. 184). Austin, TX: Pro-Ed. Reprinted with permission.)

fore, the individual must identify more than one or two words in order to respond correctly. Patients must use repair strategies if they are unable to identify the correct picture (e.g., "What about the girl?").

In performing this activity, the clinician occasionally may speak with an inappropriate behavior (e.g., while turned away from the student) or in an unfavorable listening environment (e.g., while music from a radio plays loudly in the background). In these instances, the patient can ask the clinician to avoid the speaking behavior, or request that the listening difficulty be corrected. This training thus provides practice in using facilitative communication strategies, as well as repair strategies.

Real-World Practice

In **real-world practice**, the third stage in a communication strategies training program, students practice a new skill or behavior in an everyday environment.

The final stage of the training model shown in Figure 4–1 is real-world practice. *Real-world practice* includes activities that students have performed successfully in the classroom and also some activities that require them to communicate in a setting that is highly motivating, such as the office or a social gathering. Individuals can report back to the class about their successes and problems, and they can share ideas of how to handle problems in the future.

Example of a Real-World Training Activity

Topic = Listening for Directions

Instructions: Ask a partner to hide an object somewhere in your house. Then ask your partner for directions for finding it. Only listen as the directions are told to you, and ask for clarification if necessary. After finding the object, answer the following questions:

1. Did you understand the directions?
2. Did you ask for clarification about any part of the directions? If yes, what did you say? How did your partner respond?
3. Did you have any problems in finding the object? If yes, did you ask for more information from your partner? What did you say?

SHORT-TERM TRAINING

So far we have considered procedures for conducting an intensive, relatively lengthy communication strategies training program. The clinician leads an individual or group through three distinct phases, formal instruction, guided learning, and real-world practice, using a variety of procedures and activities.

For many reasons, an extended program such as the one we have considered may not be feasible. A person may not have time to commit to a longer program, or the clinic may not have the personnel available to conduct training. In these situations, short-term approaches are available for providing brief communication strategies training. One approach is to provide materials and self-directed instruction. Another approach is to provide a short tutorial.

Materials Approach

The *materials approach* for providing communication strategies training during a brief time interval includes providing printed and recorded materials to the hard-of-hearing person about communication strategies. This might be accomplished by means of a clinic library, an audiovideo tape station, and printed pamphlets.

The library can be established in a small room adjacent to the clinic waiting room or in the waiting area itself. It might include periodicals and books about hearing loss, communication strategies, speech and auditory training activities, and assistive devices. The materials can be read in the waiting room before or after an appointment, or even checked out and returned by mail. A video cassette player also might be placed in the library or waiting room. Individuals can view videotapes about hearing loss and communication strategies.

Short Tutorial

WATCH: a brief communication strategies training program.

Another way to provide a brief communication strategies training program is by means of a short tutorial. *WATCH* is an acronym that Montgomery (1994) coined to describe his short-tutorial communication strategies training program. This program requires about 1 hour to administer. The acronym represents the following concepts:

W = **Watch the talker's mouth, not his eyes.**

A = **Ask specific questions.**

T = **Talk about your hearing loss.**

C = **Change the situation.**

H = **Acquire health care knowledge.**

The clinician discusses with the patient each of these concepts in this order.

During the "W" component, the clinician encourages the patient to focus on the talker's mouth for speechreading, as opposed to hand gestures or other items in the communication setting.

During the "A" component, the patient is taught to use specific rather than nonspecific repair strategies. A clinician might dramatize this point by speaking with a low voice or slurred speech, and then ask the person to use specific repair strategies.

During the "T" component of the program, the clinician discusses the importance of revealing a hearing loss to one's communication partners. A patient can then manage the communication interaction more effectively and implement instructional strategies.

The clinician asks the patient to identify situations in which communication is problematic during the "C." Together, they consider possible ways to overcome these problems.

Finally, the clinician provides information about health care and hearing loss resources during the "H" component of the program.

A short program such as WATCH may not always result in a momentous change in how a patient uses communication strategies. However, much of the program's value lies in the fact that simple ideas have been reviewed. The individual might reflect on these ideas and develop them or even become motivated to enroll in a more extended communication strategies training program.

COMMUNICATION STRATEGIES TRAINING FOR FREQUENT COMMUNICATION PARTNERS

Persons with whom the hard-of-hearing person converses with frequently also may benefit from receiving communication strategies training. A frequent communication partner may be a spouse, a son or daughter, a close friend, or a health-care provider. If the hard-of-hearing person is a child, this person may be a parent. An entire chapter in this text (Chapter 17) is devoted to instruction for parents. The goals of communication strategies training for frequent communication partners are to foster empathy for the difficulty of the speechreading task, encourage the use of appropriate speaking behaviors, learn how to tailor messages so they are easy to recognize, and learn how to repair communication breakdowns effectively.

In many ways, the topics included in a communication strategies training program for frequent communication partners mirrors the content for hard-of-hearing individuals. Table 4–3 summarizes topics that may be reviewed. Frequent communication partners can learn to present their messages with appro-

Table 4–3. Content that may be included in a communication strategies training program for frequent communication partners.

Appropriate Speaking Behaviors

Frequent communication partners may be encouraged to:

- Speak clearly and slowly.
- Speak with their faces toward the hard-of-hearing individual.
- Avoid putting objects in or near their mouths while speaking.
- Stand away from windows or bright light sources when talking to someone who has a hearing loss.

Empathy

Frequent communication partners may be asked to consider:

- The difficulty of the speech recognition task when one must rely on a degraded audio signal, perhaps with the use of filtered speech samples.
- The difficulty of the lipreading task.
- How stress and anxiety levels may rise when someone has a hearing loss, and how persons with hearing loss often may experience fatigue and desire social withdrawal.

Organized Messages

Frequent communication partners may be asked to:

- Avoid verbosity, and to use concise and syntactically simple sentences. For example, they might say, *Let's go to a movie*, rather than *I haven't really thought much about it, but I know we aren't doing much on Saturday, so maybe let's go to a movie*.
- Avoid ambiguity by using precise terminology. For example, they may say, *The sweater is Sarah's*, rather than, *It's hers*.

Comprehension

Frequent communication partners may be encouraged to:

- Ask their partner often if he or she comprehended a message.
- Ask for verification and listen to the hard-of-hearing person repeat or paraphrase what they have just said.
- Provide feedback about whether the individual correctly recognized the message.

Repair of Communication Breakdowns

The frequent communication partner may receive coaching about how to use repair strategies optimally. Following a communication breakdown, they might:

- Repeat their messages.
- Rephrase their messages, and say it in a different way. For example, the sentence, *I left* may be rephrased as *I went home*.
- Repeat a keyword, to indicate the topic of conversation. For example, if the sentence, *Tom fell down* was not recognized, the communication partner might repair the communication breakdown by saying, *Tom. Tom fell down.*

Table 4–3. *(continued)*

Repair of Communication Breakdowns *(continued)*

■ Simplify the message by using fewer words or by using more commonplace words. For example, the sentence, *Jane bought a brown bowler hat* might be simplified to *Jane bought a hat.*

■ Elaborate, by providing more information and repeating important key words. For instance if the sentence, *I cut the paper* was misunderstood, the frequent communication partner might say, *I have some scissors. I cut the paper with the scissors.*

■ Build from the known, by presenting information that can easily be recognized to establish a context. For instance, the original sentence might have been, *Please put the wallet in my purse.* In repairing a communication breakdown, the communication partner may say, *Please put the wallet* (and then point to the wallet) *in my purse* (with a gesture toward a purse).

priate speaking behaviors. For example, they can learn to speak clearly and slowly, and to make sure their faces are clearly visible so the hard-of-hearing person can speechread. Frequent communication partners also can learn to organize their messages. They can learn simple principles for message organization, such as those summarized in Table 4–3. For example, they can avoid verbosity and use semantically simple sentences. Finally, they can learn to use repair strategies (see also Chapter 17).

Communication strategies training for frequent communication partners often is provided at the same time that the hard-of-hearing individual receives training, frequently within the same class. In addition to receiving communication strategies training, they also may receive support and counseling from the speech and hearing professional about adjusting to the changes in life quality that occur because of their relatives' or friends' hearing losses. For instance, frequent communication partners often detect changes in their life quality after the patient incurs a hearing loss (Stephens & Hétu, 1991). Sometimes they report feeling stressed by excessive noise in the home, such as a loud television volume or loud speaking. They may experience annoyance, irritation, or tension as a result of this noise and also as a result of recurring misunderstandings between themselves and the person with hearing loss. Social interactions outside the home may decrease, and feelings of social isolation and loneliness may set in. The frequent communication partner also may have to assume extra tasks as a result of the patient's hearing loss, such as interpreting for the person during group conversations or acting as intermediary for the person's telephone calls. In many cases, communication strategies training, along with counseling, can enhance and accelerate the adjustment process that frequent communication partners may have to undergo.

COMMUNICATION STRATEGIES TRAINING FOR CHILDREN

Children who have hearing impairments also may benefit from communication strategies training. The program content may focus on facilitative and repair communication strategies, as we have been discussing for adults in the foregoing sections.

Facilitative and Receptive Repair Strategies

Laser video-disc based training programs and one-on-one printed programs are currently available for providing training for facilitative strategies and receptive repair strategies (Tye-Murray, 1994; Tye-Murray, Tyler, Bong, & Nares, 1992). Often, programs for children are simplified when compared to those designed for adults. For example, children might receive instruction for only three repair strategies (e.g., *say it again, tell me in a different way, what are you talking about?*), because other strategies, such as asking for an elaboration, may involve abstract concepts that are too difficult for them to grasp.

Formal Instruction

Formal instruction for children might include a review of effective listening behaviors (e.g., *pay attention, watch the talker's face, try to identify key points*) and how to ask talkers to clarify a message (e.g., *When you don't understand a message, ask the talker to say just one word. This will tell you what he or she is talking about.*). Most children will experience great difficulty in applying concepts learned during formal instruction to the give-and-take of everyday conversation. Indicating that a communication breakdown has occurred in a gracious and socially acceptable manner can be challenging for even the most accomplished conversationalists. Moreover, finding the words to instruct the talker is not easy. Children will need abundant opportunity to practice repairing communication breakdowns, and the clinician probably should reiterate formally taught concepts many times in an informal way, in many different contexts.

Guided Learning

Guided learning for children focuses the child's attention on good listening behaviors and communication strategies. The child practices the behaviors and strategies in a structured setting, via modeling and role-playing. In *modeling*, a child might watch the clinician as he or she demonstrates the desired behavior and then try to imitate it. In role-playing, as with adults, a hypothetical listening situation is created, wherein the child must listen and use communication strategies. When setting up a scene for role-playing, the speech and hearing professional should select situations that are important to the child; for example, a department store or movie theater. The props should be as realistic as possible so that the child feels as if the interactions was really occurring (Tullos, 1990).

In **modeling,** an instructor demonstrates a behavior and the student attempts to imitate it.

Real-World Practice

Once a child has practiced communication strategies in structured settings, he or she may apply them to everyday experiences. Real-world practice activities help children transfer their use of communication strategies to natural settings. Activities should require them to interact with different talkers, in a variety of contexts. Guidelines for developing real-world activities for children are presented in Table 4–4.

Expressive Repair Strategies

In addition to learning how to use facilitative and receptive repair strategies, children also can learn to use expressive repair strategies. Expressive repair strategies may be appropriate to use when the child presents a message, usually with speech, and the communication partner does not recognize it. The child then repairs the communication breakdown, perhaps by trying again using his or her best speech or by adding hand gestures.

Table 4–5 summarizes a five-step training plan of action for teaching children to use expressive repair strategies (Elfenbein, 1994). Formal instruction and guided learning can be provided during the first four steps. Real-world practice is provided in the fifth step.

In this plan, children begin by reviewing principles of basic communication processes and consider the sender-message receiver relationship and the various ways of communicating. Children may create a book about the ways people communicate, tearing pictures from old magazines for illustrations. The next step, Step 2, entails talking about communi-

Table 4–4. Guidelines for developing real-world practice activities for children.

A. Assign a real-world practice activity that the child has performed successfully during guided learning practice.

If the child is to ask someone to repeat a message following a communication breakdown, the youth first should practice asking for clarification in the classroom or clinical setting. Then the child can be asked to attempt the strategy in for example, art class. Although not necessary, the art teacher can be briefed beforehand that the child will practice repair strategies with her or him.

B. Select a communication situation in which the child will feel motivated to communicate.

For instance, a young child might be asked to use repair strategies when ordering food at a fast food restaurant.

C. Select an interaction that allows the child to experience some success.

For example, you might ask the child to interact with a familiar teacher before asking the youth to try using repair strategies with an unfamiliar store clerk.

D. Provide instructions for the activity. Present the instructions with simple language and vocabulary.

The purpose of a homework activity might be to listen for the main points of a one-paragraph narrative. The clinician might provide the following written instructions:

This envelope contains a story. Ask your mother to read it to you. Watch and listen carefully. If you do not understand the story, ask questions. Draw a picture about the story.

E. Provide a means for the child to record the experience.

In the activity described in letter D above, the record is the child's drawing.

Source: Adapted from Glennon, S. L. (1990). Homework activities for social skills training. In P. J. Schloss and M. A. Smith (Eds.), *Teaching social skills to hearing-impaired students* (pp. 85–90). Washington, DC: Alexander Graham Bell Association for the Deaf.

cation breakdown: What happens when a breakdown occurs? How can you tell that it has happened? Why did it happen? Here, children might generate a list of the ways that people signal a breakdown. Step 3 focuses on message formulation, and Step 4 focuses on introduction of expressive repair strategies. Children might play a game in which they are assigned a particular expressive repair strategy, such as mime. Communication breakdowns can be simulated, and children can implement their assigned repair strategy. The final step in the model presented in Table 4–5 provides practice in using communication repair strategies. At this time, children might talk about their feelings and responses to com-

Table 4-5. Five-step plan of action from teaching children to use communication strategies.

Step 1. Understanding basic communication processes

       A. Sender-message-receiver relationship
       B. Ways to communicate (e.g., speech, sign, writing, mime, gesture)

Step 2. Understanding communication breakdowns

       A. Definitions and examples
       B. Causes of communication breakdown
       C. Ways people signal confusion

Step 3. Message formulation

       A. Information to be transmitted
       B. Evaluation of the receiver's position (e.g., background knowledge)
       C. Evaluation of sender's abilities (e.g., speech proficiency)
       D. Environmental constraints (e.g., background noise)
       E. Social constraints (e.g., conventions of politeness and etiquette)

Step 4. Introduction of communication repair strategies

       A. Receiver's responsibilities
         1. Acknowledge confusion
         2. Identify causes of breakdown
         3. Implement receptive repair strategies
       B. Sender's responsibilities
         1. Be alert to signals of confusion
         2. Identify causes of a communication breakdown
         3. Implement expressive repair strategies

Step 5. Practice using communication repair strategies

       A. Move from sheltered environments to the real world
       B. Move from transmission of simple to complex to more complex messages
       C. Discuss feelings associated with communication breakdown

---

Source: Adapted from Elfenbein, J. (1994a). Communication breakdowns in conversations: Child-initiated repair strategies. In N. Tye-Murray (Ed.), *Let's converse: A how-to guide to develop and expand the conversational skills of children and teenagers who are hearing impaired* (pp. 123–146). Washington, DC: Alexander Graham Bell Association for the Deaf.

munication breakdown. Often, it is reassuring to learn that their classmates have experienced similar frustration and embarrassment following a communication breakdown. They can be videotaped using a repair strategy during a conversation with a school secretary or another teacher. Later, the class can view the videotape and critique the interaction.

EFFICACY OF TRAINING

Few experimental investigations have focused on the efficacy of communication strategies training. So the question remains, is training beneficial to those who receive it? Preliminary data suggest the answer to this question is *yes*. Abrahamson (1991) reported that 89% of the patients who began a 6-week communication strategies training program completed it. Attendance rates at the classes averaged 85%. Their willingness to stay with the program suggests that participants were benefitting from it. Another investigation showed that patients changed how they used repair strategies after participating in a communication strategies training program that concentrated on repair-strategy use (Tye-Murray, 1991). Following training, subjects began to use the repair strategies that they found were especially helpful during their training sessions. For example, if during the course of training an individual found that asking for the topic of conversation helped him or her to understand an unrecognized message, then the individual was more likely to begin using that strategy. Finally, Kricos and Holmes (1996) provided active listening training to a group of older adults with hearing loss. The program included both speech perception training and emphasis on use of communication strategies. Following training, subjects showed improved speech recognition and enhanced psychosocial functioning.

Little if any work has focused on the efficacy of communication strategies training for children.

FINAL REMARKS

Communication strategies training can empower many students to manage their communication environments more effectively. However, students will vary in the extent to which they benefit. Some individuals are incapable of changing their communication behaviors. Some do not have the meta-communication skills to examine their conversational styles and may not be able to monitor how they interact with their communication partners, regardless of the quality or amount of instruction. For example, an elderly woman might not use communication strategies, and might deal with communication problems with excessive aggression, but these behaviors are a part of her personality and likely will not change with aural rehabilitation intervention. In these instances, it is critical that individuals who interact frequently with the hard-of-hearing person receive instruction as well.

KEY CHAPTER POINTS

✔ A communication strategies training program should be tailored to accommodate a patient's expectations, age, socioeconomic background, life style, and particular communication problems.

✔ The content of a communication strategies training program centers around problems specifically related to hearing loss and how these problems can be minimized. Training may be provided for facilitative and repair communication strategies. Patients may also consider assertive versus nonassertive listening behaviors.

✔ One model for a training program includes three stages: formal instruction, guided learning, and real-world practice. A variety of exercises and activities can be used for each stage.

✔ A communication strategies training program for children can include instruction for the use of expressive repair strategies in addition to the use of receptive repair strategies and facilitative communication strategies.

PART II

Speech Perception

5

Assessing Hearing and Speech Recognition

Topics

- Review of the Audiological Examination
- Purpose of Speech Recognition Testing
- Patient Variables
- Stimulus Units
- Test Procedures

- Difficulties Associated with Speech Recognition Assessment
- Final Remarks
- Key Chapter Points
- Key Resources

The audiogram provides a general description of the magnitude of a person's hearing loss. However, the audiogram does not always adequately portray the communication difficulties an individual may experience nor the person's aural rehabilitation needs. This is one reason why conversational fluency and communication handicap are assessed. Speech recognition measurement also is an important element in assessing how hearing loss affects an individual's life and communication interactions. The term speech recognition refers to the reception of *speech information* through listening, lipreading, or speechreading.

In this chapter, we will focus on important considerations underlying the assessment of speech recognition. These considerations are (Figure 5–1):

■ Purpose
■ Patient variables
■ Stimuli units
■ Test procedures

Before we turn to these topics, we will begin with a brief review of the audiogram and other components of the audiological examination.

REVIEW OF THE AUDIOLOGICAL EXAMINATION

An **audiogram** is a graphic representation of hearing thresholds as a function of stimulus frequency.

A typical audiological assessment includes an *audiogram*, a determination of speech recognition threshold, and an assess-

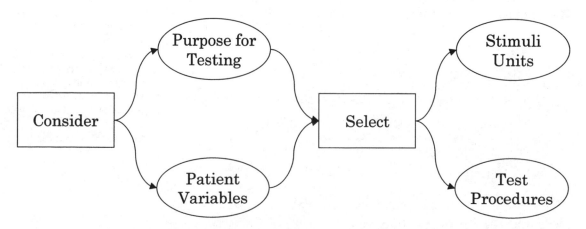

Figure 5–1. Assessing speech recognition.

ment of speech discrimination. Sometimes the examination might entail a determination of most comfortable loudness and uncomfortable loudness levels for speech as well.

The audiogram provides an objective assessment of an individual's ability to detect sounds. The test typically is performed by an audiologist, with the use of an audiometer. The audiometer presents tones, and the individual indicates when he or she hears them. The goal is to determine the softest sound level at which the tones can be detected. Tone frequencies usually include 250, 500, 1000, 2000, 4000, and 8000 Hz. The frequency of 250 Hz corresponds approximately to a "middle C" played on the piano.

The tones may be presented by *air conduction*, either through headphones or soundfield, or by *bone conduction*, through a vibrator placed behind the ear against the temporal bone. Air conduction test results indicate hearing losses that might be either *conductive* (involving the outer or middle ear) or *sensorineural* (involving the inner ear, eighth nerve, brain stem, midbrain, and/or auditory cortex) in nature. Bone conduction test results reflect only the sensorineural component. By comparing the air and bone conduction results, the audiologist can determine whether there is hearing loss stemming from a problem in either the outer or middle ear. The difference between the two sets of thresholds is termed the *air-bone gap*.

Audiological thresholds are plotted on an audiogram, where the Y-axis indicates *sound level* (loudness) and the X-axis indicates *frequency* (pitch). The *pure tone average* (PTA) is a means to summarize someone's hearing status. The pure tone average is an average of the hearing thresholds for the frequencies of 500, 1000, and 2000 Hz (Figure 5–2).

The pure tone average often is used to assign a label to the hearing loss. The following descriptors are used:

Normal: The PTA is 25 dB HL or better.

Mild: The PTA is between 26 and 40 dB HL.

Mild-to-moderate: The PTA is between 41 and 55 dB HL.

Moderate: The PTA is between 56 and 70 dB HL.

Severe: The PTA is between 71 and 90 dB HL.

Profound: The PTA is poorer than 90 dB HL.

Table 5–1 indicates the relationship between degree of hearing loss and speech recognition, as a function of the descriptors outlined above.

Air conduction: sound that travels through the air into the internal auditory canal and progresses through the middle ear, inner ear, and to the brain.

Bone conduction: transmission of sound through the bones in the body, particularly the skull.

Conductive is used to describe hearing loss that stems from an impairment in the outer or middle ear.

Sensorineural is a type of hearing loss that has a cochlear or retrocochlear origin.

Air-bone gap: the difference between air- and bone-conduction thresholds, a difference may indicate a conductive component in the hearing loss.

Sound level is the intensity of sound expressed in decibels.

Frequency: the number of regularly repeated events in a given unit of time, usually measured in cycles per second and expressed in Hertz (Hz).

Pure tone average (PTA): Average of hearing thresholds at 500, 1000, and 2000 Hz.

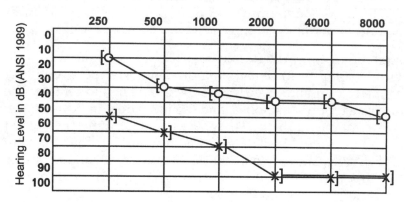

Figure 5–2. Audiogram for someone who has a PTA of 35 dB in the right ear (a mild hearing loss) and 73 dB in the left ear (a severe hearing loss).

Speech reception threshold (SRT): the lowest presentation level for spondee words at which 50% can be identified correctly.

When determining the *speech reception threshold (SRT)*, the audiologist determines the softest level at which a patient can understand simple words. In one procedure, an audiologist might ask the patient to repeat *spondees*. These are bisyllabic words that have equal stress on both words, such as *baseball*, *ice cream*, *hotdog*, and *sidewalk*. The words are presented through the audiometer, and the level is varied until the patient is able to repeat just 50% of the words correctly. This level is recorded as the SRT.

The audiological examination usually includes a test of speech recognition, in addition to the audiogram and SRT testing. For instance, the clinician might present monosyllabic words at a comfortable listening level, and expect the patient to repeat back each word. When word recognition scores are referred to in a clinical setting, they are often called *speech discrimination scores*. The term speech recognition is preferred in this text, to avoid confusion with the term discrimination when it is used in a training context, to indicate discriminating one stimulus from the next.

Speech discrimination score: the percentage of monosyllabic words presented at a comfortable listening level that can be correctly repeated.

Most comfortable loudness (MCL): level at which sound is most comfortable for a listener.

Sometimes the audiologist might want to determine the hearing level for which speech is most comfortable to listen to, and the level at which it becomes too loud. The *most comfortable loudness level (MCL)* typically is determined by asking the individual to listen to running speech. The initial presentation level may be just above the level of the SRT, and then gradually increased. The individual indicates when it is at a comfortable level, when it is too soft, and when it is too loud. The

Table 5–1. How degree of hearing loss affects speech recognition.

Hearing Loss	Effect on Word Recognition
Mild (PTA = 26–40 dB HL)	In quiet situations, speech recognition will be fairly unaffected. In the presence of noise, speech recognition by may decrease to 50% words correct if the PTA is 40 dB HL. Consonants are most likely to be missed, especially if the hearing loss involves primarily the high frequencies.
Mild-to-Moderate (PTA = 41–55 dB HL)	Will understand much of the speech signal if it is presented in a quiet environment face-to face, and if the topic of conversation is known and the vocabulary is constrained. If a hearing aid is not used, the individual may miss up to 50–75% of a spoken message if the PTA is 40 dB and 80–100% if the PTA is 50 dB.
Moderate (PTA = 56–70 dB HL)	If the individual does not use a hearing aid, he or she may miss most or all of the message, even if talking face-to-face. Will have great difficulty conversing in group situations.
Severe (PTA = 71–90 dB)	May not even hear voices, unless speech is loud. Without amplification, the individual probably will not recognize any speech in an audition-only condition. With amplification, he or she may recognize some speech, and detect environmental sounds.
Profound (PTA = 90 dB HL or greater)	May perceive sound as vibrations. An individual will rely on vision as the primary sense for speech recognition. May not be able to detect the presence of even loud sound without amplification.

Source: Adapted from Flexor, C. (1994). *Facilitating hearing and listening in young children.* San Diego, CA: Singular Publishing Group.

uncomfortable loudness level (UCL) is the threshold level at which the speech changes from being comfortably loud to being uncomfortably loud.

Uncomfortable loudness level (UCL): level at which sound is uncomfortably loud for a listener.

In Chapter 13, we will return to hearing and sound measurement when we consider noise exposure in the context of aural rehabilitation. That chapter also includes a more in-depth descriptions of how we hear.

Sound-Field Testing

Often, tests of speech recognition are presented in soundfield as opposed to under headphones. If the patient typically wears a hearing aid, he or she often wears the aid for testing. Newby and Popelka (1992) discussed the reasons for soundfield testing:

"Testing with a loudspeaker is referred to as *sound-field testing* because the sound is not confined, as it is in an earphone, but is circulated in a field about the patient's head. Unless we are talking over the telephone, or for some reason listening through earphones, all our listening throughout the day is of the sound-field type. To judge how the patient hears in a typical sound-field listening situation is the main reason that we give speech tests through a loudspeaker" (pp. 182–183).

PURPOSE OF SPEECH RECOGNITION TESTING

When designing an aural rehabilitation plan for a particular patient, you will almost always want information about his or her speech recognition skills. There are many ways to use the results of this assessment. These include the following:

■ **To determine need for amplification.** If a person demonstrates reduced speech recognition, then amplification might be considered.

■ **To compare performance with a listening aid to performance without an aid.** This can be accomplished by measuring speech recognition with and without the device.

■ **To compare different listening devices.** An individual might be tested with one listening device and then another to determine the device that affords the best performance. This is feasible when two or three devices are being compared, but becomes problematic when many devices are under consideration.

■ **To assess performance longitudinally.** There may be instances when you want to monitor speech recognition over time, and answer questions like, "Is the patient's hearing deteriorating because of use of a listening device?" or, "Has speech recognition changed as a result of auditory training?" Care must be taken that measurements are not affected by the learning of test materials with repeated administration or, in the case of children, by language growth or cognitive maturation.

■ **To determine need for speech perception training.** If an individual experiences difficulty in recognizing speech, even when using appropriate amplification, then the person may be a candidate for training.

■ **To determine placement within a training curriculum.** Not every individual begins a speech perception training program with the same tasks. People will enter training with different skill levels, and training objectives will need to be selected accordingly.

■ **To determine if expected benefit has been achieved.** One goal of providing a listening aid or providing speech perception training is to improve speech recognition. You may assess whether individuals obtained expected benefit by comparing their performance with that of a group of persons who have a similar hearing loss and/or who have received similar interventions.

The purpose may dictate the test. For instance, you may use one test for determining placement in an auditory training curriculum and another test for assessing benefit from a hearing aid. Other important variables that will influence test selection pertain to the patient.

PATIENT VARIABLES

In selecting appropriate test materials for assessing word recognition, it is important to consider variables such as cognitive/linguistic level and hearing ability, for these will affect how an individual performs on a particular test. A consideration of patient variables will help you to choose between test stimuli, response format, testing conditions, and whether to use live or recorded stimuli.

The patient must have the maturity and cognitive skills to take the test. For example, it would be inappropriate to expect a 3-year-old child to repeat a seven-word sentence, as it would be to expect an elderly person with dementia to do so. If a young child takes a closed-set test, then it might be necessary that the response items can be illustrated by pictures, because the child could not read orthographic choices.

Similarly, the test must present items that are within the linguistic competency of the individual. Otherwise, you will not know whether someone performed poorly on a test because he or she did not know the vocabulary or grammatical structures or because of hearing limitations. For example, you might ask a child to repeat the sentence, *The man ate an artichoke for dinner.* If a child is unfamiliar with the word *artichoke*, it is unlikely that the child will be able to repeat it during a speech recognition test, especially if he or she has a significant hearing loss.

The degree of hearing loss will affect test selection. For instance, if an adult just received a cochlear implant, it may be inappropriate to administer a monosyllabic word test in an audition-only condition, because the individual likely will exhibit a "floor" performance.

Sometimes you will need to consider communication mode and other disabilities. For example, if a child uses sign, the test instructions should be presented with sign, and provisions for recording the child's responses must be made (i.e., if the child signs responses, then someone must interpret them). If an individual has decreased speech intelligibility as well as a hearing loss, then the responses may have to be written.

STIMULI UNITS

Once you have identified your purpose for testing and have thought about patient variables, test selection can be made. Test stimuli that are used typically to assess speech recognition are summarized in Table 5–2. Examples of tests that correspond with each type are also listed, for both children and adults. Each kind of stimulus presents both advantages and disadvantages.

Phonemes and Phoneme Contrasts

Phoneme testing permits phonetic errors to be examined. The items may be designed to assess consonant or vowel recognition.

Test results indicate the kinds of speech features utilized during speech recognition. For example, an individual may not have scored very high on a test that presents a closed set of items such as *eemee, eenee, eesee, eebee, eepee,* and *eetee.* However, an analysis of errors may reveal that even though overall performance was poor, the individual consistently utilized the voicing feature. For instance, *eepee* may have been heard as *eetee* or *eesee,* both of which contain unvoiced elements, but

Table 5–2. Examples of word recognition tests that use phoneme, word, and sentence stimuli for children and adults. These tests typically are administered in an audition-only condition.

Test	Author(s)	Stimulus Type	Stimulus Units	Response Format	Target Population
Speech Pattern Contrast Test (SPAC)	Boothroyd, 1994	Phoneme (also includes test of suprasegmental contrasts, such as word stress)	Words and phrases	Closed set	Children over age 10 yrs
California Consonant Test	Owens and Schubert, 1977	Phoneme	Monosyllables	Closed set	Adults
Audiovisual Feature Test	Tyler, FryaufBertschy, and Kelsey, 1991	Phoneme	Rhyming words, including b, c, d, key, me, knee	Closed set (10-choice)	Children
Iowa Consonant Confusion Test	Tyler, Preece, and Tye-Murray, 1986	Phoneme	Nonsense bisyllables, including eemee, eesee, eedee, eebee	Closed set (13-choice)	Adults
Iowa Vowel Confusion Test	Tyler, Preece, and Tye-Murray, 1986	Phoneme	Monosyllables with an (hVd) format, including heed, who'd, had, head	Closed set (nine-choice)	Adults
Northwestern University Children's Perception of Speech (NU-CHIPS)	Elliott and Katz, 1980	Word	Monosyllables constructed with the most frequently occurring phonemes in the English language, such as fork, dog	Closed set (four-choice)	Children who have the receptive language abilities of age 2.6 yrs or older
Word Intelligibility by Picture Identification (WIPI)	Ross and Lerman, 1971	Word	Monosyllabic words, such as bear, pear, stair, chair, ear, hair	Closed set (six-choice)	Children

Table 5–2. (*continued*)

Test	Author(s)	Stimulus Type	Stimulus Units	Response Format	Target Population
Phonetically Balanced Kindergarden (PBK)	Haskins, 1949	Word	Monosyllabic words	Open set	Children
Northwestern University Auditory Test No. 6 (NU-6)	Tillman and Carhart, 1966	Word	Monosyllabic words	Open set	Adults
CID Auditory Test W-22	Hirsh et al., 1952	Word	Phonetically balanced monosyllabic word lists	Open set	Adults
Bamford-Kowal-Bench Sentences (BKB)	Bench and Bamford, 1979	Sentence	Sentences constructed with vocabulary familiar to 8–16 yr old hard-of-hearing children	Open set	Older children and adults
Central Institute for the Deaf (CID) Everyday Speech Sentences	Davis and Silverman, 1978	Sentences	Sentences that vary in length and structure	Open set	Older children and adults
Speech Perception in Noise (SPIN)	Kalikow, Stevens, and Elliot, 1977	Sentences	Sentences that have either high context for the last word in the sentence or low context	Open set, presented with a background of speech babble	Adults
CUNY Sentences	Boothroyd, Hanin, and Hnath, 1985	Sentences	Unrelated sentences	Open set	Adults

never as *eebee* or *eenee*, which contain only voiced elements. Thus, in designing auditory training goals, you might aim to build on this ability to utilize the voicing feature.

Although you can evaluate subjectively an individual's errors and qualitatively assess error confusions, formal statistical and mathematical analyses can be performed on the results. These provide a quantitative indication of the kinds of information that an individual utilizes during speech. Such analysis include information transmission analysis (Miller & Nicely, 1955), multidimensional scaling, and clustering.

A feature analysis of consonant phoneme confusion errors indicates which parameters of the speech signal are detected and utilized. Features that typically are included in this kind of analysis include nasality voicing, duration fication, place, and envelope (Miller & Nicely, 1955; Van Tasell, Soli, Kirby, & Widin, 1987). A commonly used consonant classification system appears in Table 5–3.

For the nasality feature, consonants /m and n/ are classified as nasal consonants. A person who appears to hear the nasality feature is probably responding to the frequencies around and below 300 Hz. Consonants that are aperiodic in nature /p, t, k, f, s, ʃ/) are grouped together for the voicing feature, while the relatively long duration consonants are grouped together for the duration feature (/z, s, ʃ/). The voicing and duration fea-

Table 5–3. An example of a classification system for consonants that may be used to classify consonant phonemes for a feature analysis. The numbers are arbitrary, and serve only to indicate the group to which a sound belongs within a feature.

Consonant	Voicing	Place	Nasality	Duration	Frication	Envelope
b	1	0	0	0	0	1
d	1	1	0	0	0	1
g	1	3	0	0	0	1
p	0	0	0	0	0	0
t	0	1	0	0	0	0
k	0	3	0	0	0	0
v	1	0	0	0	1	1
f	0	0	0	0	1	2
z	1	1	0	1	1	1
s	0	1	0	1	1	2
ʃ	0	2	0	1	1	2
m	1	0	1	0	0	3
n	1	1	1	0	0	3

tures probably relate to temporal cues and the voice pitch. Consonants produced with steady turbulence (/v, f, z, s, ʃ/) usually are grouped together for the frication feature. This feature relates to high-frequency turbulence. The place feature, for which consonants are categorized according to whether they are produced in the front, middle, or back of the vocal tract, is cued by spectral or frequency changes over time, particularly in the region of the second vowel formant (see Chapter 7). Finally, the envelope feature reflects time-intensity variations in the audio signal. To recognize words, persons must detect and utilize at least some of these features in the signal. A feature analysis indicates how well a patient can distinguish these cues from one another. We will revisit the topic of features in Chapters 7 and 9 when we consider designing objectives for auditory and speechreading training.

An advantage of using phoneme stimuli is that performance is relatively independent of an individual's vocabulary level. It is not important that individuals be familiar with the test stimuli, and indeed, the stimuli are often *nonsense syllables*, such as *eesee* and *eeteee*. This same advantage can become a disadvantage if you are testing young children, who often must be tested with vocabulary that they know.

Nonsense syllables: syllables of speech that have no meaning.

A principal disadvantage of using phoneme stimuli is poor face validity. We do not communicate with these kinds of stimuli typically, and it is not straightforward how recognition relates to conversational speech understanding. For instance, nonsense syllables do not require individuals to organize streams of information into linguistically meaningful chunks, nor to process speech information with the same rapidity as ongoing speech.

Features and Cues

When considering speech recognition, the terms features and cues often are used. Dorman (1993) defines them as follows: "The term 'cue' refers to a specific aspect of an acoustic signal that has been demonstrated to be important for recognition of a phonetic segment, or for distinguishing between two phonetic segments. The term 'feature' generally refers to articulation, and not to a particular acoustic cue. Thus, the feature 'place of articulation' encompasses sounds with extremely different acoustic signatures. For example, the place cues for voiced stop-consonants reside in transient bursts and formant transitions of brief duration, but the place cues for fricatives reside in long duration fricative noises which differ greatly in frequency and in amplitude. This must be kept in mind when sorting through the results of studies that report on the reception of features by . . . patients." (p. 146)

Words

The most commonly used stimuli for assessing speech recognition are monosyllabic words (Martin & Morris, 1989). Many word lists are designed to be *phonetically balanced*, meaning that the words include phonemes in the same proportion in which they occur in spoken English. Most word lists are comprised of monosyllables that have the phonemic structure of consonant-vowel-consonant (e.g., *cat* or *man*). These stimuli generally are difficult to recognize, more so than phrases or simple sentences.

One advantage in using real words is that they have somewhat higher face validity than phonemes. We communicate with words in daily conversation. The tests are also easy to score, and allow a wide range of skill levels to be assessed. Responses from a word test can be scored by percent of words repeated verbatim, or percent of phonemes correct (e.g., if the word is *bat*, and an individual responds *pat*, two of the word's three phonemes are scored as correct). The reasons that percent phoneme scores are sometimes computed are to obtain a fine-grain understanding of an individual's performance, and to provide a different vehicle for comparing test results. For example, two people might achieve the following scores on the same test:

Person 1: 30% words correct, 40% phonemes correct

Person 2: 30% words correct, 65% phonemes correct

Even though the individuals erred an equal number of times in repeating the words, Person 2's errors better approximate the target than do Person 1's error responses. Thus, the second person may have better listening ability than the first person.

As with phonemes, word stimuli may not reflect very well how an individual performs in everyday listening situations because we typically listen to connected discourse. For instance, words are presented rapidly during conversation. We do not pause to think about the identity of each word as it is spoken, as one does when taking a test of isolated word recognition. Research suggests that, during normal conversation, we might receive speech at between 140 and 180 words per minute (Miller et al., 1984). It is possible for two people to perform similarly on a word test, in which the demands of fast on-line processing are not great, and yet function differently in everyday conversation. Another problem in using words as test stimuli may arise if the test-taker has a language delay because performance on word tests may be influenced by vocabulary. A child who has a limited vocabulary may perform poorly simply because he or she is unfamiliar with the test words.

Phrases and Sentences

A speech recognition test may consist of a series of unrelated phrases or sentences. For instance, the test may commence with the sentence, *The cook cut the apple*, and then continue with, *The boy and girl walked to school*, which is contextually unrelated to the first sentence. Alternatively, the test may present sentences centered on a common theme. For instance, before the test begins, the individual may be informed, "The sentences you will hear concern activities to do at the lake." The first sentence may then be, *We paddled a canoe*. The second sentence may be, *We went for a swim this morning*, and so forth. Performance will be better for topic-related than unrelated sentences.

Sentence stimuli have high face validity because we typically communicate with phrases, sentences, and paragraphs. As such, performance on a sentence test may better reflect how a person performs in the real world than performance on a phoneme or isolated word test. Sentences have the following features, which are characteristic of everyday speech:

Prosodic cues are provided by intonation, rate, and duration of speech sounds.

■ *Prosodic cues:* When we listen to speech, we attend not only to individual sounds, but also to intonation, rate, and duration cues, and these help us to identify words and understand meaning. For example, an individual may be presented with a complete sentence, but because of hearing loss, the person may hear only, *mmm mm-mm mmm?* Even though the individual receives a gross approximation of the message, there is still enough information to know that a question is be-

ing asked, and that the question contains four syllables, and possibly, enough information to know that it
contains three words.

■ *Contextual information:* The words in a sentence provide contextual redundancy. Recognition of some
words facilitates recognition of other words. If an individual hears, *Mary closed the* _____, it is possible
to deduce that the final word is a noun, based on
grammatical context, and that the word might be *door*,
based on semantic cues.

■ *Coarticulation:* When words are spoken in succession
as in a sentence, they blend together and vary as a
function of what precedes and follows. For example,
the schwa sound in the word *the* will sound different if
the word *blue* follows than if the word *green* follows.
These coarticulation effects provide redundant cues for
word recognition.

Contextual information
facilitates recognition of
other words.

Coarticulation, subtle
differences in sounds when
words are spoken in
succession in sentences,
provide clues for word
recognition.

Even though sentences have these features of everyday
speech, they also pose some disadvantages for assessment.
One disadvantage of using sentence-level stimuli is that performance can be influenced by linguistic knowledge and familiarity with the topic. For example, a young child with limited grammatical knowledge may not perform as well as an
older child who has good language skills, even though the two
children might have similar perceptual skills. Memory also
may affect results. If you present a 10-word sentence to a 5-
year-old child, the child may forget the beginning of the sentence by the time you present its end.

Sentence tests are usually scored by computing a percent words
correct score, although sometimes they are scored for percent
phonemes correct. In order for a word to be scored as correct,
it must be repeated verbatim. If the sentence is, *The girls walked
to school*, and a person responds, "The girl walked to school,"
that sentence is scored as four out of five words correct. The
omission of /s/ from *girls* makes it an incorrect repetition.

Selection of Test Stimuli

There are no cookbook procedures to follow when deciding
which test stimuli to use. However, one guiding principle is
that the measures chosen should inform you about how an individual performs in natural situations, and should be independent of confounding factors such as vocabulary and grammati-

cal knowledge, cognitive abilities, and memory (Boothroyd, 1991). Often, clinicians opt to use a test-battery approach, using more than one test so that the aggregate presents different kinds of speech units.

TEST PROCEDURES

We have now considered tests and test selection. First, you must decide your purpose for testing, then you must consider characteristics of the test-taker, and then decide on the test stimuli. Once a test has been selected, decisions must be made about the protocol that will be followed for administering the test. In this section, we will turn our attention to test procedures. Considerations for assessing speech recognition include the test condition, the type of response set, and whether testing occurs with live voice or recordings.

Test Condition

Tests of speech recognition can be administered in one of three conditions (Figure 5–3):

Audition-only: presentation of only an auditory signal in testing.

■ *Audition-only:* Only the auditory signal is presented, usually at a normal or moderately loud conversational level.

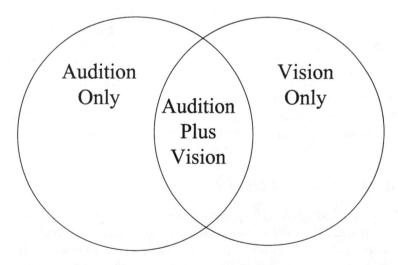

Figure 5–3. The test conditions used for speech recognition testing.

■ *Vision-only:* Only the visual signal is presented, usually showing the head and neck of the test talker (this is a lipreading condition).

■ *Audition-plus-vision:* Both the auditory and visual signals are presented (this is a speechreading condition).

Vision-only: presentation of only a visual stimulus in testing.

Audition-plus-vision: presentation of both auditory and visual signals simultaneously, as in speechreading.

Audition-Only

The audition-only condition is most frequently used for speech recognition assessment because it relates most directly to hearing ability. The signal may be presented in quiet or in the presence of noise.

The sound level for presenting the speech stimuli is often at a normal or moderately loud conversational level (60–70 dB SPL). Alternatively, the level might be set at about 30 to 40 dB above the patient's SRT. When this latter level is chosen, we say that the stimulus is 30 to 40 dB sensational level (SL). The intent of using sensation levels is to liken functional listening levels across patients.

Noise may be introduced to increase the difficulty of the listening task and/or to gain a better understanding of how the person performs in the real world. The noise signal may be talker babble (e.g., six people read text, and their speech signals are overlaid to create a signal noise source) or masking noise (which sounds like a radio off-station). Sometimes the competing noise signal is semantically meaningful. A meaningful competing signal might be used to determine how well an elderly individual can tune out distracting competitors.

When a speech recognition test is performed in the presence of noise, the audiologist records the *signal-to-noise ratio (SNR)*, which indicates the difference between the sound level of the signal and the sound level of the noise. Thus, if the signal is presented at 40 dB and the noise is presented at 30 dB, the SNR is +10 dB.

Signal-to-noise ratio (SNR): the level of a signal relative to a background of noise.

Vision-Only

Sometimes a test of speech recognition is administered in a vision-only condition. The visual signal typically is comprised of the talker's head and shoulders, with the talker facing the patient head-on. The talker should be well-lit, so his or her face is fully visible and not in shadows. The talker usually is placed before a plain, nondistracting background.

Audition-Plus-Vision

Usually, performance for a particular individual will be optimal for an audition-plus-vision condition. This condition is used when best performance is desired or when hearing is so poor that the auditory signal provides only a supplement to lipreading.

Both the vision-only and audition-plus-vision conditions are employed when one is interested in accessing speechreading enhancement and/or determining goals for speechreading training. *Speechreading enhancement* is computed by comparing speech recognition scores in a vision-only condition to scores obtained in an audition-plus-vision condition. The greater the difference between the two scores, the greater the amount of enhancement provided by the auditory signal. Sometimes speechreading enhancement is expressed as a ratio, and is computed by dividing the speech recognition score in a vision-only condition by the speech recognition score obtained in an audition-plus-vision condition.

Speechreading enhancement: the difference or ratio between speech recognition performance in an audition-only condition and an audition-plus-vision condition.

Hearing Loss Can Be Difficult to Detect in a Good Speechreader

Sometimes mild or moderate, and even severe hearing losses go undetected in children because they are proficient speechreaders. Some children may mispronounce some sounds or words, but their parents and teachers do not readily associate their articulation problems with hearing loss. Jeffers and Barley (1971) related the following incident:

> "Richard, age five, was [a child whose hearing loss went undetected]. The parents suspected that his younger brother had a hearing loss, but had no idea that Richard might also be similarly involved. His speech was excellent for his age, and his comprehension and recall vocabularies, larger than average. His loss was discovered through a whim of the audiometrist who decided that she might as well check Richard's hearing at the same time that she was testing his brother. Richard was found to have a binaural hearing loss of 42 dB [for the pure tone average of 500, 1000, and 2000 Hz] . . . and to be severely hard-of-hearing (60 dB or greater) for a good part of the consonant range. A year later his first grade teacher evinced complete disbelief regarding the loss and almost convinced

the parents that a misdiagnosis had been made. On a test of speech intelligibility without speechreading given at normal conversational level, he made a score of 48 percent, which would indicate great difficulty in understanding. With speechreading, his score was 84 percent, indicating good comprehension." (p. 10)

A few tests are available for assessing speechreading and speechreading enhancement. Tests for children include the Craig Sentences and the Craig Words (Craig, 1964). Tests for adults include the Iowa Sentence Test (Tyler, Preece, & Tye-Murray, 1986) and the City University of New York (CUNY) sentences (Boothroyd, Hanin, & Hnath, 1985). The latter two tests include sentences that are stored on laser videodisk.

The CHIVE (Children's Visual Enhancement Speech Test)

Assessing speechreading enhancement can be problematic. Individuals vary widely in their vision-only word recognition. For instance, in a test comprised of sentences, one person might recognize 90% of the words using only the visual signal, and another person might not recognize any of the words. The first person has a "ceiling effect" and has little room for improvement when the auditory signal is added. The second person has a "floor effect," and may not be helped when a degraded auditory signal is added.

Another difficulty that can arise when attempting to assess speechreading enhancement, particularly with regard to children, is that the individual's linguistic skills can greatly influence performance. For instance, a child with good linguistic skills will recognize more words in a sentence than a child with poor linguistic skills, all other factors being equal.

The CHIVE (Tye-Murray & Geers, 1997) is a test of speechreading enhancement for children, specifically designed to minimize ceiling and floor effects and to eliminate the effects of syntactic factors and minimize the effects of semantic factors on performance. It is comprised of 40 words. Half of the test words are highly likely to be recognized in a vision-only condition and half are less likely to be recognized. The test affords these advantages: (1) Ceiling and floor effects are minimized and (2) it is appropriate for testing a diverse group. The complete test is presented in the Key Resources at the end of this chapter.

Response Format

Another important issue to consider when testing speech recognition is what kind of response format will be used to elicit responses. Many standardized tests have an *open-set* format. This means that no response choices and no contextual cues are provided. The materials are not familiar to the patient, and have never been practiced, say during training.

An **open-set** task or test does not provide choices.

Closed-set tests often are used with cochlear-implant users and with children. These tests provide a limited set of response choices, and are easier than open-set tests. The members and the size of the response set can be selected to test features of speech recognition and to vary test difficulty. For example, if a teacher is interested in determining whether a new cochlear implant user utilizes suprasegmental cues, the response choices when the test word *ball* is spoken might be *ball, ice cream,* and *tricycle,* words that vary in duration and stress pattern. On the other hand, if the teacher is testing an experienced cochlear-implant user, the response set might be *ball, bill, bowl,* and *bell,* which will require the child to attend to more fine-grained segmental cues. The task will be more difficult when there are four response choices as opposed to only three.

A **closed-set** task or test provides fixed choices.

Live-Voice Versus Recorded Test Materials

The next issue to consider in regards to selecting speech-recognition test materials is whether testing will be performed *live-voice* or whether *recorded stimuli* will be used. As the terms imply, test items can be presented by a live talker or they can be presented via a playback system, such as a tape recorder or compact disc player. The advantages of using live voice are that no playback equipment is required, and the talker can adjust the rate of stimulus presentation to meet performance needs. Many young children are more comfortable with a live-voice test paradigm than a recorded-voice paradigm.

Despite these advantages, there are even more disadvantages associated with using live voice rather than recorded speech. Live talkers can introduce variability from one test session to the next, and from one test site to another. Talkers have different speaking styles, and they may vary in their style from one day to another. For instance, test talkers may vary on any of the following variables:

- **Voicing frequency:** Female test talkers usually have high pitches, and may be more difficult to understand than male test talkers, who have characteristically low-pitched voices. Most people have better hearing in the lower frequencies than the mid and high frequencies.
- **Intonation:** Sentences spoken with appropriate and expressive intonation are generally easier to understand than ones spoken with a monotone or inappropriate intonation. Thus, a test talker who uses more voice inflection while speaking the test sentences will be easier to understand than a test talker who uses less inflection.
- **Speech rate:** Rapidly spoken speech is more difficult to recognize than moderately slow speech. One test talker may speak slowly while another may speak more quickly.
- **Clarity of articulation:** Clearly articulated speech is easier to recognize than conversational or mumbled speech. Test talkers may vary in their ability to speak clearly.
- **Physical characteristics:** In an audition-plus-vision or vision-only condition, talkers who have pronounced lip and jaw displacement, no facial hair, and expressive facial movements will be relatively easier to speech-read or lipread.

It is important that talker characteristics not confound test results. Otherwise, you will not be able to monitor an individual's performance over time, nor compare his or her performance to that of other people who have been tested in other clinics. In today's world, many audiology clinics and other hearing-related settings rely exclusively on recorded materials to assess speech recognition. Live-voice testing is becoming increasingly rare.

Synthesized and Altered Speech

Most recorded test materials present speech spoken by an adult talker, speaking as clearly as possible. However, there are two other kinds of recorded materials that sometimes are used to assess word recognition, synthesized speech, and altered speech.

Synthesized speech is created with a computer or other technological apparatus and not by a human vocal tract. Synthesized speech may be used if the tester wants to determine how a pa-

Synthesized speech is created with a computer not the human vocal tract.

tient utilizes a specific cue for speech recognition. For example, a series of acoustic waveform samples may be created so that there is a systematic variation in the voice-onset time for /b/ in the word *bat*. The tester then might determine at what step in the continuum the patient hears the word *bat* versus *pat*.

Altered speech is human speech that is recorded and then altered in some way.

Time-compressed speech is speech that has been accelerated by removing segments of the waveform and then compressing the remaining segments together without changing its frequency composition.

Expanded speech is recorded speech that is altered by duplicating small segments of the signal so that it sounds like a slow speaking rate.

Filtered speech is passed through filter banks for the purpose of removing or amplifying frequency bands in the signal.

Low-pass filtered speech has been passed through filter banks that removed the higher, but not the lower, frequencies.

High-pass filtered speech has been passed through filter banks that removed the lower, but not the higher, frequencies.

Altered speech is human speech that is recorded and then altered in some way, usually by means of a computer software package. Altered speech may be time-compressed, extended, or filtered. *Time-compressed speech* has been digitized and then processed so that small segments are periodically deleted from the ongoing signal waveform. When it is played back, time-compressed speech sounds like natural speech produced at a fast speaking rate. Conversely, *expanded speech* is created by duplicating small segments of the signal so that the speech sounds as if it were produced with a slow speaking rate. *Filtered speech* is created by passing the speech signal through filter banks. *Low-pass filtered speech* includes the lower but not the higher frequencies, whereas *high-pass filtered speech* includes the higher but not the lower frequencies. Altered speech sometimes is used when the tester is interested in how well the patient can recognize speech when the auditory system is challenged.

In sum, synthesized speech and altered speech often are used to examine the effects of specific acoustic cues on speech recognition or to create a difficult speech listening condition. These stimuli might be used to address the following questions:

■ Does an individual utilize the plosive burst cue when distinguishing a /t/ from a /s/?
■ Even though a young and aged person have similar hearing thresholds, is the older person less able to understand time-compressed speech, which is a more taxing listening task?

DIFFICULTIES ASSOCIATED WITH SPEECH RECOGNITION ASSESSMENT

There are several problematic issues that should be considered when attempting to evaluate speech recognition and the effects of training on speech recognition performance. Three of the more significant issues include:

- Learning effects
- Test-retest variability
- Clinical significance

Learning Effects

Montgomery and Demorest (1988), among others, noted that clients often learn the test items when they are presented more than once, even when several weeks separate the test periods. Thus, because of *learning effects*, performance improves for reasons other than an aural rehabilitation intervention, such as receipt of speech perception training. For example, suppose someone was presented with the sentence, *The boy and girl are walking to school* during a speechreading test and recognized the words, *The boy* _____ _____ _____ *walking* _____ _____. If the patient repeated the test 3 months later, he or she might recognize all of the words, because he or she re-membered the sentence remnant, and used that information as contextual cues for identifying the rest of the sentence. Even recognizing the sentence rhythm and syllabic pattern might trigger recall. You may not think it is possible to remember di-alogue for that length of time, but one simply need reflect how the words of a song learned in grade school come back after many years of not hearing it, often after just hearing the first couple words.

Learning effects: performance on a test improves as a function of familiarity with the test procedures or items, not as a result of a change in ability.

Test-Retest Variability

Another difficulty related to assessing speechreading perfor-mance is that patients, especially children, vary in their perfor-mance from day to day. Thus, a patient may achieve a score on one day, take it on another day, and achieve a different score, even though it is the very same test. There may be several fac-tors that contribute to *test-retest variability*. One reason for this relates to the individual. For example, on some days a child may be highly motivated to perform well, whereas on others, the child may be restless and uninterested. As such, scores may improve or decrease over time, not as a result of training but rather, as a result of fatigue, interest, and mood.

Test-retest variability is a measure of the consistency of a test from one presentation to the next.

The nature of the test also may contribute to variability. Most tests are inherently variable, such that simply taking the test two times will yield somewhat different results, even if all testing parameters are held constant. If a test presents a closed-set of choices, the patient may perform better on one day than another as a function of chance.

Test-Retest Reliability

An issue closely related to variability is *test reliability*. Reliability of a test relates to the extent that test results are repeatable, and the level of reliability is expressed in terms of a standard error of measurement. Mendel and Danhauer (1997) define reliability as follows:

> Reliability concerns the extent to which measurements are repeatable by the same individual using different measures of the attribute, by the same individual using different measures of the attribute, or by different people using the same measure of the attribute without the interference of error (Bilger, 1984). Reliability can be expressed in terms of the standard error of measurement. If a listener is given the same test many times, the score determined from an average of the test scores would approach some value (that is, the true score) more and more closely. The degree to which a single test score approximates the true score determines the reliability of the test." (pp. 10–11)

Finally, test conditions can affect variability (Dowell, Brown, & Mecklenburg, 1990, p. 199). Changes in any of the following variables can shift test scores:

■ *Mode of presentation:* e.g., changing from live-voice to recorded stimuli may result in a decline in scores.
■ *Location:* e.g., changing from a sound-treated booth to a clinic office may also lead to decreased performance.
■ *Talker:* e.g., someone who is familiar versus unfamiliar, and someone who is male rather than female will typically be easier to understand.
■ *The number of times an item is repeated:* e.g., presenting a test item twice, or as often as an individual requests, usually leads to better performance than presenting it only once.

Use a Conservative Interpretation

"As with auditory discrimination ability, performance on speechreading tests can vary from day to day or moment to moment depending on alertness, motivation, fatigue, and so on. If we consider that a particular speech test may have an expected reliability of ±15% when performed in the [audition-only] condition and similar reliability when performed as a speechreading task, then the same test as an auditory-visual task may only be reliable within a range of 40% (±20%) due to the addition of the variances in the combined condition. This will also depend on the actual scores obtained and the assumptions made about the variance in the combined condition. This suggests that caution should be exercised in assessing performance based on [audition-plus-vision] test scores. For reliable assessment, it is necessary to have a complete battery of testing and to minimize any controllable sources of variance." (Dowell, Brown, & Mecklenburg, 1990, p. 199)

Clinical Significance

Another difficulty associated with speech recognition assessment relates to clinical significance. It sometimes is difficult to determine whether a small change in performance is clinically significant. For instance, an individual might recognize 30% of the words in a sentence test prior to receiving speechreading training. Afterwards, the person might recognize 36% of the words. In this instance, the hearing professional must determine whether speechreading has improved in a meaningful way.

Solutions

There are no easy solutions to the kinds of problems associated with speech recognition assessment that we have just considered. Some have tried to bypass them in a variety of different ways. We will consider some of these efforts in this section.

Learning Effects

One way in which the learning problem has been addressed is with the use of *equivalent lists*, that is, sets of sentences that are presumed to be equally difficult to recognize. Equivalency is usually established by playing the separate tests to a large group of subjects. If on average, the subjects recognize an equal number of words on each list, then the lists are said to be equivalent.

Equivalent lists contain items that are presumed to be equally difficult to recognize.

The problem with this tactic is that the lists may be equivalent when some listening devices are used but not others (Tyler,

1993). For instance, a group of hearing aid users may perform similarly on two lists of test items, whereas a group of cochlear-implant users may not. Similarly, equivalency may vary with the configuration of hearing loss, such that a group of individuals with a sloping mild-to-moderate loss will not perform like a group of individuals who have a flat severe hearing loss. List equivalency also may vary as a function of test condition. For example, two lists may be equivalent when presented in a vision-only but not in an audition-plus-vision test condition.

Some researchers have tried to minimize learning effects by constructing tests that have a large number of items, say 100 or more sentences (Tyler, Preece, & Tye-Murray, 1985). With so many test items, it is thought that patients may be less likely to remember them, even with repeated testing. However, there is little empirical data available to support this assumption.

Test-Retest Variability

Performance variability has been addressed by devising tests that require repeated testing on two consecutive days. The Repeated Frame Sentence test is presented in the Key Resources as an example (Tye-Murray, 1993). If a client performs similarly on both days, we can assume scores reflect ability. On the other hand, if scores differ markedly, extraneous variables such as motivation may be affecting the test results.

Clinical Significance

A within-subject statistical procedure (Tye-Murray, Tyler, Woodward, & Gantz, 1992) has been used to compare post-training performance to pretraining performance to establish whether a change is statistically significant. The number of words repeated verbatim in each sentence of a pretraining test can be compared to the number of key words repeated verbatim in the same sentence following training. A paired t-statistic can be computed using all sentences in a list. Although statistical significance does not necessarily equate with clinical significance, it does indicate whether or not a change is robust.

FINAL REMARKS

In this chapter, we have considered in a general way how to assess individuals' ability to recognize speech. We have not focused on particular tests, rather, we have focused on the principles that must be considered when choosing a test for a particular individual. The results of speech recognition testing are invaluable when designing an aural rehabilitation plan.

KEY CHAPTER POINTS

✔ A typical audiological assessment includes an audiogram, a determination of speech recognition thresholds, and an assessment of speech discrimination/recognition. The audiogram by itself does not always adequately reflect the magnitude of a patient's communication difficulties.

✔ You might assess speech recognition abilities for any number of reasons. For instance, you might be interested in evaluating a patient's need for amplification or assessing the patient's performance over time.

✔ Patient variables, such as the cognitive/linguistic skill of the test taker, will influence selection of test materials. For example, you would not select a sentence test for evaluating a three-year old child.

✔ Test stimuli may be phonemes, words, phrases, unrelated sentences, or topically-related sentences. Each kind of stimulus offers advantages and disadvantages.

✔ Once you have selected your test materials, you can make decisions about test procedures. For example, you might opt to present the stimuli in an audition-only condition, using live-voice and background noise.

✔ Patients may learn the items in a test with repeated testing.

✔ Test-retest variability sometimes is an important issue. Some people, especially children, may vary in their performance from day-to-day.

KEY RESOURCES

The CHIVE Sentence Test

Description: The CHIVE is comprised of three word lists. Each list is to be administered in a different condition. Each list contains 20 words. Experiments have determined that 10 words in each list are "easy," meaning that the majority of people can identify them using only vision alone, and 10 words are "difficult," and only a minority of people can lipread them. The words are within the vocabulary level of 7- to 9-year-old children with profound prelingual hearing losses (Tye-Murray & Geers, 1997). Here, the words are organized by difficulty level. In practice, they are presented randomly within the list.

List A (Audition-plus-vision)

Easy:	*Difficult:*
1. telephone	11. ten
2. elephant	12. hug
3. mouth	13. rock
4. fish	14. talk
5. newspaper	15. sit
6. hamburger	16. cat
7. warm	17. full
8. thumb	18. sing
9. chair	19. birthday cake
10. ship	20. map

List B (Vision-only)

Easy:	*Difficult:*
1. family	11. line
2. remember	12. neck
3. basketball	13. kill
4. bath	14. kiss
5. beautiful	15. dinosaur
6. ice cream cone	16. sock
7. look	17. juice
8. shoe	18. foot
9. light	19. math
10. cheese	20. Mickey Mouse

List C (Audition-only)

Easy:

1. grandfather
2. fall
3. policeman
4. farm
5. ball
6. butterfly
7. push
8. love
9. hear
10. chocolate

Difficult:

11. down
12. plate
13. six
14. good
15. hill
16. tall
17. sun
18. car
19. pull
20. vegetable

The Repeated Frame Sentence Test

Description: "Lists A and B are presented in an audition-plus-vision condition and lists C and D are presented in a vision-only condition. Lists A and C are completed on one day and lists B and D on the next day. Speechreading training begins thereafter. On completion of the training program, the tests are administered again during a 2-day period. The tests are scored by the number of key words repeated verbatim.

By testing on two separate days, some information about performance variability is obtained. Also, two scores within a test condition are available. Before audiovisual speech recognition performance is considered to be improved, scores on both lists A and B must improve following training; likewise for visual speech recognition and lists C and D.

The lists in the The Repeated Frame Sentence Test each contain 24 sentences, with six sets of four. Each set of four sentences share syntactic structure and differ only in two or three key words. The keywords within are interchangeable and are approximately equally probable in the sentence context. They also have the same number of syllables. The use of sentence sets is meant to minimize the learning effects associated with repeated testing. For instance, if the patient recognizes the words *in the sky* in list A, the key words will not be known due to prior to the list. *Three stars, ten birds, six clouds,* and *eight clouds* are all possible elements of the test sentence. The sentences within a list are randomly presented.

Posttherapy performance on a test list is compared to pretherapy performance using a within-subject statistical procedure (Tye-Murray, Tyler, Woodworth, & Gantz, 1992). The number of words correct in each sentence is tabulated and then a paired t statistic is computed, with the sentences paired to compare performance pre- and post-therapy. A paired t-test is appropriate because the same sentences are presented before and after aural rehabilitation therapy. Since a list contains 24 sentences, each t-test statistic has 23 degrees of freedom" (p. 129–130).

The Repeated Frame Sentence Test

"The sentences are presented in random order, but are presented in sets of four here, with each set corresponding to one sentence frame. Key words are italicized. Whether the list is presented in audition-plus-vision or vision-only mode is noted in parentheses" (p. 141).

List A (Audition-plus-vision)

1. The *boat* is *fast*.
2. The *train* is *slow*.
3. The *plane* is *big*.
4. The *bike* is *small*.
5. A *lunchbox* is on the *bed*.
6. A *balloon* is on the *desk*.
7. A *baseball* is on the *chair*.
8. A *pencil* is on the *floor*.
9. The *snake* is looking for *food*.
10. The *cat* is looking at the *moon*.
11. The *bear* is looking at the *tree*.
12. The *frog* is looking at the *bug*.
13. *Three stars* are in the sky.
14. *Ten birds* are in the sky.
15. *Six clouds* are in the sky.
16. *Eight kites* are in the sky.
17. The *silly* dog is *sleeping*.
18. The *funny* dog is *playing*.
19. The *ugly* dog is *sitting*.
20. The *pretty* dog is *eating*.
21. *Pick* up your *hat*.
22. *Put* on your *coat*.
23. *Put* on your *shoes*.
24. *Take* off your *boots*.

List B (Audition-plus-vision)

1. The *queen* is *nice*.
2. The *king* is *mean*.
3. The *nurse* is *thin*.
4. The *dog* is *bad*.
5. Her *mom* is in the *bedroom*.
6. Her *friend* is in the *backyard*.
7. Her *dad* is in the *kitchen*.
8. Her *aunt* is in the *bathroom*.
9. *Grandma* is eating a *hotdog*.
10. *Mother* is eating a *cookie*.
11. *Grandpa* is eating a *pancake*.
12. *Father* is eating an *apple*.
13. The *silverware* and *plates* are on the table.
14. The *potatoes* and *forks* are on the table.
15. The *bananas* and *bowls* are on the table.
16. The *hamburgers* and *knives* are on the table.
17. I *want* the *soup*.
18. I *cook* the *eggs*.
19. I *need* the *meat*.
20. I *like* the *peas*.
21. Point to your *hair* and *nose*.
22. Point to your *arms* and *face*.
23. Point to your *hands* and *ears*.
24. Point to your *eyes* and *feet*.

List C (Vision-only)

1. The *pen* is in the *bowl*.
2. The *book* is in the *bag*.
3. The *key* is in the *jar*.
4. The *ball* is in the *room*.

5. The *football* is *outside* the box.
6. The *money* is *under* the box.
7. The *candy* is *inside* the box.
8. The *whistle* is *behind* the box.
9. *Drink* the *juice.*
10. *Buy* the *milk.*
11. *Stir* the *tea.*
12. *Pour* the *pop.*
13. The *lady* is washing the *shirts.*
14. The *teacher* is washing the *dress.*
15. The *farmer* is washing the *pants.*
16. The *woman* is washing the *dish.*
17. The *car* is *yellow.*
18. The *truck* is *blue.*
19. The *kite* is *dirty.*
20. The *bike* is *little.*
21. The boy has a *pink* and *blue* bike.
22. The boy has a *white* and *green* bike.
23. The boy has a *brown* and *green* bike.
24. The boy has a *black* and *red* bike.

List D (Vision-only)

1. *Five boys* are in the water.
2. *Two ducks* are in the water.
3. *Four fish* are in the water.
4. *Nine boats* are in the water.
5. I see a *rabbit* and a *cow.*
6. I see a *turkey* and a *pig.*
7. I see a *turtle* and a *mouse.*
8. I see a *chicken* and a *horse.*
9. A cat is *running* in the *street.*
10. A cat is *waiting* in the *house.*
11. A cat is *walking* in the *grass.*
12. A cat is *standing* in the *yard.*
13. *Get* some *cake.*
14. *Take* some *pie.*
15. *Have* some *lunch.*
16. *Make* some *bread.*
17. The *cowboy* is *tall.*
18. The *mailman* is *mad.*
19. The *doctor* is *short.*
20. The *fireman* is *sad.*
21. A *boy* is *making* the paper airplane.
22. A *man* is *watching* the paper airplane.
23. A *clown* is *throwing* the paper airplane.
24. A *girl* is *making* the paper airplane.

Source: From Tye-Murray, N. (1993). Aural rehabilitation and patient management. In R. S. Tyler, (Ed.), *Cochlear implants: Audiological foundations,* (p. 141). San Diego, CA: Singular Publishing Group. Reprinted with permission.

6

Listening Devices and Related Technology

Topics

- Hearing Aids
- Cochlear Implants
- Assistive Listening Devices (ALDs)

- Final Remarks
- Key Chapter Points
- Key Resources

After a patient receives a comprehensive audiological assessment, and before he or she receives speech perception training, appropriate listening devices must be selected and fitted. These systems may include a hearing aid or a cochlear implant, and/or assistive listening devices (ALDs). The provision of appropriate technical devices is an essential element in the aural rehabilitation plan, whether the patient is an adult or a child. These instruments can minimize conversational difficulties, and maximize the use of residual hearing for daily functioning.

The objectives for providing an individual with a listening device are twofold (Gudmundsen, 1997):

1. **to make speech audible, without introducing distortion or discomfort, and**
2. **to restore a range of loudness experience.**

In optimal circumstances, the three kinds of listening devices that we will review in this chapter can be selected and fitted to achieve the two objectives just listed.

This chapter presents an introduction for readers who are unacquainted with listening devices and a key-points review for those who are familiar with them. We will discuss both related terminology and categories within device types.

HEARING AIDS

Prior to the 20th century, there were three ways to help a hard-of-hearing person hear better (Gudmundsen, 1997): (1) speak loudly, (2) talk right into the person's ear, or (3) provide the person with an ear horn, speaking tube, trumpet, or other similar device. The advent of electronic hearing aids has revolutionized the methods available to assist hard-of-hearing persons to hear more. To appreciate the relatively rapid advances that have occurred in hearing aid technology in the last 1½ centuries, it is worthwhile to review Table 6–1. This table highlights some of the landmark events that have occurred in hearing aid design.

Two major trends are evident in modern hearing-aid design: miniaturization and enhanced signal processing. Over time, hearing aids have become smaller. Early hearing aids were so

Table 6-1. Some landmark events in the history of hearing-aid technology and marketing. Siemens, Oticon, Telex, Beltone, Maico, Dahlberg, Miracle-Ear, Widex, Starkey, Argosy, Microtronic, Philips, and Danavox are companies that manufacture hearing aids.

1847: Siemens is founded in Germany by Werner von Siemens. Makes many improvements in telegraph, telephone, and electric transmission systems.

1890: National Carbon Company is founded, and later becomes Eveready Battery Co.

1904: The company that later becomes Oticon is founded by Hans Demant to import American hearing aids to Denmark.

1910: Siemens makes its first hearing aids for employees, offering them to the public in 1912. Early aids are hand-carried.

1914: Siemens introduces a small hearing aid receiver fitted close to the auditory canal, with sound carried via an animal membrane.

1919: Siemens makes the first audiometer.

1924: Siemens patents first compact carbon microphone amplifier for use in pocket hearing aids.

1929: Siemens builds first wearable tube amplifiers with improved response and loudness.

1940: Maico introduces its first wearable hearing aid (made in three parts) incorporating miniature vacuum tubes.

1941: Maico introduces tone adjustments for fitting various hearing losses.

1944: Beltone introduces first all-in-one hearing aid, the Mono-Pac.

1953: Maico markets first completely transistorized hearing aid.

1955: Dahlberg introduces the Miracle-Ear, the first electronic hearing aid designed to be worn in the ear. That same year, Dahlberg introduces innovative BTE and eyeglass instruments and begins providing private-level hearing aids to Sears Roebuck. Siemens' first transistor hearing aid introduces the telecoil.

1961: Siemens introduces Auriculina, the first BTE with frontal sound pick-up.

1962: Miracle-Ear IV is first hearing aid to use integrated circuitry.

1967: Siemens develops a BTE with push-pull amplifier, and introduces the Fonator speech/auditory training instrument. Widex introduces a sound hook to reduce wind noise.

1971: Maico patents dephasing microphone that offers directional hearing.

1972: Starkey establishes right of return policy for its custom full-concha hearing aids.

1976: Danavox is first hearing aid manufacturer to launch a direct audio input system. Siemens introduces BTE with input compression.

1979: Oticon introduces E24V, the first hearing aid with a user-operated switch to choose between omni- and directional microphones.

1982: Argosy Electronics releases the CCA, the industry's first successful in-the-canal instrument.

1986: Beltone's new Suprimo hearing aid, offering three custom integrated circuits and eight fitting controls, is a long step toward a fully programmable instrument.

1988: Philips introduces infrared remote-controlled ITEs and ITCs.

(continued)

Table 6–1. *(continued)*

1989: Maico offers the first programmable hearing aid.

1991: Philips introduces the first very-deep-canal instrument, the XP Peritympanic.

1992: Danavox introduces DFS Genius, a digital system for suppressing feedback.

1995: Oticon announces DigiFocus, the first 100% digital ear-level hearing aid. Maico offers the first programmable CIC.

1996: Telex introduces SoftWear, a completely soft-shelled hearing aid.

1997: Argosy introduces Quadrasound, a proprietary microchip providing access to four separate signal processors within each hearing instrument. Widex introduces first digital signal processing instrument in a CIC model. Telex introduces the AcuSound, the first hearing aid to split the incoming signal into two channels based on the signal's amplitude.

Source: Adapted from the "A timeline of the hearing industry." *The Hearing Journal, 50,* pp. 54–70.

large and cumbersome so as not to be portable. These tabletop electrical aids often were used only in educational settings where teacher and students might sit around a shared table. The early portable aids were not much of an improvement over the tabletop devices. They were housed in large cases that had to be carried on the body or with the hand and were operated with vacuum tubes. In the last few decades, there have been rapid advances toward miniaturization, so now it is possible to use a hearing aid and have it be completely invisible, unless someone looks directly into the ear. Probably the primary factor spurring this trend toward miniaturization is cosmetic concerns on the part of the users.

Along with miniaturization, there has been another trend evident in hearing-aid designs, and that is a growing sophistication in their *signal-processing* capabilities (ability to alter the signal in some way, usually according to a processing algorithm), all in virtual real time. Some of the advances related to developments in signal-processing include the following:

Signal processing involves manipulation of various parameters of a signal.

Some hearing aids have **multiple memories** that allow the speech signal to be processed in more than one way.

Multiple memory hearing aids allow the user to select the processing strategy according to the listening environment.

Noise reduction is the difference in the sound pressure level (SPL) of a noise measured at two different locations.

■ *Multiple memories,* so that a patient might adjust the hearing aid one way when listening in quiet and another way when listening in noise, to maximize sound quality and speech reception. Hearing aids that provide access to different amplification characteristics sometimes are referred to as *multiple memory hearing aids*.

■ *Sophisticated noise reduction circuits,* so that the hearing aid amplifies speech and not undesirable background noise.

■ *Acoustic feedback cancellation*, so that hearing aids will not "whistle" when sound escapes from the receiver.

■ *Programmability*, which allows the audiologist to set gain, frequency response, and other electroacoustic properties of the hearing aid. This feature may be especially attractive if the user is experiencing a progressive hearing loss, and the hearing aid must be altered over time to accommodate the changing listening needs.

■ *Digital processing*, so that the signal is converted from analog to digital form, processed to achieve a target signal, and then converted back to an analog signal.

■ *Multiple channels*, a signal processing technique wherein the signal is filtered into frequency bands, so that some bands (usually the high-frequency bands) receive more gain than other bands (usually the low-frequency bands).

Although these trends are indicative of evolving designs, there are some constancies in the components that make up a hearing aid, no matter what the style or special features.

Hearing-Aid Components

Hearing aids are comprised of three fundamental components: a microphone, an amplifier, and a receiver (Figure 6–1). The acoustic signal enters the *microphone* from the environment, and is converted into an electrical signal. The signal then is passed to the *amplifier*, where it is amplified. The amplified signal goes to the *receiver*, is converted back to an acoustic signal, and then is delivered to the patient's external auditory canal.

The hearing aid also carries *batteries*, which provide power for its operation. Batteries come in at least five sizes (denoted by the following codes, from largest size to smallest: AA, 675, 312, 13, 230, or 10). Batteries may be mercury or zinc, with zinc batteries lasting about twice as long as mercury. Although battery life is dependent on a number of factors, such as the kind of battery it is, the style of hearing aid in which it is used, and the volume control setting, a zinc battery will last about 1 to 4 weeks.

Acoustic feedback cancellation is a feature that avoids the annoying squeal produced by hearing aids when the microphone picks up the amplified sound from the hearing aid and reamplifies it.

Programmability in a hearing aid means that several parameters of the instrument, such as gain, are controlled by a computer.

A hearing aid that uses **digital processing** converts the signal from analog to digital form, processes the signal to achieve a target, and then converts the signal back to an analog form.

A hearing aid that uses **multiple channels** filters the signal into frequency bands so that some bands (usually the high frequency bands) can receive more gain than others.

A **microphone** is a transducer that converts an audio signal into an electronic signal.

An **amplifier** increases the intensity of sound.

A **battery** is a cell that provides electrical power.

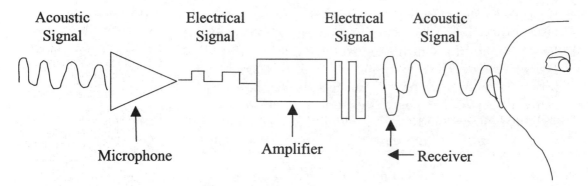

Figure 6-1. Schematic of a hearing aid.

Microphones

Microphones are designed to respond to sound, without distorting it or introducing extraneous noise. The microphone converts the audio signal into an electrical signal.

Directional microphones are more sensitive to sound originating from in front of the user than sound coming from behind the user.

Omnidirectional microphones are sensitive to sound coming from all directions.

There are two general types of microphones: directional and omnidirectional. *Directional microphones* are designed to respond primarily to sound originating from in front of the user, and not from the back. *Omnidirectional microphones* respond to sound originating from all directions. Directional microphones are most common in behind-the-ear instruments, which we will consider shortly, and are meant to enhance the signal-to-noise ratio for the user. For instance, a directional microphone will pick up the speech of a talker who stands in front of the user, but not from two individuals who speak about something else in the back of the room. As such, directional microphones are often desirable for listening in noisy situations.

Amplifiers

The **gain** of a hearing aid is the difference in decibels between the input level of an acoustic signal and the output level.

An amplifier is also a component in all hearing aids. Amplifiers increase the level of the signal. *Gain* describes the amount of amplification provided by an amplifier, and is defined as the difference between the hearing aid's input and output. For instance, if an input signal is 30 dB SPL and the output is 60 dB SPL, the gain of the hearing aid is 30 dB.

Amplifiers may be classified as one of two types: peak-clipping or compression. These terms refer to their mode of limiting the output of the signal, so that it is not so loud as to be uncomfortable to the user nor does it have the potential to cause a noise-induced hearing loss. The goal of peak clipping or compression is to limit the *maximum power output (MPO)* of the hearing aid, which is the maximum output level a hearing aid will put out in response to a very loud input signal.

Maximum power output (MPO): the maximum intensity level that a hearing aid can produce.

An amplifier with a *peak-clipping* circuit provides a constant or linear amount of gain (or amplification) across a range of input levels. There is a one-to-one relationship between the input and output, so that the sound is amplified by a consistent amount until it reaches a saturation level. At this *saturation level*, sound coming into the amplifier is so loud, that the amplifier begins to "clip" or cut off the peaks of the signal. Although this effectively limits the level of the audio signal, it also introduces distortion; therefore, sound quality decreases. Figure 6–2 presents an example of the relationship between input and output levels of the hearing aid in a peak-clipping system

Peak-clipping is a method of limiting hearing aid output in which a constant or linear amount of gain is provided across a range of input levels until it reaches a saturation level, at which the amplifier begins to "clip" off the peaks of the signal.

Saturation level: point at which an amplifier no longer provides an increase in output compared to input.

A nonlinear amplifier system usually functions with a *compression* circuitry. The use of compression has three purposes. One purpose of compression is to limit the maximum output of the hearing aid, so that sound is never so loud as to cause discomfort to the user.

Compression is a nonlinear form of amplifier gain used to determine and limit output gain as a function of input gain.

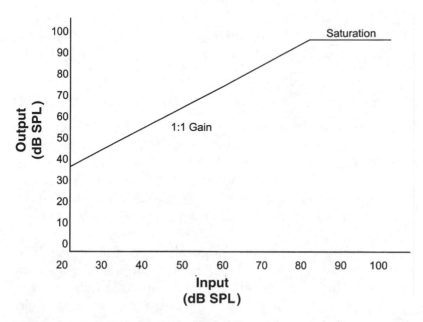

Figure 6–2. Input/output loudness function for a hearing aid that uses peak-clipping to limit output.

Dynamic range is the difference in decibels between an individual's threshold of sensitivity for a sound and the level at which the sound becomes uncomfortably loud.

A second purpose of compression is to provide a range of sounds to the user within the person's dynamic range. *Dynamic range* is defined as the difference between a person's threshold for sound and the level at which the sound causes discomfort. In many persons with significant hearing loss, dynamic range is reduced, and may be only 40 dB or less.

A third purpose of compression circuitry is to provide a varying amount of gain (amplification) of the speech signal as a function of the input level. Thus, soft sounds are amplified more than moderately-loud sounds.

The point on an input-output function where compression is activated is termed the **kneepoint**.

In a compression circuitry, sound may be amplified in a linear fashion until it reaches a level of incoming intensity that triggers the compression function. At this point, often referred to as the *kneepoint,* the signal is amplified to a lesser degree, and never amplified beyond a preselected level. This kind of output limiting is used most commonly in today's hearing aids. Figure 6–3 presents the relationship between input and output of a hearing aid that has a compression circuit, and indicates the kneepoint. There are different kinds of compression circuits. For example, the *K-AMP circuit* provides more gain for high frequencies than low frequencies at low-intensity input levels, but not for high-intensity input levels. *Mulitiband compression* permits different degrees of compression and output limiting for different frequency bands in the incoming signal, so that the growth of loudness in a signal can be controlled, and the signal can be shaped to maximize speech recognition.

A **K-AMP circuit** is designed to provide more gain for moderate-level sound, no gain for high-intensity sound, and compression limited for the highest level sound. It often also provides more amplification for the high frequencies.

Multiband compression is a method of shaping the loudness growth of a signal to maximize speech for the listener using different degrees of compression and output limiting for different frequencies.

Earmolds

In addition to a microphone, amplifier, and receiver, some hearing aids require the use of earmolds (whereas the casing actually replaces the earmold in many other kinds of hearing aids). Earmolds deliver sound from the receiver to the ear and help hold the hearing aid in place. Earmolds are custom-made to fit into the ear canal of the user. An earmold attaches to plastic tubing, which leads to the hearing-aid receiver. It can be constructed in a variety of configurations, to suit the needs of the individual user. For instance, some earmolds fill the entire concha of the ear while others consist only of a half-ring that anchors it within the concha. The former style of earmold might be used for a severe or profound hearing loss, the latter for a mild loss.

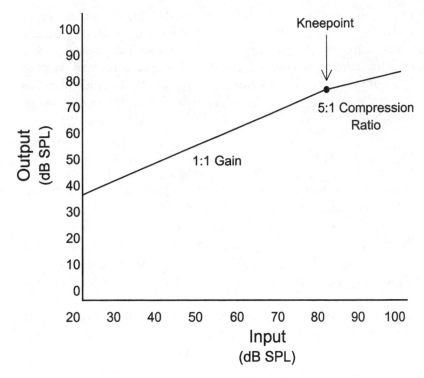

Figure 6–3. Input/output loudness function for a hearing aid that uses compression circuitry to limit output.

Other Features of Hearing Aids

In addition to the components previously shown in Figure 6–1, some hearing aids have additional features. These include an on-off control, a volume control, a telecoil, and a remote control.

On-Off Control

The *on-off control* may be a small switch that moves back and forth to turn the hearing aid off when not in use and on when the hearing aid is needed. The on-off control also may be incorporated into the volume control wheel. When a hearing aid does not have an on-off switch, the hearing aid is activated by inserting the battery.

On-off control: a small switch that moves back and forth to turn the hearing aid off when not in use and on when needed; may be incorporated into the volume wheel.

Telecoil

The *telecoil* is a special circuit that enhances telephone communication. The telephone receiver emits electromagnetic signals, which are picked up by the hearing-aid telecoil. The hear-

A **telecoil** is an induction coil that receives electromagnetic signals from a telephone or loop amplification system.

ing-aid microphone thus is bypassed. The signal picked up by the telecoil is amplified and transduced to an audio signal, and then delivered to the ear. If the hearing aid has an on-off switch, it may include a *T* position for *telecoil* and an *M* position for *microphone*, so the user can switch on the telecoil before using the telephone. An *MT* option on the on-off switch allows for simultaneous use of both the telecoil and microphone.

Volume control

The **volume control** on a hearing aid is used to adjust its ouput; may be manual or automatic.

A *volume control* allows the user to adjust the level of amplification. It usually is a rotating wheel. When a hearing aid does not have a volume control, it typically has a screw-set control that the audiologist can adjust with a screw driver.

Remote Control

A **remote control** is a hand-held device that permits adjustments in the volume or changes in the program of a programmable hearing aid.

A *remote control* is a hand-held device that can serve two purposes. First, it can be used to program the electroacoustic properties of a hearing aid. Second, a remote control can be used to switch the hearing aid from one channel to another, to adjust the volume, and to turn it off and on.

Hearing-Aid Styles

Now that we have considered the basic components of a hearing aid, let us now review the ways in which the components can be packaged to function as a listening device. There are six general styles of hearing aids. These are body aids, eyeglass aids, behind-the-ear aids (BTE), in-the-ear aids (ITE), in-the-canal aids (ITC), and completely-in-the-canal aids (CIC).

Body Aids and Eyeglass Hearing Aids

Body hearing aid: a hearing aid worn on the body and including a box worn on the torso and a cord connecting to an ear-level receiver.

The *body-aid* casement is about the size of a deck of cards, and is worn on the torso. The casement leads to a custom-made earmold by means of a long cord. The body-worn casement houses the microphone, amplifier, and receiver. Body aids may provide powerful amplification, and are useful for severe and profound hearing losses. They also have large controls, so they can be used by individuals who have reduced manual dexterity. Body aids are durable and can be harnessed to a young child, so that the likelihood of it being lost or damaged may be reduced.

Despite these advantages, body aids are not used very often today. They are relatively bulky and highly visible. The placement of the microphone on the chest rather than near the ear also may decrease a user's ability to localize sound. They sometimes are used with children who have a pinna that cannot support a behind-the-ear hearing aid, and children who do not have an external ear canal. For these latter children, the body aid may be attached to a *bone-conductor*, which delivers sound through the skull.

Like body aids, eyeglass hearing aids are rarely prescribed any more (Figure 6–4). In an *eyeglass aid*, the microphone, amplifier, and receiver are housed in the temple of the glasses. In principle, they function much like a BTE. The microphone is near the ear, and the receiver directs sound through tubing, into an earmold placed within the user's concha. Although an eyeglass aid presents the advantage of reduced hardware (i.e., the user wears only one prosthesis and not two), it also presents many disadvantages. These disadvantages include the fact that eyeglass aids are heavy, often unattractive, and a need for repair means a loss of eyeglasses.

Behind-the-ear (BTE) Hearing Aids

The *behind-the-ear hearing aid* components are built into a small shell that fits behind the pinna (Figure 6–5). The hearing-aid case is connected to an earmold by a small plastic tube. This is probably the most flexible style of hearing aid because it can be fitted with many available options, such as a powerful telecoil circuit. In addition, an earmold can be constructed to accommodate the user, which may be desirable for several reasons. For instance, if a child suffers from chronic otitis media, then he or she might not

A **bone-conductor** is a vibrator or oscillator used to transmit sound to the bones of the skull by means of vibration.

In an **eyeglass hearing aid**, the hearing aid is housed in the temple of a pair of eyeglasses.

The style of hearing aid known as a **behind-the-ear (BTE)** hearing aid is worn over the pinna and coupled to the ear by means of an earmold.

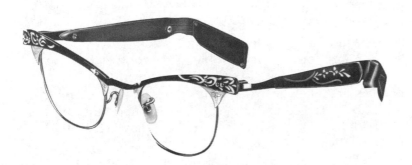

Figure 6–4. An eyeglass hearing aid. (Photograph courtesy of Central Institute for the Deaf)

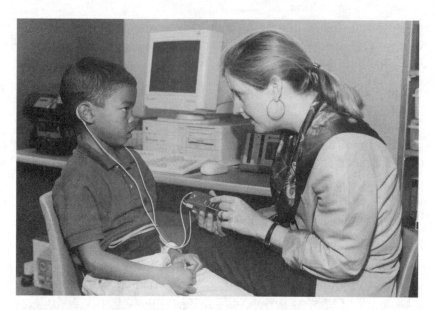

Figure 6–5. A behind-the-ear hearing aid. In this picture, an audiologist is fitting a personal FM trainer to the child's hearing-aid. The audiologist holds the FM receiver, which connects to the child's hearing aid by a cord. (Photograph by Patti Gabriel, courtesy of Central Institute for the Deaf)

be able to use a device that occludes the ear canal, as does an in-the-ear (ITE) aid. If a child is still growing, the earmold can simply be recast when the ear outgrows the existing one. With smaller hearing-aid styles, such as ITEs, a new hearing aid must be recast as it becomes too small to accommodate a child's growing skull. Other advantages of BTEs include the following:

- When used with a soft earmold, a BTE affords greater safety than all-in-the ear hearing aids. This is important especially for children, who may be at high risk for being hit in the ear, say, by a ball in gym class.
- A BTE has the capability of direct audio input, so it can be hardwired to an assistive listening device.
- BTEs have few problems with feedback.
- There are fewer repair problems than other hearing-aid styles.
- BTEs are relatively easy to clean, because the earmold can be detached and washed. This is important for individuals who perspire a lot, or who have wax build-up or chronic otitis media.
- A BTE can be used with a nonoccluding earmold, which may be important if the individual has chronic otitis media or is unable to have an occluded ear canal for other reasons.

BTEs may be undesirable if the patient is concerned about cosmetics, as they typically are visible, unless covered by long hair.

In-the-Ear (ITE) and In-the-Canal (ITC) Hearing Aids

ITEs and ITCs are hearing-aid styles that fit completely in the external ear. A primary difference between the two styles is that the ITC fills less of the concha than the ITE. The two styles of listening devices must be custom-fitted to the user's ear. The audiologist takes an earmold impression of the ear and then sends the impression to the manufacturer for construction of the aid. The casings of ITEs and ITCs house all of the hearing-aid components, and no additional tubing or earmold is necessary. These two styles are the most widely dispensed hearing aids in today's market, probably because of cosmetic reasons. Figure 6–6 presents a photograph of an ITE aid in the ear.

ITCs may offer some disadvantages as compared to BTEs, even though they are less noticeable. They may not be able to provide as much amplification and often do not have room for hearing-aid options, such as telecoils or volume controls. They also tend to be more expensive.

An **in-the-ear (ITE) hearing aid** fits into the concha of the ear.

An **in-the-canal (ITC) hearing aid** fits in the external ear canal, only partially filling the concha.

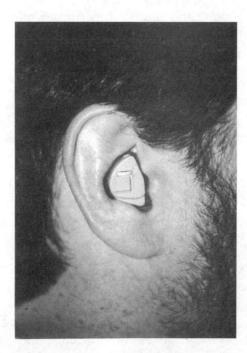

Figure 6-6. An ITE hearing aid. (Photograph courtesy of Central Institute for the Deaf)

A **completely-in-the-canal (CIC) hearing aid** fits entirely within the exteral ear canal.

Completely-in-the-Canal (CIC) Hearing Aids

CICs are worn completely inside the ear canal and do not occupy the concha. They are inserted and removed from the ear canal by means of a short clear cord attached to the hearing-aid casement. CICs are so small that options often are not available, such as an on-off switch, a volume control, and a telecoil. Nonetheless, they offer many advantages. They tend to be easy to insert and remove, often more so than trying to insert an earmold, as with a BTE aid. Some people report a better sound quality with CICs than with other styles, which is due in part to the absence of an *occlusion effect*. An occlusion effect may occur with most other hearing aid styles. An occlusion effect, caused by plugging the ear canal, may result in speech sounding as if the individual is "listening inside of a barrel." The advantages of CICs can be summarized as follows (Mueller, 1994; Staab, 1992):

In the **occlusion effect**, low-frequency sound in bone-conducted signals is enhanced as a result of closing of the ear canal.

■ Easy to handle
■ Reduction of an occlusion effect
■ Reduction of feedback
■ Improved sound localization
■ Less electronic gain is needed than with other styles, because the volume between the end of the hearing aid and the tympanic membrane (eardrum) is minimal
■ Elimination of wind noise
■ Better cerumen control than with styles that fill the ear canal
■ Enhanced telephone use without the need for additional assistive listening devices
■ Virtually invisible to others when inserted into the user's ear canal
■ Greater high-frequency gain

Binaural Versus Monaural Fitting

Sometimes, the audiologist will recommend that a patient receive two hearing aids instead of one. Even though two hearing aids are more expensive than one, and may require more effort to maintain, binaural amplification fitting offers many advantages over a monaural fitting, including the following:

■ *Elimination of head shadow:* With one hearing aid, sound coming from the unaided side of the head may be attenuated by as much as 12–16 dB, especially high frequency sounds. Use of two hearing aids allows sound to be received on both sides of the head.

■ *Loudness summation:* When sound is received by both ears, a summing of the two signals results. Thresholds for sound may improve by 3 dB or more, as compared to monaural thresholds in either ear.

■ *Binaural squelch:* Listening performance will be better in noise when the user wears two hearing aids instead of one. This improvement in signal-to-noise ratio may be 2 or 3 dB.

■ *Localization:* A normally hearing person is sensitive to interaural differences in a sound's intensity and phase and this allows him or her, in part, to localize the sound source. A monaural hearing-aid fitting disrupts these cues, whereas binaural hearing aids serve to preserve this localization ability.

Attenuation of sound to one ear because of the presence of the head between the ear and the sound source is called the **head shadow** effect.

Loudness summation: a summing of the signals received by each earresulting in a 3-dB advantage for binaural over monaural hearing.

Binaural squelch: improvement in listening in noise when wearing two hearing aids instead of one, resulting in a 2-3 dB improvement in signal-to-noise ratio.

Localization: the ability to locate the source of a sound in space due to the normal ear's sensitivity to interaural differences in phase and intensity.

Selecting a Hearing-Aid Style

A consideration of hearing-aid styles leads to the question, "How do you determine which style to provide to a particular individual?" There is no pat answer to this question, but the selection of a particular style of hearing aid often is dependent upon the degree of hearing loss, the patient's preference, the cost of the device, the person's age and lifestyle, and his or her physical status.

Degree of Hearing Loss

As part of a hearing-aid evaluation, an audiologist will obtain an audiogram. The magnitude and configuration of an individual's hearing loss will then help to determine the style of hearing aid selected.

Table 6–2 indicates optimum style options as a function of degree of hearing loss. For example, if an individual has a profound hearing loss, a CIC device is not appropriate because it will not provide enough amplification for the person's listening needs.

The recommendations listed in Table 6–2 are generalizations, and audiologists sometimes select these aids even if they are not optimal for the hearing loss because of other considerations, such as user preference.

Table 6–2. Recommendations for hearing-aid style as a function of degree of hearing loss.

Style	Hearing Loss for Which Use Is Optimal	Hearing Loss for Which Use Is Appropriate But Not Optimal
Body aid	All degrees, although usually used for severe and profound losses	
Eyeglass aid	All degrees	
BTE	All degrees	
ITE	Mild through severe	Severe-to-profound; not recommended for profound
ITC	Mild through moderate	Moderate-to-severe; not recommended for severe or profound
CIC	Mild	Moderate; not recommended for severe or profound

User Preference

Probably as important as the magnitude and configuration of the hearing loss in selecting a hearing-aid style is the preference of the user. The audiologist will talk with the patient, and carefully consider his or her preferences and prejudices concerning hearing-aid styles. If user preferences are not considered, the hearing aid may not be used. For example, if an audiologist provided someone with a BTE, and the individual turned out to be too self-conscious to wear it, than the BTE probably was an inappropriate selection on the audiologist's part.

Costs

A closely related issue to preference is cost. CICs and digital hearing aids are the most expensive hearing aids. It is important to explore an individual's financial resources to purchase certain hearing-aid styles early on in the selection process. Those styles that are deemed too expensive then cannot be considered further.

Lifestyle

Lifestyle is also an important factor to consider during the selection process. For instance, a physician or nurse who often uses a stethoscope, and does not want to use one with a built-in-amplifier, may best be served by a CIC, because this style can be used with a stethoscope. A person who uses the telephone for a good part of the working day may opt for a BTE that has a powerful telecoil circuitry.

Physical Status

Physical status is an important consideration when selecting a hearing-aid style. Physical status includes an individual's manual dexterity and the condition of the ear. It is important to assess a person's gross and fine motor skills and to evaluate how well the individual can move his or her hands, fingers, and arms. Both fine and gross motor skills are necessary for putting on and taking off a hearing aid. In addition, fine motor control is necessary for manipulating the controls, changing batteries, and for inserting and removing the hearing aid from the ear. If a person has poor skills, it might be best to consider a BTE, a body aid, or an assistive listening device such as a hand-held amplifier. We will revisit this issue of manual dexterity in Chapter 12, when we consider older adults.

An examination of the ear will indicate whether an individual has chronic ear infections or a deformity in the ear canal. Children often have chronic otitis media. If an ITE is prescribed, secretions might damage the device. Hence, this is one reason a BTE may be more appropriate. A deformed or nonexistent ear canal also may limit (or preclude) the use of certain styles of hearing aids.

In addition to the health of the ear and physical malformations, the curve of the ear canal may influence the selection of hearing-aid style. If the individual has a straight ear canal, without a bend, then he or she probably is not a good candidate for a CIC. The device will not stay in place. Similarly, if the individual has a shallow concha, an ITC aid may be difficult to keep in the ear.

Saturation sound pressure level (SSPL): The maximum sound pressure level that can be delivered by a hearing aid with its volume full-on.

Loudness discomfort level (LDL): the level at which sound is perceived to be uncomfortably loud.

Uncomfortable loudness level (UCL): the level at which sound is perceived to be uncomfortably loud; loudness discomfort level.

SSPL-90 curve: electroacoustic assessment of a hearing aid's maximum level of output signal, expressed as a frequency response curve to a 90 dB signal, with the hearing aid volume control set to full on.

Hearing-aid test box: an off-the-ear determination of SSPL-90 in which the hearing aid is connected to a 2-cc coupler to simulate the human ear canal, an input signal that sweeps across the frequencies at 90 dB SPL is input, and the aid's output is measured.

Gain/frequency response: the difference between the amplitude of the input signal and the amplitude of the output signal across frequencies.

Prescription procedures: Fitting hearing aids by using a formula to calculate the desired gain and frequency response.

Electroacoustic Properties

In addition to selecting a hearing-aid style, certain decisions must be made concerning the electroacoustic properties of the hearing aid. These properties affect how the hearing aid processes the audio signal. These properties include saturation sound pressure level and gain/ frequency response:

■ *Saturation sound pressure level (SSPL)*: This term refers to the maximum sound pressure level that can be delivered to the ear, when the volume control is turned full on and the input signal is 90 dB SPL. This value is determined in order to ensure that the hearing aid's maximum power does not exceed the user's *loudness discomfort level (LDL)*, also called *uncomfortable loudness level (UCL)*. The LDL is the threshold at which sound becomes so loud that the hearing-aid user cannot tolerate it, even for a brief exposure. An *SSPL-90 curve* is obtained by measuring the hearing aid's output in a hearing aid test chamber called a *hearing-aid test box*. The hearing aid is connected to a 2-cc coupler that simulates the human external ear canal volume. An input signal then is presented that sweeps across frequencies, at 90 dB SPL. The output of the hearing aid is measured.

■ *Gain/frequency response*: The difference between the amplitude of the input signal and the amplitude of the output signal across frequencies is referred to as the gain/frequency response of a hearing aid. Typically, a hearing aid for an individual is adjusted to deliver the greatest amount of gain for those frequencies for which the individual has the poorest thresholds.

Selecting the Hearing Aid and Assessing Benefits

Selection of hearing aids typically are based on the audiogram, which indicates the degree of hearing loss and the configuration. Sometimes, a formula for gain is applied (e.g., Bryne & Dillon, 1986), which is a formula used to compute the desired amount of amplification at each frequency. This strategy is referred to as *prescription procedures*.

Two objective procedures also may be used to assess benefit. The first is the use of a speech recognition task (see Chapter 5). Patients take a speech recognition test with and without their hearing aid, and amount of improvement in percent words correct on their performance is computed. The second procedure involves *probe microphone technology*. A small flexible tube is inserted into the ear canal and positioned near the eardrum. The tube connects to a microphone, which records the decibels of power delivered by the hearing aid at the end of the ear canal. These measures are called *real-ear measures*. Although these measures do not indicate how well an individual can hear when wearing the hearing aid, results indicate whether the prescribed gain at each frequency, also called the *target gain*, is being delivered by the hearing aid.

A subjective procedure to assess hearing-aid benefit is the use of a questionnaire or an inventory. The patient may complete a checklist about what he or she can or cannot hear with the hearing aid, and may indicate satisfaction with the device. We will revisit the use of questionnaires for this purpose in Chapter 11.

Probe microphone: a microphone transducer that is inserted in the external ear canal for the purpose of measuring sound near the tympanic membrane.

Real-ear measures: use of a probe microphone to measure hearing aid gain and frequency response delivered by a hearing aid at the tympanic membrane.

Target gain: the gain prescribed for each frequency of a hearing aid, against which the actual hearing aid output is compared.

Hearing-Aid Orientation

Once the audiologist receives the prescribed hearing aid from the manufacturer, the patient returns to the clinic to be fitted with the device. At this time, benefit also is assessed, and the patient receives a *hearing-aid orientation*. The hearing-aid orientation includes the following services:

■ The audiologist describes the function of each part of the hearing aid, and ensures that the patient can adjust any controls.
■ The patient practices inserting and removing the hearing aid, and inserting and removing batteries from the hearing-aid battery compartment.
■ The audiologist reviews the limitations of amplification, and why the particular hearing aid was selected.
■ The patient and audiologist determine an appropriate use-pattern for the first few weeks of using the new hearing aid.
■ The patient learns how to trouble-shoot the device.
■ The patient receives printed information about the hearing aid and warranty.

Hearing aid orientation (HAO) is the process of instructing a patient (and a family member) to handle, use, and maintain a new hearing aid.

COCHLEAR IMPLANTS

Not all hard-of-hearing individuals have the potential to benefit from using a hearing aid. For instance, someone who has little, if any, residual hearing will probably never recognize the audio speech signal, no matter how it is processed nor how much it is amplified. Another intervention available besides a hearing aid is the cochlear implant. Cochlear implants, virtually unheard of 30 years ago, are now commonplace.

A Brief History

Although cochlear implants are a relatively new development, scientists have long been tantalized by the idea of providing sound sensation by means of electrical stimulation. One of the first recorded attempts in history to stimulate the ear electrically occurred in 1790, when Volta inserted metal rods into each of his ears. The rods were connected to 30 or 40 of his newly invented electrolytic cells. With one deft move, Volta delivered approximately 50 volts to himself. The results were staggering. He perceived a sensation similar to "a blow to the head," followed by "a sound like the boiling of a viscous liquid" (Luxford & Brackmann, 1985, p. 1). The experiment was not repeated.

The more recent history of cochlear implants hails back to 1957, when two French surgeons stimulated a deaf adult by placing an electrode directly on his auditory nerve (Djurno & Eyries, 1957). The patient reported hearing a sound like "crickets chirping," or "a roulette wheel spinning" (Luxford & Brackmann, 1985). Reports of this work filtered to the medical communities in the United States and Australia. Shortly thereafter, in the 1960s and 1970s, much activity was aimed toward the development of wearable devices. Names often associated with this work are Dr. William House of Los Angeles, California and Dr. Graham Clarke of Melbourne, Australia.

By the 1980s there was widespread use of cochlear implants among adults, and they were in exploratory use with children. The Food and Drug Administration (FDA) approved multi-channel cochlear implants in 1990 for children, and now cochlear implants are considered as a treatment option for both adults and children who have profound hearing loss. Increasingly, individuals who have severe hearing loss also are considered as candidates for implantation.

The primary candidacy requirements for implantation are the presence of irreversible severe or profound sensorineural hearing loss and good general health. As we shall learn in Chapter 17, children usually are at least 2 years of age before receiving a cochlear implant, although in February, 1998, the FDA approved the Cochlear Corporation cochlear implant for implantation in children who are as young as 18 months of age. In Australia, infants may be as young as 6 months of age at the time of implantation (Clark, 1997). Adults can be of any age, even in the eighth or ninth decade of life (Spitzer, 1997).

Overview

Cochlear implants are comprised of internal and external components (Figure 6–7). The internal components are implanted in the skull, in close proximity to the inner ear. The *internal components* typically include an internal receiver, which is placed on the mastoid bone, and an electrode array, which is inserted into the cochlea. These components are not visible after implantation, but are covered by skin and hair. The user may have a small incision scar and a slight convex protrusion behind the pinna.

In a cochlear implant, the **internal components** are implanted within the skull.

The external components include a microphone, connecting cables, a speech processor, and a transmitter. The microphone and transmitter typically are worn behind the ear, and the speech processor often is worn on the chest, similar to a body hearing aid. However, some newer cochlear implants have speech processors that can be worn behind the ear, like a BTE (Clar, Cowan, & Dowell, 1997). Figure 6–8 presents a picture of a young student who recently received a cochlear implant.

The microphone of a cochlear implant picks up sound from the environment, converts it to an electrical signal, and then

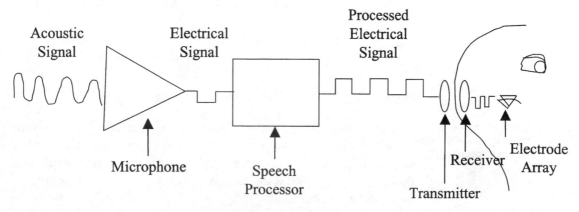

Figure 6–7. Schematic of a cochlear implant.

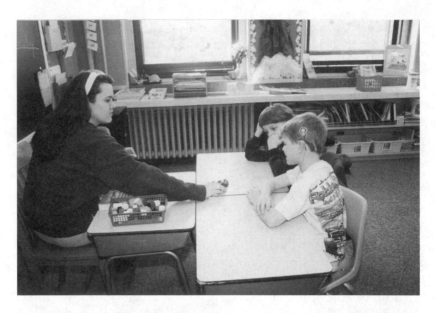

Figure 6-8. A young boy wearing a cochlear implant. The microphone is worn behind his ear like a behind-the-ear hearing aid. The external transmitter is held against his head by magnetic induction. This child has only been using the device for a short time, and his scar from surgery is still visible, near the base of his skull. (Photograph by Kim Readmond, Central Institute for the Deaf)

Speech processor: the component of a cochlear implant where the input signal is modified for presentation to the electrodes in the electrode array.

delivers it via connecting cables to the speech processor. The *speech processor*, as the name implies, processes the signal. Each cochlear-implant design utilizes a speech processing strategy, or algorithm, for determining how the signal is processed. The signal may be digitized, filtered, and then segmented, so that different components of the signal are presented to different electrodes in the electrode array.

The processed electrical signal leaves the speech processor and then is delivered to the electrode array, via a transmitter and an internal receiver. The transmitter often is worn outside of the head and delivers the signal to an internal receiver. The transmitter may be held in place by a magnet. From the internal receiver, the electrical signal passes on to the electrode array.

Electrode array: inserted into the cochlea, a wire that carries the implant's electrode pairs.

The *electrode array* is a small wire, inserted into the cochlea, usually through the round window. The electrode array carries electrode pairs. The electrode pairs, which are tiny exposed balls or rings on the wire, are comprised of positive and negative polarity contacts, between which passes current. The current stimulates the fibers of the auditory nerve.

Most cochlear implants in use in the United States today are *multichannel* devices. This means that the electrode pairs in the electrode array present different information to different regions of the cochlea. In the normal ear, different frequencies of the auditory signal excite different neurons along the cochlea. The goal of a multichannel system is to simulate the normal cochlea and present high-frequency components of the signal to the basal end of the cochlea and low-frequency components of the signal to the apical end.

Multichannel: more than one channel. Often used to describe cochlear implants that present different channels of information to different parts of the cochlea.

Although there are some variations in the processing strategies used by different models of cochlear implants, many current cochlear implants utilize an *interleaved pulsatile stimulation* algorithm. In this design, each electrode pair in the electrode array is designated to represent different frequency bands. The audio signal is processed and delivered to the electrode array by spreading pulses, in a nonsimultaneous manner (hence, they are interleaved) across the electrode pairs, from high to low or from low to high frequencies.

Interleaved pulsatile stimulation: a cochlear implant processing strategy in which trains of pulses are delivered across electrodes in the electrode array in a nonsimultaneous fashion.

ASSISTIVE LISTENING DEVICES (ALDS)

Hearing aids and cochlear implants are listening devices that may be worn during almost all working hours, and in almost all communication settings. ALDs usually are used in specific situations, such as when listening in a public hall or conversing in a restaurant when other kinds of listening devices are either inadequate to permit good communication or are not desirable to the patient (Table 6–3). Compton (1995) suggested that ALDs should address one or more of four communication needs. The four basic communication needs for most people include: (1) face-to-face communication, (2) broadcast and other electronic media, (3) telephone conversations, and (4) sensitivity to alerting signals and to their environmental signals. In selecting ALDs for a particular individual, you will want to consider the person's communication demands in the home, community, and/or school environments. Table 6–4 presents a list of situations in each of these settings in which use of an ALD may be appropriate (Compton, 1995). The Key Resources section lists sources for obtaining ALDs.

ALDs are especially useful when the audio signal is presented at a distance or when the listening conditions are less than ideal. In such conditions, a hearing aid or cochlear implant may

Table 6–3. Situations in which a person may use an assistive device.

Kind of Communication	Possible Situations or Purposes
Live, face-to-face	Restaurants, meetings, places of worship, concerts, lectures, automobile, courtroom, classroom
Broadcast or recorded media	Radio, television, movie theaters, dictation machines
Telecommunications	Telephones, intercoms
Environment	Doorbells, smoke detectors, telephone rings, appliance timers, babies' cries, children's voices, alarm clocks

Table 6-4. Situations in which use of an assistive device might be appropriate.

Home

    One-on-one conversation
    Group conversation
    Television reception
    Radio reception
    Reception of environmental signals such as the door bell

Community

    Medical treatment (visiting a physician, dentist, hospital)
    Working
        Office conversation
        Lectures
        Telephone communication
        Conferences and group meetings
        One-on-one meetings
    Traveling and recreation
        One-on-one conversation
        Conversation in the car
        Television reception
        Reception of warning signals
    Restaurants
    Public spaces

School

    Communication with the teacher
    Communication with classmates
    Speech-language therapy

not be adequate to maximize an individual's listening potential. Because the microphone of a hearing aid or cochlear implant is at the level of the individual's ear, it may not pick up sound emanating from a distant source and/or may deliver not only the desired audio signal, but also any competing background noise to the listener.

Conditions that might compromise a listening environment, and where an ALD may be especially helpful, include the following (Flexor, 1997):

■ *Ambient noise*: noise that is present in a room when it is unoccupied. This noise may emanate from open windows, air handling systems, computers, fluorescent lighting systems, or piped-in music.

■ *Reverberation*: echoes caused by sound rebounding off surfaces such as walls, floors, and ceilings. Rooms that have high ceilings, hardwood floors, and plaster walls tend to be highly reverberant, whereas those that have carpet and heavy draperies tend to have less reverberation.

■ *Background noise*: is undesirable noise that masks the auditory signal of interest. For instance, in a classroom, the teacher's voice may be the target signal, and the rattling of paper and the shuffling of feet might be undesirable background noise.

Ambient noise: noise in a listening environment.

Reverberation: prolongation of an auditory signal by multiple reflections in a closed environment, the amount of echo in a closed space.

Background noise: extraneous noise in an environment that masks the signal of interest.

In principle, ALDs work by collecting sound from the sound source (e.g., the talker's mouth) and delivering it to the user's ear. In this way, the audio signal is presented at an audible level, with a favorable signal-to-noise ratio, with minimal ambient noise, without the effects of reverberation, and with little background noise. ALDs can be categorized as one of two kinds: wireless and hardwired (Figure 6–9).

Wireless Systems

As the name implies, a wireless system does not use wire between the microphone and the unit that delivers the signal to the user's ear. Sound is transmitted from the sound source to the individual by means of radio waves or infrared signals. These kinds of systems may be used when the individual is far from the sound source, for example, in a religious service or when attending a theater play. A wireless system picks up the audio signal, either through a microphone placed near the

No ALD

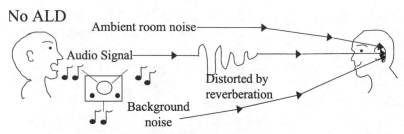

ALD, sound picked up through a microphone

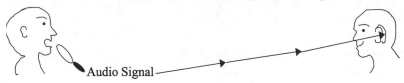

ALD, sound picked up by direct audio input (DAI)

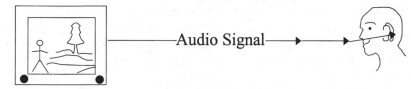

Figure 6–9. Schematic of an assitive listening device. In the top third of the figure, no assistive listening device is used, and the signal is distorted by reverberation and masked by background noise. In the center and bottom of the figure, sound is relayed from the source to the listener by means of an assistive listening device. In the center of the figure, sound is picked up through a microphone, whereas in the bottom of the figure, sound is picked up by direct audio input.

Direct audio input (DAI): a hard-wired connection that leads directly from the sound source to the hearing aid or other listening device.

sound source or by means of a direct electrical plug-in. The sound is then converted into an electrical signal by a transmitter and delivered through the air to a receiver worn by the user, either by means of radio waves or infrared (invisible light). The signal may be delivered to the ear either via earphones or through the individual's hearing aid, if it is a body aid or a BTE. Delivery through the hearing aid is accomplished in one of three ways: by means of a *direct audio input (DAI)* to the individual's hearing aid, by use of the hearing aid's telecoil circuitry, or by use of the hearing-aid's microphone.

FM Systems

Wireless systems can be further classified as FM, infrared, induction loop, or simple amplification. *FM (frequency modulation) systems* utilize radio waves to transmit sound from the source to the user.

FM systems are commonly used in classroom settings, and may be described either as a personal FM trainer or a sound-field FM system. When using a *personal FM trainer*, the teacher wears a wireless microphone (Figure 6–10), usually on a cord around her neck or clipped onto her shirt. The teacher's speech is frequency modulated on radio frequency carrier waves and transmitted through the classroom to the child, who wears a receiver. Often, the receiver connects to the child's hearing aid by a cord. If there is more than one hard-of-hearing child in the classroom, then each child wears a receiver and may receive the teacher's signal.

Personal FM trainer: a listening device in which the speaker wears a wireless microphone and the speech is frequency modulated on radio waves transmitted through the room to the listener who wears a receiver.

A sound-field FM system operates similarly to a personal FM trainer. A *soundfield FM system* differs from the personal system because the sound is transmitted to loudspeakers that are positioned throughout the room, usually two in the back of the room and one near the front. There, the signal is converted to an audio signal and played into the environment, as with a standard public address system. A child's personal hearing-aid microphone picks up the signal. Whereas a personal FM trainer offers better signal-to-noise ratios, the sound-field system is advantageous because it can be beneficial for an entire class,

Soundfield FM system: a listening system, similar to the FM trainer, in which sound from a microphone is transmitted to loudspeakers that are positioned throughout the room.

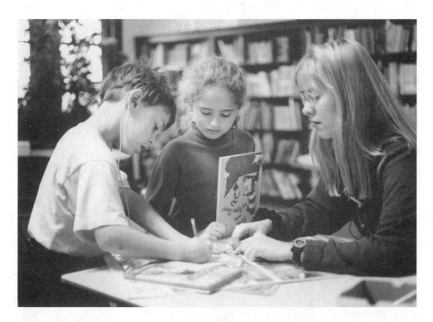

Figure 6–10. A teacher wearing a personal FM trainer microphone clipped to her sweater. The young boy wears an FM receiver that has a hard-wired connection to his behind-the-ear hearing aid. (Photograph by Kim Readmond, Central Institute for the Deaf)

even for those children who do not have a hearing loss, who may have a fluctuating conductive hearing loss, who use a cochlear implant, or who have a unilateral hearing loss (Flexor, 1997). FM sound-field systems also do not require a hard-of-hearing child to wear a special FM receiver. Hence, the child wears less hardware.

Other situations in which FM systems may be used besides the classroom setting include group lectures, one-on-one communication situations, and in the car.

Infrared systems

Infrared system: an assistive listening device that broadcasts from the sound source to a receiver/amplifier by means of infrared light waves.

Infrared systems operate similarly to FM units, but use infrared signals to transmit sound. A transmitter/emitter sends the signal encoded in infrared light waves to a wireless receiver, which contains a photo detector diode. A photo detector diode picks up the infrared signal and converts it back to the audio signal. An individual may either wear an infrared receiver that inputs directly into the ears, or may receive the signal through a DAI or by activating the hearing-aid telecoil switch. Common situations in which infrared systems are used include television watching and movie theaters. Infrared systems are not appropriate for outdoors, as sunlight interferes with transmission. The infrared signals also cannot travel through walls.

Induction Loop Systems

Induction loop systems: a system that works by running a wire around the circumference of a room or table that conducts electrical energy from an amplfier and thus creates a magnetic field, which induces the telecoil in a hearing aid to provided amplified sound to the user.

The third kind of wireless system is the induction loop system. For an *induction loop system* to operate, a loop of wire must be placed around the circumference of a room. Sound is pick up by means of a microphone or a direct input (e.g., a television direct connection). Sound is converted into electrical signals, and fed through the loop. Electromagnetic energy is broadcast throughout the room and can be picked up by a hearing aid when the telecoil circuit is activated. The listener must sit either inside of the loop of wire or beside it. Some religious settings, classrooms, and theaters have permanent loop systems in place. There are portable induction loop systems so that any room can be optimized for communication. A variation of the large area loop system is the *neckloop*, which is a wire that can be worn around the neck.

Simple Amplification

Simple amplification systems merely amplify the audio signal so that it may be more audible to the person with hearing loss. The most common implementation of simple amplification systems is in telephones. *Telephone amplifiers* either replace the telephone handset or clip onto existing handsets. Replacement handsets have built-in amplifiers, so that the signal is amplified before it is delivered to the user's ear. Often, these kinds of handsets have volume controls; therefore, they may also be used by persons who have normal hearing.

Simple amplification systems merely amplify the audio signal so that it is more audible to a person with hearing loss.

Telephone amplifiers amplify sound from a telephone receiver.

Hardwired Systems

The other kind of assistive listening device can be described as hardwired. *Hardwired assistive listening devices* connect the sound source to the listener by actual wire. A microphone may pick up the audio signal (Figure 6–11) or there may be a DAI jack that plugs into a piece of equipment, such as a television. The audio signal is converted into an electrical signal. It travels through the connecting wire, terminating at the user's hearing aid, headphones, or a neckloop. This system provides a favorable signal-to-noise ratio to the user and, usually, an adjustable amount of signal amplification. These kinds of systems are used most often for listening to television, radio, or music. However, such systems are not widely used because they require the user to be tethered to the sound source.

Hardwired assistive listening devices: devices that are directly connected by wires.

I Need to Make a Call

In addition to using a telephone amplifier, hard-of-hearing individuals have at least two other options available for using the telephone. These options include the following:

Text telephones (TTs): A telephone terminal comprised of a telephone, a keyboard, and a message display screen. The telephone handset fits into the terminal cradle. Both parties must have a terminal set. They communicate by

(continued)

Text telephones consist of a telephone, a keyboard, and a message display screen. The telephone handset fits into the terminal cradle. Both parties communicate by typing their messages.

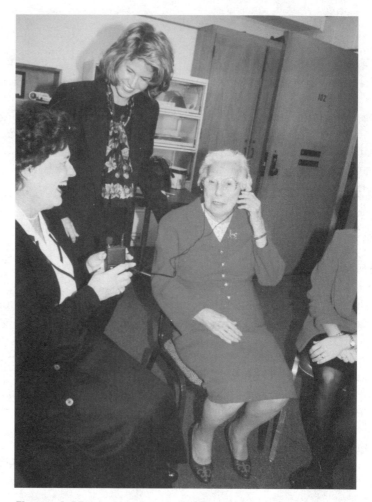

Figure 6-11. A woman and her daughter are learning to use a hard-wired assistive listening device, while a clinician (standing) provides encouragement. The daughter speaks into a microphone, while the woman listens through headphones. This kind of assistive listening device is often used in automobiles and restaurants. (Photograph by Kim Readmond, Central Institute for the Deaf)

Relay system: used by persons with significant hearing loss to use the telephone; individual contacts a relay operator who serves to transmit messages between the caller and person called by means of teletype and/or voice.

typing their messages to one another. The messages are displayed on the message display screen. TTs are sometimes referred to as telecommunication devices for the Deaf (TDDs).

Relay systems: All states provide relay systems as a service for their hard-of-hearing residents. A trained operator serves as an intermediary in a telephone conversation. The hard-of-hearing person communicates with the operator via a TT (and possibly voice), while the normally-hearing person communicates with the operator via voice. To place a call, the initiator contacts a relay operator, who in turn contacts the recipient of the call.

Other Kinds of Assistive Devices

Other assistive devices are available that cannot be classified as wireless or hardwired assistive listening devices per se. These devices are those that allow access to the environment and communication through modalities other than hearing. One of the most commonly used examples of assistive devices include television *closed-captioning* devices, which provide a written text to match the spoken words on a television program. Another example is a vibratory pager, which allows individuals to receive pages. Instead of emitting auditory beeps, a *vibratory pager* vibrates against the user to signal a call. Other examples include:

■ Vibrating alarm clocks, where a vibrator might be placed under the user's pillow.

■ Flashing alarm clocks, where a flashing lamp or strobe light might signal the alarm.

■ A doorbell signal coupled to a lamp, which flashes when the doorbell is rung.

■ A smoke detector, where light flashes signal the presence of smoke.

■ A baby cry alert systems, where a parent can be signaled if a baby begins to cry in another room.

FINAL REMARKS

In this chapter, we have reviewed some of the fundamental aspects of the most widely used technology in aural rehabilitation. We concentrated on hearing aids, cochlear implants, and assistive listening devices. There is one other kind of listening device available for individuals who for some reason cannot use a hearing aid or cochlear implant, and who are not well-served by assistive listening devices. This device is a tactile aid.

Tactile aids permit sound awareness by delivering vibrotactile sensation to the user's skin. Most devices look like a body aid, but instead of having a long cord leading to an earmold, they have a cord leading to a vibrotactile or electrotactile array.

Closed-set captioning: Printed text or dialog that corresponds to the auditory speech signal from a television program or movie.

Vibratory pagers: instead of emitting audible beeps the pager vibrates against the user to signal a call.

Tactile aids: aids that transduce sound to vibration and deliver it to the skin for the purpose of gross sound awareness and gross sound identification.

These arrays may be placed against the chest or strapped to the wrist. When sound occurs in the environment, the device microphone picks it up. The signal is transduced into an electrical signal and then delivered to the vibrotactile or electrotactile array, where the skin is stimulated. Some of the more sophisticated devices present a spectral display to the skin, and thus may provide some information about the spectral characteristics of the signal. These devices serve primarily as a supplement to lipreading, and rarely permit the user to recognize speech without the visual signal. With the advent of cochlear implants, they are not used by many people today.

KEY CHAPTER POINTS

✔ The objectives for providing an individual with a listening device are to make speech audible, without introducing distortion or discomfort, and to restore a range of loudness experience.
✔ Hearing aids, cochlear implants, and assistive listening devices are the primary listening devices available to hard-of-hearing persons. Tactile aids are used by a small number of people, primarily those who cannot benefit from the more commonly used devices.
✔ Two major trends in modern hearing-aid design are miniaturization and enhanced signal processing.
✔ Hearing aids have three fundamental components: a microphone, an amplifier, and a receiver. They also have a power source. Microphones may be directional or omnidirectional. Amplifiers may use peak-clipping for output limiting or compression.
✔ There are six general styles of hearing aids. Selection of style is dependent on the degree of hearing loss, user preference, costs, patient lifestyle, and the patient's physical status.
✔ Cochlear implants provide sound sensation by means of directly stimulating the auditory nerve. Candidacy requirements for implantation include the presence of irreversible severe or profound sensorineural hearing loss and good general health. Children usually must be at least 2 years of age.
✔ Most hearing aids in use today in the United States are multichannel devices and utilize an interleaved pulsatile stimulation algorithm.
✔ Assistive listening devices are used to address communication needs related to face-to-face communiction, broadcast and other electronic media, telephone use, and sensitivity to environmental signals and stimuli. General categories of devices are wireless and hardwired.

KEY RESOURCES

Sources for Assistive Listening Devices.

American Loop Systems
43 Davis Road, Suite 2
Belmont, MA 02178

Audio Enhancement
12613 South Redwood Road
Riverton, UT 84065

AT&T National Special Needs Center
2001 Route 46
Parsippany, NJ 07054

Audiometrics
5145 Avenida Encinitas, Suite B
Carlsbad, CA 92008

Centrum Sound
215809 Stevens Creek Blvd.,
Suite 209
Cupertino, CA 95014

Custom All Hear Systems
20833 67th Ave. West, Suite 101
Lynnwood, WA 98036

Dahlberg, Inc.
4101 Dahlberg Drive
Golden Valley, MN 55422

Hear You Are
4 Musconetong Ave.
Stanhope, NJ 07874

Hal-Hen
P.O. Box 6077
Long Island City, NY 11106

Hearing Aid Center (HAC) of America
HARC Mercantile LTD.
3130 Portage Rd.
P.O. Box 3055
Kalamazoo, MI

Hi-Tec Group International
801 N. Cass Avenue #021
Westmont, IL 60559

Lifeline Amplification Systems
55 South 4th Street
Platteville, WI 53818

Phonic Ear, Inc.
3880 Cypress Drive
Petaluma, CA 94954-7600

Precision Controls, Inc.
14 Doty Road
Haskell, NJ 07420

Quest Electronics
510 South Worthington St.
Oconomowoc, WI 53066

Radio Shack
Fort Worth, TX 76102

Silent Call Corporation
P.O. Box 16348
Clarksont, MI 48016

Sonic Alert
209 Voorheis
Pontiac, MI 48053

Telex Communications, Inc.
9600 Aldrich Avenue South
Minneapolis, MN 55420

Ultratec, Inc.
6442 Normandy Lange
Madison, WI 53719

Wheelock, Inc.
273 Branchport Ave.
Long Branch, NJ 07740

7

Auditory Training

Topics

- Candidacy for Auditory Training
- Four Design Principles
- Developing Analytic Training Objectives
- Developing Synthetic Training Objectives
- Formal and Informal Auditory Training

- Interweaving Auditory Training with Other Components of Aural Rehabilitation
- Benefits of Auditory Training
- Final Remarks
- Key Chapter Points
- Key Resources

The goal of auditory training for persons who have hearing loss is to develop their ability to recognize speech using the auditory signal and to interpret auditory experiences. Training helps them use their residual hearing to their maximum capability. During formal auditory training, you probably will not encourage individuals to watch your mouth movements as you speak. In fact, you may obscure your mouth, either by covering it or by sitting out of view (Figure 7–1).

Persons should be fitted with appropriate amplification before starting an auditory training program. A hearing aid (or cochlear implant) makes some speech sounds more audible. Auditory training will not change hearing sensitivity, but will enhance a person's ability to utilize whatever sound is available. By ensuring that individuals have the best amplification system possible, you will increase the raw material they have to work with and enhance their potential to benefit from training.

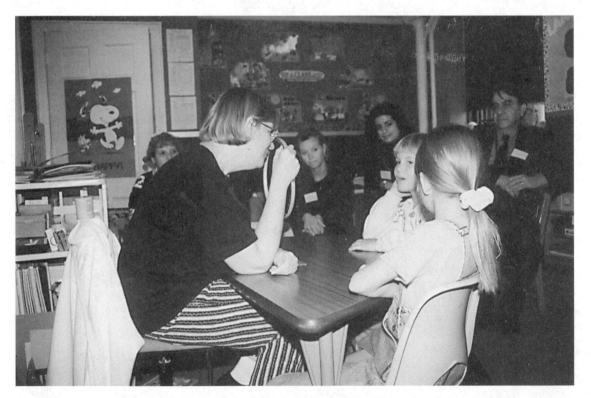

Figure 7-1. Formal auditory training. During a typical auditory training exercise, a teacher may cover her mouth movements with a mesh screen held within an embroidery hoop. The teacher does not use her hand because this would attenuate the level of her speech (Nidday & Elfenbein, 1991). (Photograph by Kim Readmond, Central Institute for the Deaf)

Historical Notes

The procedures and techniques we use to provide auditory training have evolved gradually over time. Pollack (1970) notes that the value of using residual hearing has long been realized. Archigenes in the 1st century and Alexander in the 6th century both were know to hold ear trumpets to their ear in order to intensify the speech signal. Reports of analytic training exercises date back to as early as 1791, when Ernaud designed analytic exercises for his deaf pupils. In 1805, Jean Marc Gaspard Itard, at the Paris Institute for the Deaf, provided drill training to children, asking them to discriminate one spoken utterance from another using only their residual hearing. Toynbee noted in 1860 that deaf individuals could learn to attend to their muted voices for the purposes of modulating speech production.

A seminal event in the history of auditory training in the United States occurred when Dr. Max Goldstein left his native St. Louis in 1893 to study with Dr. Adam Politzer, an otologist, and Professor Victor Urbantschitsch, an educator of the deaf, for 2 years in Vienna. Dr. Goldstein returned to St. Louis, convinced that children with significant hearing losses could learn to talk and to listen. He founded the Central Institute for the Deaf and promoted auditory and speech training for deaf children both nationally and internationally.

Rapid advances in technology during the 20th century have increased the potential importance of residual hearing. After World War II, personal hearing aids became more effective and smaller in size so that they could actually be worn throughout the day. At this time, auditory training became a meaningful component of aural rehabilitation for a large segment of the hard-of-hearing and deaf populations. Clarence Hudgins worked with children at Clarke School for the Deaf in Northampton and conducted research that ultimately demonstrated that children who received amplification could increase their speech recognition through listening training (Erber, 1982). Raymond Carhart (Carhart, 1960) developed auditory training procedures for veterans returning from World War II; many of whom had incurred noise-induced hearing losses from weapons exposure.

The advent of cochlear implants in the latter part of the 20th century has led to an explosion in the development of auditory training materials and methods. Computers and training packages founded on sound theoretical underpinnings (Moog, Biedenstein, & Davidson, 1995; Stout & Wendle, 1992) have changed the complexion of auditory training.

CANDIDACY FOR AUDITORY TRAINING

Auditory training typically is provided to children who either incurred a hearing loss before acquiring speech and language (i.e., children who are prelingually deafened) or who incurred their hearing loss afterwards (i.e., children who are postlingually deafened). Children who have prelingual and profound losses may have no memory of how speech sounds and may have limited language skills and world knowledge. Thus, they cannot draw on memories of how speech should sound nor utilize acquired knowledge for interpreting the degraded auditory signal. During auditory training, these children first must learn to attend to the auditory speech signal, and eventually must learn to relate the auditory signal to their vocabulary.

Children who have more hearing, or children who lost their hearing after acquiring some speech and language, often have a larger vocabulary and greater familiarity with grammar and may be better able to deduce meaning from the auditory speech signal, at least initially. The presence of more residual hearing, especially for the mid and high frequencies, portends good progress in auditory skill development. These children will probably begin with more difficult tasks than children who have prelingual, profound hearing losses.

It is less common for adults to receive auditory training. Adults who receive training typically are those who have experienced a recent change in hearing status. For example, someone who has just received a cochlear implant may receive auditory training to accelerate the learning process that often occurs during the first months following implantation (Figure 7–2). Someone who has incurred hearing loss following trauma or use of ototoxic drugs may receive training in order to adjust to his or her radically altered listening state. Speech through a listening device may sound different from how they remember it, and they must learn to interpret what they hear.

FOUR DESIGN PRINCIPLES

Many auditory training curricula are organized according to four design principles (Table 7–1). These four design principles are followed in developing and ordering training objectives. You may note that, in some ways, the principles we will review in this chapter parallel the considerations for assessing speech recognition that we reviewed in Chapter 5.

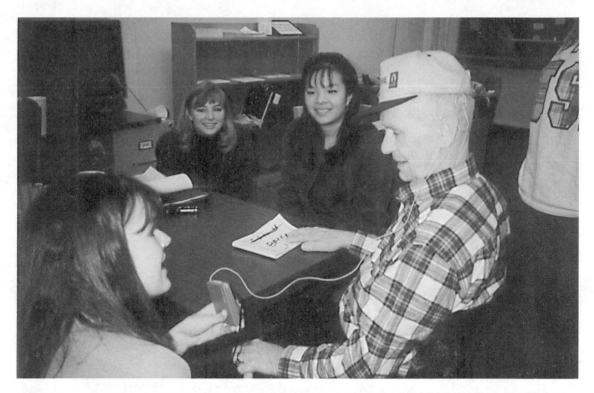

Figure 7-2. Auditory training for adults. Adults who may benefit from auditory training are those who have recently received a cochlear implant. (Photograph by Kim Readmond, Central Institute for the Deaf)

Table 7-1. Four design principles by which activities in an auditory training curriculum may be developed and organized.

A. Auditory Skill	**D. Difficulty Level**
Sound Awareness	Response Set
Sound Discrimination	closed
Identification	limited
Comprehension	open
	Stimulus Unit
	words
B. Stimuli	phrases
Phonetic-level	sentences
Sentence-level	Stimulus Similarity
	Contextual Support
	Task Structure
C. Activity Type	highly structured
	spontaneous
Formal	Listening Conditions
Informal	

Auditory Skill Level

The first consideration in designing an auditory training curriculum pertains to the person's hearing abilities. Results from an audiological assessment often are used to assign a student to one of four auditory skill levels (Erber, 1982):

■ Sound awareness
■ Sound discrimination
■ Identification
■ Comprehension

As Figure 7–3 indicates, these levels are not discrete benchmarks in auditory development but, rather, represent a continuum of skills. A person may be able to perform some activities associated with a sound discrimination level and some activities associated with identification at about the same time. In this section, we will consider the four stages through use of a case study. Table 7–2 presents auditory training activities that may be appropriate for each stage.

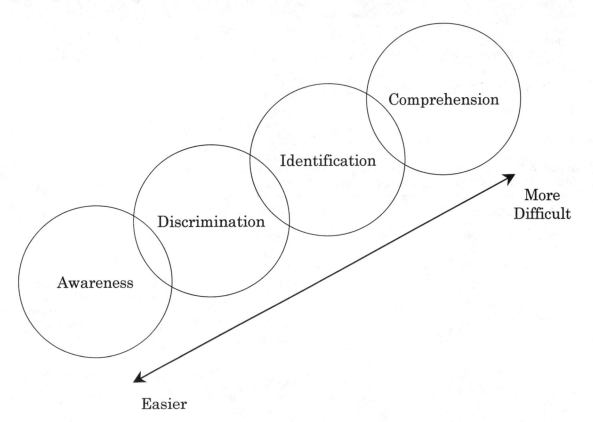

Figure 7-3. Four levels of auditory skill development. Auditory skill levels do not represent discrete benchmarks.

Table 7-2. Auditory training activities that are appropriate for each stage of auditory skill development (for children).

Sound Awareness

Play Peek-a-boo.
Play musical chairs.
March to the beat of a drum.
Push the toy car whenever the clinician says "Vrrrrm."

Sound Discrimination

Play game with toy animals ("The cow says 'moo', the sheep says 'baaa'").
Respond to the command ("Give me a crayon"/"Draw").
Play same or different game ("boy boy" "toy boy").
Repeat what you hear ("ma ma ma"/"pa pa pa").

Identification

Play the game Candyland and listen for the names of the colors.
Play with sets of postcards or stickers ("Show me the cat").
Play 'o Fish' with cards ("Give me your sevens"; "Give me your twos.").

Comprehension

Listen to a read-aloud story.
Play *I Spy*.
Play *20 Questions*.

Elizabeth Jenkins was born with a profound, bilateral hearing loss. Shortly after her fifth birthday, she received a cochlear implant. During the first few weeks of device use, Elizabeth did not respond spontaneously to sound. For instance, one night her father dropped a stack of plastic dinner plates near the room where Elizabeth was playing. Elizabeth did not turn around to see what had happened. When a telephone rang a few minutes later, she continued playing without a glance toward the sound source.

Several weeks elapsed before Elizabeth consistently demonstrated *sound awareness*, wherein she was aware when sound was present and when it was absent. Spontaneous response to sound began to occur once Elizabeth realized that sound has meaning, and that action often produces sound.

Sound awareness is the most basic auditory skill level, awareness of when a sound is present and when it is not.

Elizabeth entered the next auditory skill level, *sound discrimination*, during the latter part of her first year of cochlear implant use. Elizabeth now could recognize when two sounds were the same and when two sounds differed, although she could not necessarily associate meaning with the two sounds

Sound discrimination is a basic auditory skill level in which the listener is able to tell whether two sounds are different or the same.

or name them. For instance, she could indicate that an "Eeeeeeeeeeeeeee" spoken by her teacher was different from an "Eh."

Identification is a basic auditory skill level in which the listener is able to label some auditory stimuli.

After about 12 months of cochlear implant use, Elizabeth entered into the *identification* level of auditory skills development and began to label some auditory stimuli. If her mother asked for a blue crayon, she could pick the blue crayon from a box of four other crayons. This skill relates to an awareness that objects have names, and names have auditory representations. At the identification stage, there were some occasions when Elizabeth imitated someone's utterance, but did not comprehend what the utterance meant.

Comprehension is a higher auditory skill level in which the listener is able to understand the meaning of spoken messages.

More than 2 years elapsed before Elizabeth begin to demonstrate some of the listening behaviors associated with the *comprehension* level of auditory skill development, in which she understood the meaning of spoken messages. This stage requires not only advanced auditory skills but some knowledge of vocabulary and grammar as well. At this time, Elizabeth's mother could ask a question with her face not visible and expect that Elizabeth might answer it appropriately, especially if the question was supported by linguistic and environmental context.

Children with significant residual hearing and adults who have had normal hearing before incurring a hearing loss may not progress through these four stages of auditory skill development in the same way as Elizabeth did. For instance, an adult cochlear-implant user will be aware of the presence or absence of sound the first time that the device is turned on, and likely will have some speech discrimination skills (Dorman, 1993). A child who has some residual hearing, or who has incurred a hearing loss gradually over time, also will demonstrate more advanced listening skills.

DASL

Gayle Stout and Jill Van Ert Windle, authors of one of the most popular auditory training curricula for children in print (*The Developmental Approach to Successful Listening* II [DASL], 1992), have developed a placement test. This test determines whether a child should begin an auditory training program with sound awareness tasks or more advanced listening tasks. The following description summarize some initial items:

Sound Awareness

1. The tester beats a drum while standing behind the child. The child must raise a hand when he or she hears the beats. A child who consistently responds correctly is aware of the presence of low-frequency sound.

2. The tester speaks a syllable, /ba/, with mouth covered, and the child must indicate when the syllable is spoken. A child who responds to speech consistently is aware of speech in a structured listening setting.

3. The tester familiarizes the child with several different noise makers. The child must listen and indicate when the teacher sounds a noise maker and when the teacher stops the sound. This task taps into the ability of the child to detect the presence and absence of environmental sound stimuli.

Stimulus Units

The second design principle of many auditory training curricula, after a consideration of auditory skills level, pertains to the stimuli used in the training activities. Although a particular program might emphasize one more than the other, most auditory training curricula include both analytic and synthetic kinds of training activities (Figure 7–4).

During an analytic training activity, students' attention is focused on segments of the speech signal, such as syllables or phonemes. More emphasis is placed on utilizing acoustic cues, such as the presence or absence of voicing in the words *coat* and *goat* than on gaining meaning from the speech signal. Presumably, one's ability to recognize these segments in isolation will carry over to real-world communication tasks, allowing them to recognize connected discourse better.

During synthetic training, individuals learn to recognize the meaning of an utterance, even if they do not recognize every sound or word. They do not perform an analysis of the signal on a sound-by-sound or syllable-by-syllable basis.

Analytic 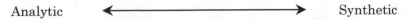 Synthetic

Figure 7–4. Analytic and synthetic training. The distinction between analytic and synthetic training activities is a continuum.

There is no clear dichotomy between analytic and synthetic training; rather, this is a continuum, and listening activities will gravitate from focusing attention on acoustic cue recognition to focusing attention on understanding the gist of a message. In the same lesson, a student might perform analytic training activities and then switch to synthetic activities.

Activity Kind

A third design principle by which many auditory training curricula organize component activities relates to the nature of the training activity (Table 7–1), whether it is more formal or informal. Formal kinds of training activities occur during designated times of the day, usually with a one-on-one lesson between clinician and student, or in a small group of students. *Formal training* activities often are highly structured and may involve drill. Students may receive reinforcements for performing a formal training task. For instance, a clinician may speak a series of words without letting the student watch. The student then repeats each word. After every successful repetition, the student drops a coin into a bank. In this example, the speaking of a series of words represents a drill activity. The collecting of coins represents a reinforcement activity.

An *informal training* activity occurs as part of the daily routine, and often is incorporated into other activities, such as conversation or academic learning. For instance, a wife may alert her husband when a horn honks or a bird sings after he receives a cochlear implant. She is using informal instruction to draw his attention toward sound, and to place names on particular sound patterns.

Except when students are very young, the optimal auditory training program includes both formal and informal training activities. Children who are very young should receive primarily informal training. Programs for adults tend to include more formal than informal activities.

Hierarchy of Listening Tasks

Warren Estabrooks (1994) presents an example of how training stimuli can be ordered to create a hierarchy of listening tasks, once the student (who, in his example, is a child) has reached the comprehension stage of listening. This hierarchy is listed below, beginning with the easier stimuli and ending with the more difficult stimuli.

- Familiar expressions/common phrases
- Single directions/two directions
- Classroom instructions
- Sequencing three directions
- Multielement directions
- Sequencing three events in a story
- Answering questions about a story: closed set and open set
- Comprehension activities/exercises in noisy environments
- Onomatopoeic words (p. 58).

Difficulty Level

The final design principle of the four listed in Table 7–1 in which training programs are organized relates to the level of difficulty inherent in the training activity. There are at least six ways to vary training difficulty, and to advance students from one skill level to the next (Figure 7–5).

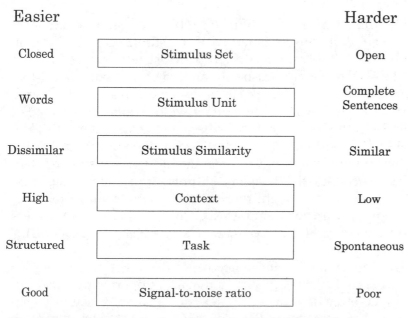

Easier		Harder
Closed	Stimulus Set	Open
Words	Stimulus Unit	Complete Sentences
Dissimilar	Stimulus Similarity	Similar
High	Context	Low
Structured	Task	Spontaneous
Good	Signal-to-noise ratio	Poor

Figure 7-5. Ways to vary the difficulty of the training task.

The first way to vary the level of difficulty is to vary the size of the stimuli set used for listening tasks. The size of the response set can be varied from a closed set, to a limited set, to an open set. As we noted in Chapter 5, a closed set means that the student is presented with a limited set of known choices. For example, a child might be ask to recognize numbers from a closed set consisting of the numerical digits *one, two, three,* and *four*. A *limited set* is one defined by situational or contextual cues. For example, the set may include words pertaining to Halloween, but the student is not briefed about the specific words that might occur during a training exercise. An open set has few inherent constraints; a wide assortment of words are possible as response choices. As a student progresses from closed to limited to open response sets, the listening task becomes more difficult.

A second way to modulate training difficulty is to vary the stimulus unit. A clinician might employ sentences rather than words and phrases. Students typically perform training activities with words or phrases more easily than with sentences. For instance, a student more likely will identify the word cat, from the response set of *cat-mouse-dog* than to identify the sentence, *That's a cat over there,* from the response set of, *That's a cat over there, That's a mouse over there,* and *That's a dog over there.* When using sentences as training stimuli, those with simple syntactic structure typically are more difficult to recognize than those with complex structure.

The third way to vary difficulty relates to stimulus similarity. The similarity or dissimilarity of the stimuli can be varied in order to alter training difficulty. Most teachers begin with stimuli that differ acoustically and, later, present stimuli that are similar. For instance, initially, when the two items in a training stimulus pair differ, they will be quite dissimilar. For instance, a clinician may say the three syllable phrase, "How are you?" and then the single syllable, "Hi." As an individual progresses through auditory training and acquires more listening experience, the items in a stimulus pair will become more similar. The pair might represent a voicing contrast (e.g., *bee* versus *pea*), a vowel contrast (e.g., *team* versus *Tim*), or a stress contrast (e.g., *MY dog went home* versus *My dog went HOME*).

The fourth way to influence difficulty level of training involves context. Speech stimuli that are supported by either linguistic or environmental context are relatively easy to recognize. For instance, *I had Wheaties for breakfast* is easier to

A **limited set** of stimuli is defined by situational or contextual cues.

recognize if the talker is standing in the kitchen holding a box of cereal than if the talker is speaking in the office lounge.

A fifth way to increase training difficulty is to move from structured listening tasks to spontaneous tasks. A student may acquire the skill to recognize a word during a structured activity, but may still not recognize it when it occurs in spontaneous conversation. If you prime a child to listen for his or her name and then speak it, the child will be more likely to respond to it than if you happen to say the name while the child is engaged in a quiet activity.

Finally, in addition to varying response set, stimulus unit, stimulus similarity, contextual support, and task structure, training difficulty also can be adjusted by altering the listening environment and/or the presentation of the stimuli. For instance, background noise, such as the playing of music, may be introduced to decrease the signal-to-noise ratio and increase the difficulty of the listening task. The level of the speech may be varied, either by the talker speaking more or less softly or by moving closer to or farther from the student.

You will want to adjust the level of training difficulty so that students are challenged but not frustrated. As a general rule of thumb, when providing formal auditory training, the level of difficulty should be increased if someone responds correctly to training stimuli 80% of the time or more. The difficulty level can be decreased if the person responds correctly to less than 50% of the training items.

DEVELOPING ANALYTIC TRAINING OBJECTIVES

At the onset of an auditory training program, a hierarchy of specific training objectives is developed. In developing a hierarchy, you will consider an individual's current skill levels, then consider in which sequence the person might best acquire more advanced listening skills and how to promote them. This process yields a well thought-out plan of action. It is not written in stone, however, and can be modified over time, according to the person's progress.

If someone has few auditory skills, training typically begins with developing an awareness of sound. If the student is very young, the child may have to learn that sound has meaning and that it is often the byproduct of an action. Children who have just acquired listening potential, such as a child who has received a cochlear implant, may not realize this important relationship between sound and activity. Nonspeech stimuli may be used to teach these concepts, such as those listed in Table 7–3.

Once sound awareness has been established, early auditory training activities may involve gross discrimination of loudness, pitch, and rate, as in the following examples performed with a xylophone:

■ **Loudness:** Strike a xylophone softly, and ask the student whether the sound is "soft" or "loud."
■ **Pitch:** Play a rising octave, and ask whether the sound is going "up" or going "down."
■ **Rate:** Strike a rapid series of notes, and ask whether the pattern is "slow" or "fast."

Once these kinds of tasks are mastered, then analytic and synthetic training activities might be introduced.

Two kinds of training objectives often are targeted with analytic training: vowels and consonants. Vowels usually are more intense than consonants and have more energy in the low frequencies, so are perceived more readily. For this reason, training for vowel recognition usually begins before training for consonant recognition. It is helpful to review the acoustic properties of vowels and consonants before attempting to design specific training objectives and lesson materials.

Table 7–3. Objects that may teach children about the relationship between action and sound. Developing the concept that sound has meaning and action often results in sound production. A young child who has had little experience with the auditory signal may need to develop these concepts before moving on to more challenging auditory tasks. By manipulating such items as listed in this table, the youngster may develop these important concepts.

■ Hammer and peg toy	■ Computerized game
■ Toy drum	■ Water faucet
■ Piano	■ Hair dryer
■ Vacuum cleaner	■ Whistle

Vowel Auditory Training Objectives

Vowel auditory training objectives typically are designed to contrast vowels that have different formants. *Vowel formants* are the result of resonances in the vocal tract that cause some frequencies to have more energy than other frequencies. For instance, if you blow into a long, rounded bottle, you will produce a low-pitched sound because the bottle's shape enhances the resonance of sound waves associated with low pitches. On the other hand, blowing into a short, tubular bottle will produce a high-pitched sound. This bottle's shape enhances the resonance of sound waves associated with high pitches. In a similar fashion, the way you shape your mouth when you speak a vowel determines the vowel formants.

Vowel formants are resonances in the vocal tract that cause some frequencies to have more energy than other frequencies.

Each vowel can be distinguished by at least two characteristic formants. These are called the first and second formants. The combination of these two formants causes each vowel to sound different from every other vowel.

How wide you open your mouth determines the first formant. If you vocalize with your mouth relatively opened, you will produce a vowel that has a high-frequency first format. The vowel /a/ in *sod* is associated with an open mouth position and also has a high first formant compared to most other vowels. More closed mouth openings, such as that associated with the vowel /u/ in *blue*, produce low-frequency first formants.

Whether the tongue body is more forward or backward in the mouth greatly determines the frequency of the second formant. Moving your tongue more forward, as when saying /i/ in *seed*, will result in a higher frequency second formant. Moving your tongue body back towards the throat, as when saying /u/, will produce a lower second formant. Approximate first and second formant values for the vowels of English appear in Table 7–4 (Peterson & Barney, 1952).

Training may begin with developing vowel awareness, especially if the student is a very young child, and has little experience with the auditory signal. Toys such as farm animals may be used. The child listens as the cow makes a *moooo* sound, the lamb makes a *baaah* sound, and the chick says *cheeeep* (Ling, 1976).

Once the student demonstrates vowel awareness, vowel training objectives might require students to discriminate between vowel stimuli, and then to identify them. Initially, contrasts will concern vowels that differ in first formant information. For

Table 7–4. Typical first and second formant frequency values for the vowels of English, spoken by an adult male talker.

Vowel	Example	First Formant (Hz)	Second Formant (Hz)
/i/	heat	270	2290
/ɪ/	hit	390	1990
/ɛ/	head	530	1840
/æ/	hat	660	1720
/a/	hot	730	1090
/ɔ/	hall	570	840
/ʊ/	hook	440	1020
/u/	who	300	870
/ʌ/	hut	640	1190
/ɚ/	hurt	490	1350

instance, a student might determine whether the words *meet* and *mat* are the same or different. Most persons with hearing loss are more likely to have residual hearing in the low frequencies than the high frequencies; therefore, first formant contrasts may be more perceptually salient than contrasts which include vowels differing in their second formants. As training progresses, students can discriminate and identify vowel stimuli that differ on the basis of second formant information, such as *bee* and *boo*. Table 7–5 presents a sample hierarchy of vowel auditory training objectives (Stout & Windle, 1992; Tye-Murray & Fryauf-Bertschy, 1992). These objectives were developed for a child who uses a cochlear implant, and who has demonstrated consistent sound awareness.

Table 7–6 presents examples of word pairs that might be used for achieving the first three objectives. In typical discrimination exercises, like those required for the first three objectives, a student may sit before two pictures, for example, one of a key and one of a bee. The clinician might say one of the words, and the student is to point to the correct word. If the student is younger, he or she may place a coin or a piece of cereal on the picture. This provides visible reinforcement, and student and clinician can count the number of markers placed, once the task is completed.

Designing Consonant Auditory Training Objectives

Consonant auditory training objectives often are designed to contrast three features of articulation: place, voicing, and manner (see also Chapter 5). Table 7–7 presents a list of consonants grouped together according to these features.

Table 7–5. A sample hierarchy of vowel training objectives.

The student:

1. Will discriminate vowels that differ in first formant information, using a two-item response set; for example, *meat* from *mat*.
2. Will discriminate vowels that differ in second formant information, using a two-item response set; for example, *bee* from *boo*.
3. Will discriminate words that have vowels with similar first and second formant information, using a two-item response set; for example, *mate* from *mit*.
4. Will identify words with different vowels, using a four-item response set; for example, *beet* from the response set of: *beet*, *boot*, *bat*, and *bet*.
5. Will identify words with different vowels, from an open set of vocabulary.

Table 7–6. Vowel and word pairs that can be used for achieving the first three analytic auditory training objectives for vowels.

Objective 1: The student will discriminate vowels that differ in first formant information, using a two-item response set.

Vowel pairs:

/u/ versus /ɜ/, /æ/, /ʌ/, or /a/   /ɪ/ versus /ɛ/, /æ/, /ʌ/, or /a/
/ʊ/ versus /ɛ/, /æ/, or /a/   /ɪ/ versus /ɛ/, /æ/, /ʌ/, or /a/

Word pairs:

shoe/shop	tune/ten	pin/pig
bee/bat	tooth/tap	moon/men
boot/bat	shoe/shut	put/pet
book/back	put/pot	bead/bed

Objective 2: The student will discriminate vowels that differ in second formant information.

Vowel pairs:

/ɪ/ versus /u/   /ɔ/ versus /e, ɚ/
/o/ versus /e, ɚ/   /a/ versus /æ/
/e/ versus /ɚ/   /ʊ/ versus /ɪ/

Word pairs:

bee/boo	low/lay	low/learn
fawn/fern	hot/hat	book/bit
me/moo	shock/shake	lock/lake
coat/cake	beet/boot	pot/pat

Objective 3: The student will discriminate vowels with similar first and second formant information.

Vowel pairs:

/o/ versus /ɔ/   /ɛ/ versus /e/
/aɪ/ versus /ɪ/   /a/ versus /ʌ/
/e/ versus /ɪ/

Word pairs:

pen/pain	hot/hut	ship/sheep
get/gate	hog/hug	fit/feet
ship/sheep	show/shawl	chip/cheap
tin/teen	wet/wait	net/knit

Table 7–7. A listing of consonants grouped together according to the features of place of articulation, voicing, and manner of articulation.

A. Consonants classified by manner of articulation

Stops: /p, t, k, b, d, g/
Fricatives and affricatives: /f, v, ð, h, s, ʃ, z, dʒ, tʃ/
Nasals: /n, m/
Glides and liquids: /w, j, r, l/

B. Consonants classified by voicing

Voiced: /b, d, g, v, z, m, n, l, w, j, r/
Unvoiced: /p, t, k, tʃ, f, θ, h, s, ʃ /

C. Consonants classified by place of articulation

Bilabial: /m, p, b, w/
Labiodental: /f, v/
Linguadental: /θ/
Alveolar: /t, d, s, z, n, l/
Velar and palatal: /k, g, ʃ, j, tʃ, h/

Place of articulation: classification of a speech sound according to where in the vocal tract it is produced (e.g., bilabial).

Place of articulation refers to where in the mouth the primary constriction occurs for the particular sound. Traditional place classifications include:

■ **Bilabial,** such as /m/ in *man,* wherein the two lips meet to produce the sound.
■ **Labiodental,** such as /v/ in *van,* wherein the lower lip and upper teeth contact.
■ **Linguadental,** such as /θ/ in *thumb,* wherein the tongue tip contacts the upper teeth.
■ **Alveolar,** such as /d/ in *dot,* wherein the tongue tip approximates or contacts the roof of the mouth just behind the front teeth.
■ **Palatal,** such as /ʃ/ in *ship,* wherein the midsection of the tongue body approximates or touches the roof of the mouth.
■ **Velar,** such as /g/ in *glove,* wherein the back of the tongue approximates or touches the roof of the mouth.

For training purposes, consonants that traditionally are considered palatal may be grouped together with velar consonants.

Voicing: classification of a speech sound according to whether it is produced with or without voice (e.g., /b/ versus /p/).

The *voicing feature* is used to classify sounds according to whether the vocal cords vibrate during the constriction phase of production. For example, /p/ is classified as an unvoiced sound whereas its cognate /b/ is classified as a voiced sound.

Manner of articulation is used to classify consonants by the kind of articulatory movements required to produce the particular sound. Consonants can belong to one of five manner groups:

■ **Stops**, such as /p/ and /d/. Stops are produced by completely closing the vocal tract at some point, and allowing pressure to build up behind the constriction. The constriction is released quickly, resulting in a burst of air. Stops are soft sounds, and can be produced with or without voicing.

■ **Nasals**, such as /m, n/. They are produced by lowering the velum and allowing air to flow through the nasal cavities. The nasal consonants tend to have high energy in the low frequencies, and they are louder than stops or fricatives.

■ **Fricatives**, such as /f, s/. These sounds are produced by forcing the breath stream through a small constriction in the mouth, which results in a turbulent airflow. Fricatives tend to have a hissing sound. They are louder than stop consonants, and longer in duration. They may be produced with or without voicing.

■ **Affricatives**, such as /tʃ/. They are produced by combining a fricative with a stop, as in chop. For training purposes, fricatives and affricatives are sometimes grouped together.

■ **Glides**, such as /w, j, l/. Glides are produced with slow, opening articulatory gestures. For instance, notice that when you say the word *lot*, your mouth opens more slowly than when you say the word *tot*. The first word begins with a glide whereas the second word begins with a stop consonant. Glides also are louder than either stops and fricatives, and are always produced with voicing.

The easiest features to distinguish for most hard-of-hearing persons, even those with significant hearing loss, are voicing cues, and manner cues that signal whether or not a consonant is a nasal. Many individuals can distinguish *bat* from *pat* (a voicing distinction) and *bat* from *mat* (a manner distinction signaling nasality). These distinctions are easiest to hear because voiced sounds and nasals are comparatively loud, and they have energy in the low frequencies.

The most difficult cues to hear are those that relate to the place feature. This is because these cues are conveyed by mid- and high-frequency information, and many hard-of-hearing individuals have their greatest hearing loss for these frequencies. Many students will not be able to distinguish *pea* from *tea* from *key* through listening alone.

Knowledge of articulatory features, and how easily they can be heard, will help you to order your auditory training objectives. Early auditory training exercises might include consonant stimuli that differ in manner and voice and/or place of production, such as *tap* and *map*. The sounds /t/ and /m/ differ in terms of manner of articulation, place of articulation, and voicing. Later exercises might require students to identify consonants that differ in place of production but share voice and manner. For instance, they might distinguish between words such as *bag*, *tag*, and *gag*. These words are similar in their acoustic properties. Table 7–8 presents a sample hierarchy of consonant auditory training objectives for young cochlear implant users (Tye-Murray & Fryauf-Bertschy, 1992).

Table 7–9 presents consonant and word pairs that exemplify the kinds of contrasts and words that might be utilized in achieving the first four objectives. When possible, at least five different sets of words should be presented for each consonant pair when using a discrimination task.

Table 7–8. A sample hierarchy of consonant auditory training objectives.

The student:

---

1. Will discriminate nasal versus non-nasal unvoiced consonants that differ in place of production; for example, *mean* from *teen*.
2. Will discriminate nasal versus non-nasal voiced consonants that differ in place of production; for example, *map* from *gap*.
3. Will discriminate unvoiced fricatives versus voiced stops that differ in place of production; for example, *son* from *gun*.
4. Will discriminate unvoiced fricatives versus unvoiced stops that differ in place of production; for example, *sea* from *key*.
5. Will identify words in which the consonants share manner of production from a four-item and then six-item response set; for example, *sat* from the response set of: *sat, fat, shot*, and *van*.
6. Will identify words in which the consonants are all either voiced or unvoiced from a four-item and then six-item response set; for example, *cat* from the response set of: *cat, pat, tap*, and *sack*.
7. Will identify words in which the consonants share place of production from a four-item and then six-item response set; for example, *pat* from the response set of: *pat, mat, bat*, and *fat*.
8. Will identify words in an open-set format, where the words are familiar vocabulary words.

Table 7-9. Consonant and word pairs that can be used for achieving the first four analytic auditory training objectives.

Objective 1: The student will discriminate nasal versus non-nasal unvoiced consonants that differ in place of production.

Consonant pairs:

/m/ versus /ʃ, s, t, k, tʃ, h, f/
/n/ versus /p, k, f, h, ʃ/

Word pairs:

meat/seat	milk/silk	near/fear
net/pet	news/shoes	no/so
man/fan	neat/feet	might/fight
may/say	no/toe	nap/tap

Objective 2: The student will discriminate nasal versus non-nasal voiced consonants that differ in place of production.

Consonant pairs:

/m/ versus /d, g, l, w, r/
/n/ versus /b, g, w, r/

Word pairs:

nail/rail	nine/wine	note/goat
mail/whale	mice/dice	kneel/deal
make/rake	knot/dot	make/lake
nail/bail	mow/dough	nap/lap

Objective 3: The student will discriminate unvoiced fricatives versus voiced stops that differ in place of production.

Consonant pairs:

/f/ versus /d, g/
/s/ versus /b, g/
/h/ versus /b, d/
/ʃ/ versus /b, d/

Word pairs:

fun/gun	sell/bell	same/game
shoe/do	heart/dart	shed/bed
she/bee	hay/day	hat/bat
sack/back	song/gone	fall/doll

Objective 4: The student will discriminate unvoiced fricatives versus unvoiced stops that differ in place of production.

Consonant pairs:

/f/ versus /t, k/
/s/ versus /p, t/
/h/ versus /p, t/
/ʃ/ versus /p, t/

Word pairs:

fall/tall	shell/tell	sing/king
fan/tan	sand/can	fat/cat
same/came	show/toe	shine/pine
fin/tin	phone/cone	soil/coil

Cycling: coming back to a training objective that has been achieved with some success in order to provide reinforcement and additional learning.

Cycling

A student does not necessarily have to meet one training objective before progressing to the next one. Vergara, Miskiel, and Oller (1994) described an auditory training program that utilizes cycling. "*Cycling* involves presenting a skill within a specified time period and then moving on to another objective . . . For example, after targeting one objective for two weeks, the teacher may choose to move on to another objective returning to the original objective at a later date . . . Cycling provides the opportunity for students to process new concepts. For example, after an initial introduction, children are provided with opportunities to experiment with a particular task so that at the time of the second presentation, they may experience a higher level of success" (p. 58). Cycling is a potent means to build listening skills and is effective in helping students overcome a plateau in their listening performance.

DEVELOPING SYNTHETIC TRAINING OBJECTIVES

In this section, we will consider synthetic training objectives. Depending on the student's skill level, synthetic training objectives might begin with very simple discrimination activities that involve suprasegmental aspects of speech. *Suprasegmental* aspects, sometimes referred to as prosodic features, include intonation, stress, duration, and loudness (see Chapter 16). During training, you might ask a child to move a toy car at a fast or slow pace, depending on whether you quickly bark, *go-go-go-go* or leisurely intone, *Gooo—Gooo—Gooo*. You might speak one of two student's names with a conversationally loud voice or a whisper, and ask that the named student imitate your production.

Suprasegmentals are prosodic aspects of speech, including variations in pitch, rate, intensity, and duration, that are superimposed on phonemes and words.

Once these kinds of tasks are mastered, the program can address objectives like those listed in Table 7–10 (Tye-Murray & Fryauf-Bertschy, 1992b). Students can discriminate and later identify multiword utterances such as I'm going home from single word utterances, such as home. This will require them to attend to information about the number of syllables in the phrase. Table 7–11 presents long and short training pairs that can be used for achieving the first objective listed in Table 7–10,

Table 7–10. A sample hierarchy of synthetic auditory training.

The student:

---

1. Will discriminate multiword utterances from single-word utterances, using a closed response set; for example, *How are you today?* from *Hi!* Later, he or she can be asked to discriminate long words from short words; for example, *Halloween* from *cat*.
2. Will discriminate a spondee from a one-syllable word; for example, *ice cream* from *shoe*. Later, he or she can be asked to discriminate a spondee from a two-syllable word; for example, *There's a toothbrush* from *There's a pony*.
3. Will discriminate between words having the same number of syllables; for example, *That's my cat* from *That's my dog*.
4. Will identify simple words from a four-item and then a six-item response set; for example, *cat* from the response set of *cat*, *dog*, *elephant*, and *camel*.
5. Will identify picture illustrations from a closed-set, after hearing one-sentence descriptions.
6. Will follow simple directions and answer simple questions, using a closed response set.
7. Will listen to two related sentences, and then draw a picture about them; for example, he or she might draw a picture after hearing, *The boy is playing. He has a ball.*

Table 7–11. Long and short training pairs that can be used for achieving the first synthetic auditory training objectives listed in Table 7–10.

The student will discriminate multiword utterances from single-word utterances:

- How are you/Hi
- See you later/Bye
- Santa Claus/tree
- Motorcycle/car
- Beat the drum/clap
- The cat in the hat/dog
- . Give me the crayon/draw
- A box of cookies/milk

---

and Table 7–12 presents two-syllable spondees that can be used for achieving the second objective listed in Table 7–10.

The next step may be for students to identify simple words from a closed set of choices; for instance, the word *Tom* from the response set of *Tim*, *John*, *Don*, and *Tom*. As skills progress, the size of the response set can be increased from four to six choices.

Comprehension activities can begin with a closed-set format and move to a more open-set format. Young students might be

Table 7-12. Examples of word pairs that can be used for the second objective listed in Table 7–10 for synthetic auditory training.

The student will discriminate a two-syllable from a one-syllable word:

Airplane/pop
Milkshake/cup
Flashlight/cake
Hotdog/bun
Pancake/plate
Snowball/ice
Toothbrush/teeth
Popcorn/bowl
Sandwich/gum

---

asked to, *Show me your nose; Show me your ears; Show me your mouth*, and *Show me your hair*. Later, they may be asked to draw a picture, step by step, without knowing what directions might occur, for example, *Pick up a blue crayon* (the student demonstrates comprehension by picking it up), *Draw a circle* (the student demonstrates comprehension by drawing the circle), *Put a fish in the circle* (the student draws a fish), and so forth.

If students are adults, a comprehension task might be to listen to a recorded passage and then to answer written questions. Afterwards, they listen to the passage a second time, reading a transcript of the passage while listening. The second presentation provides additional listening practice and allows them to check the accuracy of their answers to the questions.

FORMAL AND INFORMAL AUDITORY TRAINING

Once training objectives have been formulated, they can be pursued with formal and informal instruction.

Formal Auditory Training

General guidelines for conducting formal auditory training are presented in Table 7–13 (Tye-Murray, 1993a). Training activi-

Table 7–13. Guidelines for conducting formal auditory training.

A. Training stimuli should become more challenging to discriminate over time.

Many hard-of-hearing individuals can determine whether a sound is nasalized or voiced and, less often, whether the sound has frication. They have difficulty in distinguishing place of articulation. In initial training, students may be asked to discriminate between sounds that differ in manner and voice. In late training, they can discriminate between sounds that differ only in place.

B. A variety of talkers should speak training items.

Students learn that the same sounds or words can be acoustically different when repeated or when spoken by different talkers. This realization allows them to generalize what they learn in training to a variety of talkers. Tape recorders, VHS tapes, and digitized speech samples can be used to present stimuli.

C. Many, many training items should be presented during a relatively short period of time.

Concentrated training focuses students' attention on listening and maintains their interest, leading to fast learning. Adherence to this guideline means that training reinforcements are provided sparingly, since they may be time consuming and distracting.

D. Nonspeech training stimuli should be used only with young students who are prelingually deaf, and only for a short period.

Nonspeech stimuli develop two important concepts: First, sound conveys meaning and second, action often produces sound. The child might turn on and off a water faucet or clap hands. The exception to this guideline is the student who is interested in developing his or her ability to appreciate music.

E. An auditory training exercise can include both analytic and synthetic level stimuli.

Occasionally the student's attention is focused on recognizing speech sounds and single words or phrases, and occasionally on recognizing words in a meaningful context.

F. Training progresses from closed-set to open-set response modes.

Early in training a young student might be asked to color a shape red and need to choose between a red or blue crayon (closed-set). Later, the student might be asked to select the red crayon, when crayons from an entire box are available as options (open-set).

G. Ten to 15 minutes a day should be devoted to formal auditory training, preferably at the same time everyday.

Training thus becomes a part of the daily routine.

H. Formal training objectives should be pursued informally throughout the day.

When opportunity arises during conversation or academic instruction, the student can be presented with listening tasks that reinforce the formal auditory training objectives.

I. Training activities must be engaging and interesting.

Otherwise, the adult may simply pass through the motions of training without receiving benefit; the child may not cooperate.

ties and materials should be appropriate for students' age, gender, language skills, and everyday experiences. For instance, a young boy might respond to materials that concern soccer. An adult might enjoy materials about current news events. If possible, auditory training should occur with no more than one to three students at time, in a quiet room that offers minimal distractions. The optimal distance between the teacher and student is 6 to 12 inches. A sample lesson plan for an auditory training session is presented in Table 7–14.

Reinforcements

Reinforcements are often utilized during formal training activities. Reinforcements must be appropriate for the age and interests of the students. The following two lists present reinforcements that might be appropriate for young children and adolescents:

Table 7–14. An example lesson plan for an auditory training session.

Title: Snake and Ice Cream Game

Objective: The student will discriminate a nasal consonant versus non-nasal unvoiced consonant that differs in place of production.

Materials:

1. a picture of a snake to represent the /s/ sound
2. a picture of a boy about to eat an ice cream sundae to represent the /m/ sound.
3. a stack of 26 pennies for reinforcements

Procedures:

1. Introduce the picture of the snake by pointing to it and saying "sssssssss . . ." Ask the child to imitate your production. Similarly, introduce the picture of the sundae, and say "mmmmmm . . ," Ask the child to imitate your production.
2. Say each sound with your face visible. After each utterance, ask the child to point to the corresponding picture.
3. Place 13 pennies on each picture. Cover your mouth. Randomly say one sound after another. After each production, the child may pick up a penny from one of the two pictures. If the child removes a penny from the correct picture, he or she can keep it. If incorrect, the penny must be placed back on the picture.
4. Continue until all pennies are spent.

List 1: Young children

- Collecting stickers in a sticker book
- Putting features onto a Mr. Potato Head
- Placing puzzle pieces one at a time into a puzzle board
- Blowing soap bubbles
- Playing a card game or board game
- Stringing beads onto a bead necklace

List 2: Adolescents

- Earning tokens that can be used to purchase desirable privileges, such as time with a computer game
- Earning tokens that can be used to buy school supplies, such as pencils and notepads
- Earning tokens that can be used to buy extracurricular rewards, such as a gift certificate to a fast food restaurant

To make formal auditory training stimulating for children, *reinforcements* are often essential. After students complete a set number of items or perform so many activities, they receive something desirable, such as a sticker or special privilege. The following are general principals to follow when choosing and providing reinforcements (from Tye-Murray, 1992d, p. 85):

Reinforcement: something desirable provided to a student after he or she performs a training activity or performs in a desired manner.

A. The child should be able to perform a reinforcement activity quickly; he [she] should not spend more time with the reinforcement activity than with the training activity.

B. Reinforcement activities should not be too challenging or too absorbing; otherwise the child will not attend closely to the training task.

C. Activities must be varied; drawing lines on a paper may hold a child's interest for a few minutes, but the activity quickly wears thin.

D. Activities should interest the child; for example, if the child enjoys playing with money, he or she might drop coins into a bank.

E. The child should perform the reinforcement activity immediately after responding to a training item correctly.

F. Activities should be appropriate for the child's age and gender.

Special Considerations for Adults

Many adults will be reluctant to participate in an auditory training class. Hectic schedules, a long workday, and transportation difficulties are possible obstacles to participation. This state of affairs has resulted in some attempts to develop home training and programmed self-instruction procedures. Students may receive exercises they complete at home. They may listen to audio-taped cassettes or perform a listening activity with a family member or friend. They inform the teacher about their progress, perhaps by mailing a record-keeping schedule or workbook pages on a regular basis. The clinician stays in contact with the adult student, by making telephone calls or sending teletype messages on at least a weekly basis throughout the course of the home training program.

Informal Auditory Training

Informal auditory training is a powerful means of fostering listening skills because listening practice occurs in the context of meaningful communication and is not removed from situational context. Informal auditory training can enhance students' confidence in their abilities to engage in conversation and also increase their motivation to rely on hearing for communication.

When students are children, classroom teachers can incorporate informal listening practice into the academic curriculum (Nevins & Chute, 1995). For example, a classroom teacher might expect students to comprehend familiar phrases associated with the calendar. The teacher might query, with mouth hidden, "Tell me what today is," "Tell me what day it was yesterday," and "Tell me what will tomorrow be." The teacher may instruct, with face clearly visible, "Go to the chalkboard. I will say a number between 1 and 10." These instructions establish a context for recognizing her next instruction, which will be spoken while the student faces the chalkboard: "Write the number seven."

Auditory Training At Home

You might recommend informal auditory training activities to perform in the home. For example, parents can play musical chairs with their child to promote sound awareness. In making recommendations, you might also stress the importance of "fun time," and the need for a parent to be a parent rather than a teacher and the need for the child to have time to be a child.

INTERWEAVING AUDITORY TRAINING WITH OTHER COMPONENTS OF AURAL REHABILITATION

Commonly, auditory training is provided in conjunction with speechreading training and, if the student is a child, speech therapy. By interweaving auditory and speechreading training, you will build a student's associations between corresponding auditory and audiovisual representations of speech. It is common for training stimuli to be presented in the audiovisual condition before being presented in an audition-only condition. Students will recognize considerably more stimuli when they can both see and hear the talker rather than only hear the talker.

There are at least two reasons to incorporate speech production practice into auditory training. First, a child's awareness of oral representations of words may relate closely to the child's ability to identify the words auditorily. Second, by linking speaking and listening together, the child may realize that one purpose of learning to listen is to learn how to utilize auditory information to enhance speech production. Children must get in the habit of monitoring their own speech as they talk.

BENEFITS OF AUDITORY TRAINING

Some researchers have shown that auditory training improves the listening performance of adults (Alcantara, Cowan, Blamey, & Clark, 1990; Lansing & Davis, 1988; Walden, Erdman, Montgomery, Schwartz, & Prosek, 1981); other studies have not (Rubinstein & Boothroyd, 1987). Blamey and Alcantara (1994) suggested that the contradictory results may relate to different types of practice that were provided to the research subjects in the different experiments, the different kinds of listening skills that were evaluated, and, finally, to the varying level of performance of the subjects at their entry into a training program.

Little research has been performed on the benefits of auditory training per se for children. However, there is evidence that children who use aural-oral communication and rely on listening and speechreading for recognizing messages tend to perform better on tests of speech recognition than children who use simultaneous communication and rely on speech and sign language (Geers & Moog, 1992). Children in an aural/oral educational program often receive more auditory training than children in a simultaneous communication program, so one interpretation is that aural/oral children perform better on speech recognition tests because of the increased amount of auditory training they receive.

The benefit accrued from auditory training will vary greatly from one student to the next. For some students, benefits accumulate gradually over time, whereas others receive little or no benefit throughout the course of training. Often, young students progress in spurts. Listening skills improve, then plateau, and then improve more. The rate and extent of benefit may be influenced by at least two factors, the characteristics of the student and the program content.

Characteristics of the Students

Students who have more residual hearing, or who receive a significant amount of information through their listening devices, likely will achieve higher levels of auditory performance than students who have less hearing or who receive less information. The kind of listening aid that the student uses is important. Current cochlear implants allow many users to hear mid- and high-frequency components of the speech signal. They may hear more information about place and frication, as well as other parameters of speech, than individuals who have similar hearing loss and use hearing aids.

Progress also may be influenced by the student's age, motivation to receive training, age at which the hearing loss was incurred, duration of hearing loss, family situation, and the student's personality. For example, an elderly individual who has had a hearing loss for many years probably will receive less benefit from auditory training than a recently deafened adolescent. An outgoing, extroverted child who frequently interacts with children who have normal hearing might have a greater intrinsic desire to develop listening skills than an introverted child who prefers solitary activities.

Program Content

Program content also interacts with training gains. Issues related to program content include the appropriateness of the training activities, that is, whether the activities are enjoyable and motivating for the student and whether they are appropriate for helping the student meet the training objectives (Figure 7–6). The consistency with which teachers and other significant individuals in a student's life provide auditory stimulation and reinforce training objectives informally throughout the day, also will affect the amount of benefit received.

FINAL REMARKS

When individuals have hearing loss, listening skills often do not emerge spontaneously. Deliberate and systematic auditory training is required to foster listening potential. We have considered basic principles of auditory training in this chapter. Other resources for training curricula and activities appear in the Key Resources section.

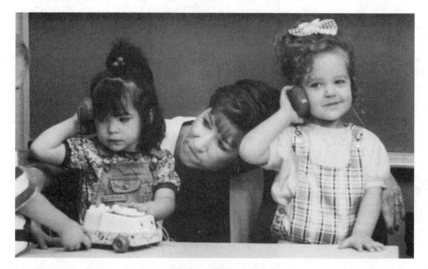

Figure 7–6. The success of an auditory training program depends in part on whether the training activities are enjoyable and motivating for the students. Activities should be age-appropriate. By Marcus Kosa, courtesy of CID

Auditory training need not be confined to speech and environmental stimuli. Some individuals with hearing loss may desire instruction that will enhance their recognition and appreciation of music. For instance, adult cochlear implant users who enjoyed music before losing their hearing often wish to begin listening again once they have received their implants. Work is currently underway in some cochlear implant programs to develop music training programs and to evaluate the efficacy of this kind of program for enhancing music enjoyment (Gfeller & Witt, in preparation).

KEY CHAPTER POINTS

✔ Usually, children with significant hearing losses receive auditory training. Adults are less likely to receive training.

✔ Most auditory training curricula are designed to progress a student from one auditory skill level to the next. The four skill levels underlying most programs are sound awareness, sound discrimination, identification, and comprehension.

✔ Many auditory training curricula include both analytic and synthetic kinds of training activities, and formal and informal activities.

✔ Difficulty of training can be adjusted by varying the size of the stimuli set used for listening tasks, the stimulus unit, stimulus similarity, context, structure, and the listening environment. As a general rule of thumb, you will want to alter the level of difficulty if a person response correctly to training stimuli 80% of the time or more, or responds correctly to less than 50%.

✔ A hierarchy of specific training objectives typically is developed at the onset of a patient's auditory training program. The objectives are targeted with both analytic and synthetic training.

✔ Analytic vowel auditory training objectives are designed to contrast vowels with different vowel formants. Consonant auditory training objectives are designed to contrast features of articulation, such as place, voice, and manner.

KEY RESOURCES

Auditory Training Curricula

The Developmental Approach to Successful Listening II (DASL), 2nd Edition, 1992.

Authors: G. G. Stout and J. V. Ert Windle

Available from:
Resource Point, Inc.
61 Inverness Drive East, Suite 100
Englewood, CO 80112

CHATS: The Miami Cochlear Implant Auditory and Tactile Skills Curriculum, 1994.

Editors: K. C. Vergara and L. W. Miskiel

Available from:
Intelligent Hearing Systems
10689 North Kendall Drive
Miami, FL 33176

Auditory Enhancement Guide, 1990.

Authors: Personnel of the Clarke School for the Deaf

Available from:
Clarke School for the Deaf
Center for Oral Education
47 Round Hill Road
Northampton, MA 01060-2199

Communication Training for Hearing-Impaired Children and Teenagers: Speechreading, Listening and Using Repair Strategies, 1993.

Author: N. Tye-Murray

Available from:
PRO-ED
8700 Shoal Creek Boulevard
Austin, TX 78758-6897

Communication Training for Hard-of-Hearing Adults and Older Teenagers: Speechreading, Listening, and Using Repair Strategies, 1997.

Author: N. Tye-Murray

Available from:
PRO-ED
8700 Shoal Creek Boulevard
Austin, TX 78758-6897

Speech Perception Instructional Curriculum and Evaluation (SPICE), 1995.

Authors: J. Moog, J. Biedenstein, and L. Davidson.

Available from:
Central Institute for the Deaf
818 South Euclid Avenue
St. Louis, MO 63110

Speechreading

Topics

- Speechreading for Communication
- Characteristics of a Good Lipreader
- The Difficulty of the Lipreading Task
- Importance of Residual Hearing
- Factors That Affect the Speechreading Process
- Oral Interpreters
- Final Remarks
- Key Chapter Points
- Key Resources

Lipreading is the process of recognizing speech using only the visual speech signal and other visual cues, such as facial expression.

Speechreading is speech recognition using both auditory and visual cues.

Before we consider speechreading training, which we will do in the next chapter, it is important to review the general topics of lipreading and speechreading. The two terms often are used interchangeably. In our discussion, we will follow the conventions of Thorn and Thorn (1989), Walden, Prosek, Montgomery, Scherr, and Jones (1977) and Lansing and Helgeson (1995). When *lipreading*, a person relies only on the visual signal provided by the talker's face for recognizing speech (Thorn & Thorn, 1989). When *speechreading*, the person attends to both the talker's auditory and visual signals, as well as the talker's facial expressions and gestures, and any other available cues. These include the setting in which the conversation is occurring or what has been discussed beforehand (Walden et al., 1977).

SPEECHREADING FOR COMMUNICATION

Persons with normal hearing routinely rely on speechreading. Consider these examples: When we are at a noisy restaurant, we understand more if we watch the talker's face while we listen. We may feel unsettled when we view dubbed foreign films, because the words we hear do not match those we see. A raised eyebrow imparts additional meaning to the question, "You're not working today?" Even infants engage in speechreading. If a 5-month-old baby hears someone phonate "eeeeeee," and simultaneously views a side-by-side projection of the same talker, on one side saying "eeeeeeee" and the other side saying "aaahhhh," the baby most likely will fixate on the visual signal that corresponds to the acoustic signal (Kuhl & Meltzoff, 1982).

A person with hearing loss will depend more on the visual signal for speech recognition than will individuals who have normal hearing. Whereas most persons can converse on the telephone with ease, or follow a news broadcast on the radio, a person with hearing loss will experience decreased speech recognition when only the auditory signal is presented. The greater the hearing impairment, the more an individual will rely on visual information for communication.

CHARACTERISTICS OF A GOOD LIPREADER

An audiologist arrives at the office on Monday morning and finds two persons waiting in the clinic area, Dr. Kevin Evans and Mr. Peter Climpton. The audiologist reads their charts and learns that Dr. Evans is a 42-year-old pharmaceutical executive who holds a doctorate degree in organic chemistry. He has had a moderate bilateral hearing impairment since the age of 16 years. Mr. Climpton is a 17-year-old male who has always had normal hearing. He recently applied for a position to work on an assembly line in a noisy factory and is required to undergo a comprehensive audiological work-up. With only this information, can the audiologist accurately predict which individual will perform better on tests on lipreading?

The answer to this question is *no*. A plethora of research has revealed that it is difficult to predict lipreading performance. Performance cannot be predicted by an individual's intelligence, educational achievement, duration of deafness (and hence, practice with the lipreading and speechreading tasks), age at hearing-loss onset, nor socioeconomic status. As such, Dr. Evans is as likely to be a better or poorer lipreader than Mr. Climpton, as vice versa. Even with additional information about their verbal abilities, cognitive skills such as visual memory and personality, the audiologist could not make an infallible prediction (see Summerfield, 1989, for a review).

A handful of variables may be somewhat predictive. For instance, on average, women lipread better than men (Dancer, Krain, Thompson, Davis, & Glenn, 1994), and young adults lipread better than elderly adults (Farrimond, 1959; Honnell, Dancer, & Gentry, 1991). There is also some evidence, albeit conflicting, that neurophysiological measures relate to performance. The latencies of recorded electrical potentials made at the cortex following stimulation of the eye by a flash of light may correlate with lipreading performance, (Shepherd, 1982; Shepherd, DeLavergne, Frueh, & Clobridge, 1977; but see Samar & Sims, 1983; Summerfield, 1992), with shorter latencies being characteristic of good lipreaders. Shorter latencies indicate more rapid transmission of neural impulses from the eye to the brain, and are unlikely to be affected by an individual's experiences, personality, or circumstances.

Some speech and hearing professionals have cited more nebulous characteristics that may relate to lipreading performance, including individuals' ability to capitalize on contextual cues, their willingness to guess, their mental agility, and their willingness to revise interpretations of a partially recognized message (e.g., Jeffers & Barley, 1971). Especially in children, linguistic and world knowledge can constrain proficiency.

Someone who has a limited vocabulary, limited knowledge of grammar, and limited world knowledge will likely experience lipreading difficulties. For instance, if a child has a limited knowledge of geography, the child will not readily recover the word missed when lipreading the sentence, "_____ *is the capital of the United States.*"

Predicting Lipreading Performance

People vary widely in their lipreading performance. Some individuals can score 80% words correct or better on a vision-only test condition, as measured by verbatim repetition of test words, whereas others score 5% or worse on the same stimuli (Bernstein, Demorest, Coulter, & O'Connell, 1991). The amount of practice in lipreading does not account for variability. Some college students who have normal hearing and who have never received lipreading training perform better on a sentence recognition test presented in a vision-only condition than adults who have an acquired hearing loss, and who have been deaf (and hence, speechreading for communicative purposes) for many years (Hanin, 1988).

THE DIFFICULTY OF THE LIPREADING TASK

If someone were to talk to you through a closed window, so you could see but not hear the person, you might recognize less than 20% of the words. Why is lipreading so difficult? The answer to this question relates to the variables listed in Table 8–1. In this section we will consider five variables that compound the difficulty of the lipreading task: visibility of sounds, rapidity of speech, coarticulation and stress effects, talker effects, and visemes and homophenes.

Visibility of Sounds

The first variable that affects the difficulty of the speech-reading task that we shall consider is the visibility of sounds. Many sounds entail minimal visible mouth movement. Woodward and Barber (1960) estimated that 60% of speech sounds are not visible on the mouth or cannot be seen readily. Words that are more visible on the face tend to begin with consonants that are made with bilabial closure (/p, b, m, w/),

Table 8-1. Factors that influence the lipreading task.

Talker	Message	Environment	Speechreader
Facial expressions	Length	Viewing angle	Lipreading skill
Diction	Syntactic complexity	Distance	Residual hearing
Body language	Frequency of word usage	Lighting	Use of appropriate amplification
Speech rate	Shared homophenes	Background noise	Stress profile
Speech intensity	Context	Room acoustics	Attentiveness
Familiarity to the speechreader		Distractions	Fatigue
Accent			Motivation to understand
Facial characteristics			Language skills
Speech prosody (intonation, stress, and rhythm)			
Objects in or over mouth			

the lower teeth pressing the upper lip (/f, v/), or the tongue tip contacting the upper teeth (/θ/). Consonants with limited visibility include sounds that are produced within the mouth, such as /k, g, t, n/. Some features of phonemes are simply not visible at all. For instance, there is no visible evidence indicating that a phoneme is either voiced (e.g., /b, d, g/) or unvoiced (e.g., /p, t, k/).

Vowels are considered not to be highly visible. They may or may not be distinguished by lip spreading (e.g., *beak* vs. *book*, where /i/ involves more lip spreading than /ʊ/), tongue and jaw height (e.g., *bit* vs. *bought*, where /ɔ/ is associated with greater tongue and jaw height than /ɪ/), and lip rounding (*boot* vs. *bet*, where /u/ is associated with more lip rounding than /ɜ/). Fortunately, even though vowels are not associated with distinctive mouth movements, they tend to be acoustically salient to individuals who have hearing loss. Vowels are relatively intense, change slowly over time in their frequency composition, and are relatively long in duration (Pickett, 1980).

Rapidity of Speech

The second factor that contributes to the difficulty of the lip-reading task is the rapidity with which words are spoken. When speaking conversationally, a talker may speak anywhere from 150 to 250 words per minute, or roughly 4–7 syllables per second, excluding time spent pausing. Whereas a typical talker may produce an average of 15 phonemes per second, the human eye may be capable of registering only about 9 or 10 discrete mouth movements in this time interval. Thus, the lipreader (speechreader) has little time to ponder the identity of a particular word, and even may not realize the occurrence of every word.

Coarticulation and Stress Effects

The third factor that contributes to the difficulty of the lip-reading task is coarticulation and stress effects, which may result in the same sound looking different depending on its phonetic and linguistic context. For example, the sound /b/ looks different in the word *boot* versus *beet*. The lips begin to round in anticipation of the following /u/ in the first case; the lips begin to spread in anticipation of the following /i/ in the second case. If an alveolar consonant follows a rounded vowel such as /u/ in the word *hoot*, the lip rounding may hide the tongue and the teeth (Benguerel & Pichora-Fuller, 1982).

Stress can also affect the appearance of a word. The word *you* looks different in the following question, depending on the talker's stress pattern:

> *What did ya do yesterday?*
> *What did YOU do yesterday?*

Talker Effects

Talker effects may confound lipreading efforts because the same sound may look different when spoken by two different people. For instance, two talkers may differ in the degree of mouth opening used for speaking the vowels in the sentence, *"That is Pat's."*

Visemes and Homophenes

After being introduced to a visiting professor, an academician launched into a lively discussion of current topics in theology. Only after several minutes had elapsed, with just lukewarm interest expressed by the visiting professor, did the academician realize that his hostess had introduced him to a *geologist*, not a *theologist*.

The fact that sounds belong to viseme groups and many words are homophenous increases lipreading and speechreading difficulty. *Visemes* are groups of speech sounds that look alike on the face (Fisher, 1968). The sounds [b, m, p] comprise a viseme. When these sounds are spoken without voice, as in *bat*, *mat*, and *pat*, they are indistinguishable on the mouth. There is some disagreement among researchers as to which sounds constitute a viseme, although all agree that there are fewer visemes than phonemes (e.g., Binnie, Montgomery, & Jackson, 1974; Erber, 1974; Lesner, Sandridge, & Kricos, 1987). Two listings of consonants grouped as visemes as compiled by two different sources appear in Table 8–2.

Visemes are groups of speech sounds that appear identical on the lips (e.g., /p, m, b/).

Table 8-2. Consonants grouped as sets of visemes. Reports from two different research groups.

Erber (1974)	Lesner, Sandridge, and Kricos (1987)
/p, b, m/	/p, b, m/
/f, v/	/f, v/
/θ, ð/	/θ, ð/
/ð, ʒ/	/ð, ʒ, dʒ, tʃ/
/w, r/	/w, r/
/l/	/l/
/n, d, t, s, z/	/t, d, s, z, n, k, g, j/
/k, g/	
/h/	

Source: Adapted from Lesner, K., Sandridge, S., and Kricos, P. (1987). Training influences on visual consonant and sentence recognition. *Ear and Hearing, 8,* 283–287; and Erber, N. P. (1974). Visual perception of speech by deaf children: Recent developments and continuing needs. *Journal of Speech and Hearing Disorders, 39,* 178–185.

Homophenes are words that look identical on the mouth.

Homophenes are words that look the same on the mouth. In the example above, *theology* looked like *geology* to the academician who was talking to the visiting professor. It is not always intuitively clear which words are homophenous and which words are not. For example, as different as the words *grade* and *yes* sound, they are nonetheless homophenous. When only the visual signal of the talker is presented, you likely cannot discriminate one word from the other. On the other hand, even though the words *boon* and *doom* sound similar, and might be confused with one another if the listening environment is noisy, you will have no problem in distinguishing one from the other if you can see the talker's face.

Somewhere between 40 and 60% of words in English are homophenous (Berger, 1972). Grammatical sentence cues and other linguistic and situational cues can decrease the confusion about word identity, and some talkers will better distinguish words on the basis of the visual signal than other talkers.

Facial Expressions and Situational Cues

The poem below, written by a young man with significant hearing loss, underscores how facial expressions and situational cues can facilitate the speechreading task.

"I looked with longing at her lips,
To scan the words appearing.
I could not make out what she said;
Alas, I have no hearing.

But how I hoped to read those lips,
To know what she was saying;
To guess that enigmatic smile
Around the corners playing.

And as I gazed upon her face
It seemed I saw a pleading.
And then I knew, the words came through;
'Lips are not *just* for reading" (Berger, 1972, pp. 61–62).

IMPORTANCE OF RESIDUAL HEARING

Persons who are most dependent on the visual signal for speech communication are those who have only a minimum of residual hearing. Even a little hearing can be helpful.

Many individuals with a severe or profound hearing loss hear only low-frequency information, even when wearing a hearing aid, and receive information only about changes in voice pitch when they listen to speech. To approximate what this might sound like, clamp your hand over your mouth and recite "Humpty Dumpty Sat on the Wall." The signal you hear as you speak does not provide enough information to allow anyone to recognize your speech in an audition-only condition. However, if someone were to hear this degraded signal and have a clear view of your mouth while you spoke, this information might dramatically improve his or her speechreading performance. An experiment by Rosen, Moore, and Fourcin (1981) demonstrated this phenomenon.

Rosen et al. (1981) asked a test talker to produce a series of nonsense syllables with varying medial consonants, such as /apa/, /ama/, /ada/, and /asa/. A laryngograph was placed on his throat, which reflected vocal fold vibration, and the output was used to develop an auditory signal that reflected the changes over time in the talker's fundamental frequency (voice pitch). When the test subjects (who had normal hearing) saw but did not hear the talker, they identified 44% of the consonants correctly. When they saw the talker speak and heard the concomitant changes in fundamental frequency, their performance improved to 72% consonants correct.

The results of this experiment help to explain why so many people with profound hearing losses are dependent on their hearing aids for successful communication. Even though they receive minimal auditory information, their ability to speechread is enhanced greatly by the amplified signal.

FACTORS THAT AFFECT THE SPEECHREADING PROCESS

How well someone speechreads in a particular situation is influenced by at least four factors. As Table 8–3 indicates, these factors are the talker, the message, the speechreading environment and situation, and the speechreader.

The Talker

The talker can increase or decrease the difficulty of the speechreading task (Table 8–4).

Table 8–3. Factors that contribute to the difficulty of the speechreading task.

- Visibility of sounds
- Rapidity of speech
- Coarticulation
- Talker variability
- Visemes and homophenes

Table 8–4. Speaking behaviors that impede the speechreading task. This list was generated during a group discussion with adults who are hard-of-hearing.

I have a difficult time speechreading when the talker:

- mumbles.
- doesn't look at me when talking.
- chews gum.
- has an unusual accent.
- has a speech impediment.
- smiles too much.
- moves around while talking.
- uses no facial expressions.
- shouts.
- has a high pitched voice.
- talks too fast.
- uses long, complicated sentences and obscure vocabulary words.
- has a beard and/or mustache.
- wears dark glasses.

Talker behaviors

A talker who uses appropriate but not exaggerated facial expressions, who speaks with clear and not mumbled speech, and who uses body language is relatively easy to speechread. The following behaviors make a talker difficult to speechread:

- Shouting
- Mumbling
- Turning away
- Speaking rapidly
- Covering the mouth with a hand
- Smiling simultaneously while talking

Familiarity

Hard-of-hearing persons will have an easier time recognizing the speech of someone who is familiar, such as a family member, than someone who is unfamiliar, because they are accustomed to the talker's mouth movements and speech patterns. There is some evidence that thin lips are easier to speechread than thick or immobile lips and that a foreign accent increases difficulty (Berger, 1972).

Gender

Talker gender influences the difficulty of the task. Females are easier to lipread than males (Daly, Bench, & Chappell, 1996). However, even though females' speech may be more recognizable when it is presented in a vision-only condition, it may not necessarily be easier to recognize in an audition-plus-vision condition, as the higher fundamental frequency of the female voice is harder for most hard-of-hearing persons to hear than the lower fundamental frequencies associated with male voices. For male talkers, the presence of facial hair, as with a mustache or beard, can impede speechreading by obscuring lip and jaw movement.

How Something Is Said Will Affect How One Speechreads It

Try this experiment. Say to a friend, without using your voice, "Oh my aching back." As you speak, use minimal facial expression and body movements. Ask your friend to guess what you have said. Chances are, the guess will be incorrect. Now mouth the phrase again, but this time, assume a pained expression and rub your back with your hand. The odds are high that the friend will quickly recognize your utterance this second time around. This experiment reveals an important principle in speechreading: *Context cues can dramatically affect an individual's ability to speechread.*

The Message

The second factor that can influence speechreading performance is the message that a talker presents. The structure and the component words affect recognition.

Structure

Some messages are easier to speechread than others, depending on their length, syntactic complexity, frequency of use, similarity to other words, and linguistic context. As a general rule, the longer the sentence and the greater its syntactic complexity, the more difficult it will be to speechread. Words that have two syllables tend to be easier to recognize than monosyllables spoken in isolation.

Frequency of Usage

Commonplace words, such as the word *sweater*, have a higher probability of being recognized than words that are used less frequently, such as the word *cardigan*. We say that the word *sweater* has a greater **frequency of usage** than *cardigan*, because it is more likely to be spoken in everyday conversation.

Frequency of usage is a measure indicating how often a particular word occurs during everyday conversation.

Neighborhoods

Words that have fewer response possibilities are also easier to recognize. For example, the word *bat* may be difficult to recognize, even though it begins with a highly visible mouth movement, because many other words are similar both visually (e.g., *bad, bet, mat, met, pat*) and acoustically (e.g., *cap, cat, scat, bad*). On the other hand, the word *telephone* is easier to recognize, even though it is less commonplace than the word *bat*, because not many words look or sound similar to *telephone*. We say that lexically easy-to-recognize words have few **lexical neighbors**, or few words that are phonemically (or visually) similar, whereas lexically difficult-to-recognize words have many neighbors (Greenberg & Jenkins, 1964; Kirk, Pisoni, & Osberger,1995).

Lexical neighbors are words that are phonemically (or visually) similar.

Context

Words that are specified by context typically are easiest to recognize. For example, the word *table* is harder to identify when embedded in the sentence *Candace will buy the _____,* than in the sentence, *Candace will set the _____ and chairs in the kitchen*. Context cues provide cues for a word missed. Although *table* and *sable* are homophenes, and are acoustically similar, you probably would not mistake one word for the other because *table* makes more sense in this second sentence context. Grammatical structure also provides contextual cues. For instance, in the sentence, *The _____ read the book*, grammatical sentence structure specifies that the missing word is a common noun (Boothroyd, 1988).

Topical Cues Can Help

Simply knowing the topic of conversation can enhance a speech-reader's performance. For example, if you allow someone to read the word *homes* before asking the person to speechread the sentence, *She just moved into a three-bedroom apartment*, the person will speechread more words correctly than if no topical word is presented beforehand (Hanin, 1988). The sentence, *I cut my finger with a knife*, will be easier to speechread if it is preceded with a related sentence such as, *I was careless with a sharp blade*, than if it is preceded by an unrelated sentence such as, *You need special watering tools* (Gagné, Tugby, & Michaud, 1991).

The Environment and Communication Situation

The third factor that can affect speechreading performance is the environment.

Viewing Angle

If the speechreader sees the talker full-face, rather than in profile or turned at an angle, the speechreader will recognize more words (Figure 8–1). If a conversation is occurring in a group setting, as in a conference held around a rectangular table, the speechreader may miss the beginnings of many utterances, as one person and then another interjects comments in the discussion, because the speechreader must locate the talker first. The individual often may not have an advantageous viewing

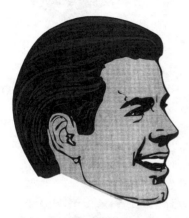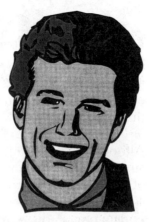

Figure 8–1. Talkers seen head-on are easier to speechread than talkers viewed in profile.

angle of the talker, particularly if the talkers turn their heads toward various participants as they speak.

Distance From the Talker

Distance from the talker also can affect performance, particularly if the speechreader is too far away to view the talker's mouth movements (Figure 8–2). A child speechreading from the back row of a classroom will not recognize as much of the teacher's spoken message as one who sits in the front row, and who has *favorable seating*. A good distance for speechreading is approximately 3 to 6 feet from the talker.

Room Conditions

A poorly-lit talker, who speaks in front of a light source so that shadows appear on the face, will be relatively difficult to speechread (Figure 8–3) and so will one who stands before a bright window in a room with no overhead lights. Light shining in the eyes of the speechreader can impair performance. Other factors that exert an effect include room reverberation, the availability of assistive devices, interfering objects, such as a support beam extending from a room's floor to ceiling, visual distractions, and room noise.

Favorable seating for speechreading includes being close enough to see the talker's lip movements, being able to see the talker full-face, rather than in profile, and having the talker's face well lit.

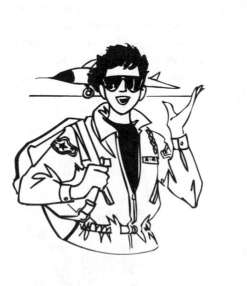 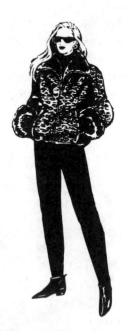

Figure 8-2. Distance from the talker will affect a person's speechreading performance. This is one reason why a child should have favorable seating in the classroom.

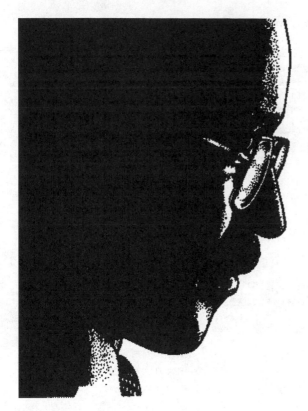

Figure 8-3. Poorly lit talkers are difficult to speechread.

Background noise. Just as with listening performance, the presence of background noise can impair someone's speechreading performance. Table 8–5 lists common sources of room noise that can interfere with the speechreading task. A noisy environment can mask speech and decrease the speechreading enhancement effect afforded by residual hearing, as well as distract the speechreader from the speech recognition task (Figure 8–4). The presence of visible movement, such as movement by others in the room or activity seen from a window, also can be distracting.

The Speechreader

Finally, variables related to the individual can affect the person's speechreading performance.

Innate Skill and Hearing Acuity

Speechreading performance relates to lipreading skill, as well as to an individual's hearing acuity. Generally, the better the

Table 8–5. Examples of noise sources common to various communication settings.

Home	Restaurants	Workplace	Classroom
Kitchen sink/running water	Dishes/ silverware	Computers	Children talking
Washer/dryer	Music	Printers	Paper rustling
Air conditioner	Guests talking	Machinery	Shoes scuffling
Furnace			Chairs moving
Vacuum cleaner			Projectors
Television			Fans, ventilators, furnace, air conditioner
Radio			Hall noise
Family members talking			
Open window/ door (lawn mower, leaf blower, traffic)			
Refrigerator			

lipreading skill and the greater the amount of residual hearing, the better the speechreading performance. However, the nature of the hearing loss also affects performance. For example, two persons may have severe hearing losses. If one has a conductive loss and the other has a sensorineural loss, the latter individual may have poorer speech discrimination, and therefore may perform more poorly on a speechreading task.

Speechreading and lipreading performance also is influenced by individuals' use of appropriate amplification and use of eyeglasses when needed. Poor visual acuity, such as that stemming from cataracts, will of course hinder performance.

Emotional and Physical State

An individual's level of stress, fatigue, and attentiveness can affect performance. For example, if the speechreader is engaged in a job interview, anxiety may impair his or her speechreading performance. A businessman may not speechread family members very well at home because he is fatigued

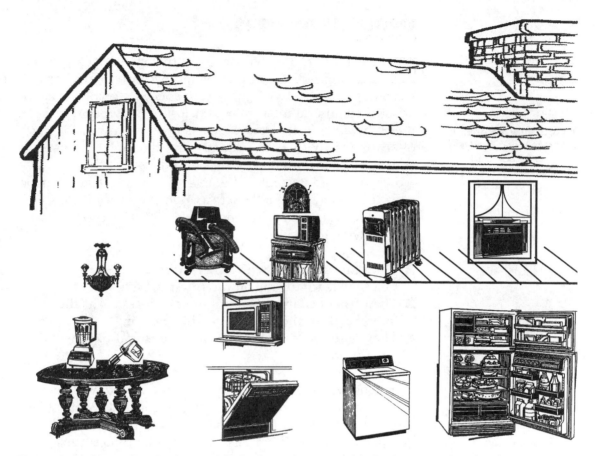

Figure 8–4. A sample of noise sources that may be present in the home environment.

from a long day of concentrating on co-workers' auditory and visual signals.

Speechreading as an Art Form

Evelyn Glennie is a classical percussionist who has a profound hearing loss. In a 1995 radio interview (KMOX, St. Louis), she was asked why she speechreads so well. Ms. Glennie replied that she approaches speechreading in the same way that many people with normal hearing listen to music. At a symphony, audience members do not necessarily attend to every note, but rather, attend to the structure of the music and the interplay of the various instruments. Similarly, Ms. Glennie explained, she does not try to speechread every word. She follows the message as it is conveyed by the words she recognizes, by what has been said beforehand, and by the talker's facial expressions, head nods, body posture and hand gestures.

ORAL INTERPRETERS

The final topic to be considered in this chapter concerning speechreading is the oral interpreter. Because many hard-of-hearing persons rely on the visual speech signal, occasions arise when an oral interpreter is helpful or even essential. An *oral interpreter* is someone who sits in clear view of the hard-of-hearing individual and silently repeats a talker's message as it is spoken, often lagging behind by only one or two words. An oral interpreter attempts to convey a talker's mood and intent. They must adhere to a Code of Ethics (1984), which dictates their professional code of behavior. This code includes the following guidelines:

An **oral interpreter** sits in clear view of a hard-of-hearing person and silently repeats a talker's message as it is spoken.

■ **They cannot share with other individuals information they learn during an interpreting assignment.**
■ **They cannot change the meaning of a message as they interpret it for the hard-of-hearing person.**
■ **They cannot add their opinions or personal commentary to a message.**

Situations where an oral interpreter may be required include meetings, lectures, churches or synagogues, and courts of law. Castle (1988) notes that group situations, panels of talkers, and question-and-answer periods may often be difficult for those with hearing loss. In these situations, speechreaders may not know where to look as speaking turns shift rapidly, and the talkers turn this way or that way as they speak. An oral interpreter in these situations can alleviate communication difficulties.

As a speech and hearing professional, you may be asked on occasion to help locate an oral interpreter for a hard-of-hearing person. Possible sources for finding one are listed in the Key Resources section at the end of this chapter.

Bisensory Perception

What we see may influence what we hear, and what we hear may influence what we see. One of the most dramatic demonstrations of this point is what has become known as the "McGurk Effect," so called because it first was described in an investigation reported by McGurk and MacDonald (1976).

McGurk and MacDonald presented discrepant auditory and visual speech stimuli to a group of normal-hearing subjects. The stimuli were consonant-vowel monosyllables. For example, a subject may have heard the syllable *ba* while simultaneously seeing someone speak *da*. For some combinations of consonants, subjects heard a third consonant that differed from the two syllables. When they heard *ba* and saw *ga*, they typically perceived the syllable *da*. These results suggest that, when we recognize speech, we integrate auditory and visual speech information as we decode the signal.

FINAL REMARKS

Intuitively we associate speech recognition with the sense of hearing. However, as we have learned in this chapter, the sense of sight also can be an important component in our everyday communication. In fact, persons with hearing loss may be very reliant on their vision for recognizing spoken messages. A topic that currently is receiving much attention in the research literature pertains to auditory-vision integration; that is, how we combine the disparate auditory and visual signal of a talker into a unified percept (e.g., Massaro, 1987). The answer to this question may have important theoretical implications for models of speech perception. For our present purposes, this is an interesting question because exploring the answer may help us design more effective speech perception training protocols.

KEY CHAPTER POINTS

✔ Even persons with normal hearing rely on speechreading to some degree.
✔ Some people are better speechreaders than others. The reasons for this are unclear. Performance cannot be predicted by such factors as intelligence or practice with the speechreading task.
✔ Lipreading is difficult. Some of the factors that may compound the lipreading task include the partial visibility or nonvisibility of many speech sounds on the face, the rapidity of speech, coarticulation, the visual similarity of many sound groups, and talker eccentricities. For instance, the

words *Bob* and *Mom* are indistinguishable on the lips. The word *hick* requires minimal visible mouth movement.

✔ A little bit of residual hearing can increase markedly one's ability to recognize speech when looking and listening simultaneously.

✔ The talker, message, environment, and state of the person affect how well the individual will recognize a spoken message. For instance, a talker who mumbles will be difficult to understand.

KEY RESOURCES

Sources for Oral Interpreters

Speechreaders may locate an oral interpreter by investigating the following resources:

■ The telephone directory, under local interpreter referral center
■ A local university or college that provides speech and hearing services
■ Programs or agencies serving hard-of-hearing adults or other persons with disabilities
■ The State Office of Vocational Rehabilitation (OVR)
■ An audiology clinic
■ An otolaryngologist's office
■ Clubs and organizations for deaf and hard-of-hearing individuals
■ Other persons with hearing loss

Speechreading Training

Topics

- Candidacy

- Traditional Methods of Speechreading Training

- Developing Speechreading Skills

- Analytic Speechreading Training Objectives

- Synthetic Speechreading Training Objectives

- Efficacy of Speechreading Training

- Oral Interpreting

- Final Remarks

- Key Chapter Points

In this chapter, we will consider speechreading training, including candidacy issues, training philosophies, training techniques, and training efficacy. At the beginning of the 20th century, speechreading training was a principal component of most aural rehabilitation programs, in large part because there were few alternative means for alleviating communication problems experienced by persons with hearing loss. We simply did not have the technology to reduce hearing difficulties. In those times, persons would attend speechreading classes and perform drill activities at home.

With the advent of hearing aids, cochlear implants, and assistive listening devices, individuals are better able to use their residual hearing. Concomitantly the popularity of speechreading training has waned, so that now it rarely is found as the sole element of an aural rehabilitation program.

CANDIDACY

Who is a candidate for speechreading training? The answer to this question depends in part on who you ask. In this text, it is suggested that children may benefit from training, especially if they use simultaneous communication (Chapter 15) and do not rely solely on speechreading for everyday communication (i.e., children who use both speech and manually coded English to communicate). Adults who have recently lost their hearing also may be candidates for training. In addition to improving their speechreading skills, they may receive psychological benefits from participating in a program, feeling that they have taken constructive action to deal with their hearing losses. Adults who have a hearing loss that is long-standing may benefit more from other types of aural rehabilitation intervention than speechreading training, interventions such as communication strategies training.

TRADITIONAL METHODS OF SPEECHREADING TRAINING

In this century, four speechreading training methods have been popular in the United States (Berger, 1972; Jeffers & Barley, 1972). These methods were advocated originally by Bruhn, the Nitchies, the Kinzes, and Bunger.

In about 1912 Martha Emma Bruhn introduced the Mueller-Walle method, a method that originated in Germany. The hallmark feature of this program was an emphasis on rapid syllable drill, such as *she-ma-flea* and *she-may-free*. Students also practiced recognizing homophenous words, using sentence context cues to distinguish between possible meanings.

Edward B. Nitchie, who published his first book, *Lip-reading Principles and Practices* in 1912, rarely employed syllable drill. Instead, he emphasized the importance of psychological processes of speechreading. Practice usually centered on sentence materials and the identification of homophenous words through contextual cues. Students sometimes practiced speechreading themselves by talking before a mirror. Training materials were presented without voice. Nitchie's text was updated by his wife Elizabeth in 1940, and it has been one of the most widely read texts on the subject in the 20th century.

Cora Kinze studied with both Bruhn and Nitchie before establishing her own school for speechreading training with her sister Rose in 1917. Not surprisingly, the sisters developed an eclectic method, combining the analytic syllable drill of Bruhn with the more synthetic exercises of Nitchie.

The Jena Method was developed by Karl Brauckmann who lived in the city of Jena, Germany and published two brief textbooks in 1925. The Jena method was introduced to the United States by Anna Bunger. A hallmark of Brauckmann's approach was its emphasis on *mimetic* and *kinesthetic* forms and sensations, and the recognition that our ability to produce speech relates to our ability to perceive it. In this method, students focus on the mouth movements of the instructor, while simultaneously speaking the training materials. Training materials include repeated syllables and then words derived from the syllables.

Mimetic means imitating or copying movements.
Kinesthetic relates to the perception of movement, position, and tension of body parts.

Some of the fundamental principles underlying these seminal training programs are evident in more modern training curricula. Students' attention typically is focused on sound identification (as in the Mueller-Walle method), as well as on recognizing the gist of a sentence (following Nitchie). Most contemporary programs recommend that training items be presented with both the auditory and the visual signals. The notions of kinesthetic awareness of one's own speech production and of lipreading one's own speech either via a mirror or videotape has enjoyed recent attention (as with the Jena method), as investigators have attempted to show that production practice enhances perception performance, with modest success (De Filippo, Sims, & Gottermeier, 1995; van Uden, 1983).

DEVELOPING SPEECHREADING SKILLS

The first class of a communication training program often is informational in nature and includes a consideration of the speechreading process. A handout like the one reprinted in Table 9–1 might be used to guide discussion among adult clients. This handout reviews factors that affect the speechreading process, and the importance of using speechreading cues maximally.

In addition to considering the principles outlined in Table 9-1, class participants also might be asked to reflect on their speechreading habits and listening difficulties. They often review rules to follow when speechreading, such as those listed in Table 9–2. For instance, although *Watch the talker's lips*, the first rule presented in Table 9–2, seems like an obvious recommendation, some people become distracted by watching the talker's hand gestures or they have a habit of listening with lowered eye gaze, instead of concentrating on the talker's mouth movements. As a result, their speechreading performance is not as good as it could be.

Finally, during an introduction to speechreading, class participants might review charts like the one presented in Figure 9–1 to identify difficult listening situations and to formulate solutions for rectifying the difficulties. They might be asked to identify which seats in Figure 9–1 present the most favorable circumstances for lipreading and speechreading, and which seats present the least favorable. This kind of activity sensitizes students to the concept of favorable speechreading conditions.

Following this kind of introduction, the class may (or may not) receive formal speechreading training. In today's world, rarely if ever do participants in an aural rehabilitation class practice lipreading (vision-only speech recognition). Rather, they practice recognizing speech using both the auditory and visual signals. As noted, children are more likely to receive formal speechreading training than adults. This is especially true for those who have received a cochlear implant. As with formal auditory training, formal speechreading training objectives can be divided into two categories: analytic and synthetic.

Table 9–1. A handout that might be distributed at an adult rehabilitation class in order to stimulate discussion about the speechreading process.

Speechreading is a process of attending to auditory and visual information to recognize a spoken message. Speechreading is not just watching others' lips to identify the words they are saying. It also consists of making the most of your hearing, and using your mind to collect all the information available to make a "best guess." Speechreading includes the following:

1. **Lipreading.** Watch the mouth movements of the talker, including the lips, jaw, and tongue tip. It is impossible to identify every word, but you can identify some words and sounds that will help you ascertain what is being said.

2. **Facial expression.** It is possible to identify people's moods or how they feel by the expression on their faces. You can also glean subtle nuances of meaning in their messages by attending to facial expressions.

3. **Gesture, posture, and movement.** What people are doing, how they are sitting, and the gestures they make give clues to what they are thinking about and what they might say.

4. **Situational cues.** You can anticipate what a person is going to talk about by the situation or place they are in and the relationships of the people present.

5. **Knowing the topic.** It is easier to follow conversation when you know what the talker is talking about. The easiest way to find out is to ask someone else who is listening. You might say, "What are we discussing?"

6. **Knowledge of language.** You might be able to make educated guesses about a particular word missed on the basis of sentence structure.

7. **Keeping informed.** Knowing what news items or subjects are of current interest to people may help you to anticipate what will be talked about. Read newspapers and magazines and watch the news on television.

8. **Emotional factors.** Keep motivated and develop self-confidence even though there will be times that you make errors.

9. **Use your hearing.** Although you have a hearing loss, you may be able to hear sounds and words that help you to identify the message or idea.

Until now, you *have* been taking advantage of these clues to some extent. One goal of this class is to make you more conscious of them so you use them maximally. Using these clues, much of the message can be predicted. Some parts of the message are less predictable (e.g., hearing a new name), making them more difficult. Therefore, you must use two kinds of information: (a) the part of the message you did understand and (b) any additional knowledge that can help you to fill in the gaps in order to figure out the whole message.

Source: Adapted from "Speechreading instruction for adults: Issues and practices," by R. Cherry & A. Rubinstein, 1988, p. 302. *Volta Review,* 90.

Table 9–2. Rules to follow when speechreading. A handout like this might be discussed during a group class.

---

1. **Watch the talker's lips.**
   This seems obvious, but often, a speechreader can be distracted by other events in the room, or the talker's hand gestures. Also, there may be a tendency to watch the talker's eyes instead of the mouth.

2. **Provide information to the talker about how to communicate with you.**
   This may include asking the talker to speak clearly and at a slightly louder than normal conversational level. The talker should not shout or exaggerate lip movements. The talker should face you when speaking, and should not chew or cover the mouth, such as with a hand.

3. **Try to ensure that the room is well-lit and that your position in the room allows for optimal speechreading performance.**
   You will want to find a seat where light does not shine in your eyes and adjust light sources so they do not cast shadows on the talker's face. Position yourself near enough to the talker so you can clearly see the talker's mouth and facial expressions.

4. **Try to minimize background noise.**
   Background noise might be minimized by ensuring that radios and televisions are turned down or off. Favorable seating, say at a table away from the kitchen in a restaurant, may also minimize background noise.

5. **Know the topic of conversation.**
   During a conversation, ask someone the topic of conversation. It is much easier to recognize a message if you know what is being discussed. If you know in advance that a specific topic will be discussed, try to learn something about it beforehand.

6. **Pay attention to context cues.**
   The situation in which the conversation occurs may provide information about what is being said. The talker's facial expressions and what has been discussed beforehand may also be informative.

7. **Keep a positive attitude.**
   Speechreading can be tiring. Stay motivated, and do not be distracted by your own anxiety and self-doubts.

ANALYTIC SPEECHREADING TRAINING

Analytic speechreading training objectives are directed toward developing vowel recognition and consonant recognition skills. The logic underlying many speechreading curricula is gradually to increase patients' reliance on the auditory signal

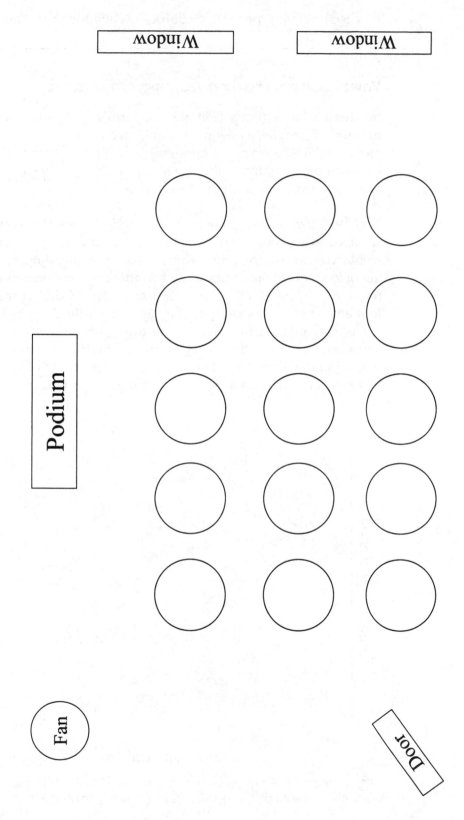

Figure 9-1. A chart that can be used when discussing listening environments and ways to minimize speechreading difficulties. Students might be asked to identify where they might sit to optimize speechreading performance.

for discriminating phonemic contrasts while they speechread (Figure 9-2).

Vowel Speechreading Training Objectives

In Chapter 7, Auditory Training, the term *vowel formant* was defined. To review, vowel formants are resonances in the mouth, which cause some frequencies of the speech signal to have more energy than other frequencies. Every vowel can be distinguished by its formant patterns.

Table 9–3 presents one possible hierarchy of analytic vowel speechreading training objectives. If a person has only rudimentary speech recognition skills, initial speechreading training objectives should focus his or her attention on distinguishing /i/, /u/, and /a/. These sounds differ both in their formant structure and in how they appear on the mouth. The /i/ is produced with a narrow mouth opening, with some spreading of the mouth corners. It has a first formant of low frequency, and a second formant of high frequency. Typically, the lips pucker and form a narrow opening when you phonate

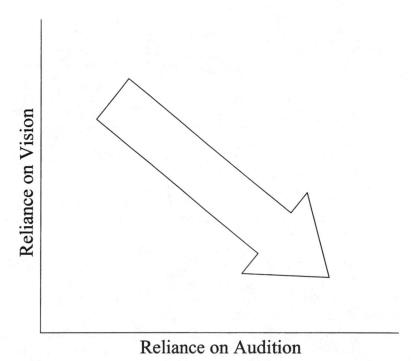

Figure 9–2. During speechreading training, patients become increasingly reliant on the auditory signal for speech recognition.

/u/, and both first and second formants have a relatively low frequency value. For /a/, the lips form a moderate opening and appear relaxed; the formants have mid-range values. Table 9–4 presents examples of word pairs that can be used in achieving the first three vowel speechreading training objectives listed in Table 9–3.

Consonant Speechreading Training Objectives

In our previous discussion concerning auditory training (Chapter 7), we considered three different types of speech features: manner, voice, and place of articulation, and noted that consonants can be characterized in terms of these three features. To review, manner denotes the type of articulatory gestures that you use to produce a particular sound. Manner categories include glides (e.g., /l/ as in *lip*), stops (such as /t/ in *top*), fricatives and affricatives (such as /f/ in *fruit*), and nasals (such as /n/ in *new*). The voicing feature indicates whether the vocal folds vibrate during the consonantal constriction, for example, /b/ is voiced whereas /p/ is not. The place of articulation feature indicates where in the mouth that the primary constriction occurs. Place designations include bilabial (such as /b/ as in

---

Table 9–3. Vowel analytic training objectives that were designed for young cochlear-implant users. These objectives are also appropriate for adults who have significant hearing loss.

The student:

---

1. Will discriminate words with /i/ and /u/; for example, *me* from *moo*.
2. Will discriminate words with /i/ and /a/; for example, *keep* from *cop*.
3. Will discriminate words with /u/ and /a/; for example, *coop* from *cop*.
4. Will identify words with /i/, /u/, and /a/, using a four-item and then six-item response set; for example, *bean* from the response set of: *bean, pot, pit,* and *pool*. The vowels in the response set may include vowels other than /i, u, a/.
5. Will identify words with /u/, /i/, and /a/ from an open set of familiar vocabulary.

Subsequent training that contrasts other vowels can be incorporated into consonant training activities.

Source: Adapted from Tye-Murray, N. (1992c). Speechreading training. In N. Tye-Murray (Ed.), *Children with cochlear implants: A handbook for parents, teachers, and speech and hearing professionals* (pp. 115–136). Washington, DC: Alexander Graham Bell Association for the Deaf.

boy), labiodental (/θ/ as in *thick*), linguadental (/f/), alveolar (e.g., /t/), palatal (e.g., /ð/) and velar (e.g., /g/).

It is fortuitous that the visual signal associated with consonant production ideally complements the auditory signal. Cues that signal manner and voice often are easier for hard-of-hearing persons to hear than are cues that signal place of articulation. For instance, someone with a severe hearing loss who uses amplification is likely to hear the difference between the words *bat* and *pat*. However, if presented with only the visual signal, these two words will be indistinguishable. In contrast, cues about place of articulation tend to be somewhat visible, but place of articulation is difficult to determine through listening alone for persons who have significant hearing loss. A hard-of-hearing individual might discriminate the words *pat* and *sat* if they can see the talker, but may not be able to discriminate them if they only hear the talker.

Table 9–4. Examples of word pairs that can be used in achieving the first three analytic vowel speechreading training objectives listed in Table 9–3.

Objective 1: The student will discriminate words with /i/ and /u/.

Word pairs:

beet/boot	see/soup	she/shoe
heat/hoot	leap/loop	peel/pool
read/root	jeep/jewel	sheet/shot
keep/coop	knee/new	geese/goose

Objective 2: The student will discriminate words with /i/ and /a/.

Word pairs:

heat/hot	keep/cop	cheap/chop
peak/pop	fear/far	deal/doll
see/sod	pea/pod	seed/sock
team/top	read/rod	jeep/job

Objective 3: The student will discriminate words with /u/ and /a/.

Word pairs:

two/top	clue/clock	goose/got
who/hot	pool/pot	suit/sock
juice/job	dew/dog	clue/clock
boot/box	room/rot	moose/moss

A list of consonant speechreading training objectives appears in Table 9–5. The first speechreading consonant training objectives may involve discriminating consonants that differ in place of production, and that share either voice or manner (Table 9–5). For example, a student may be asked to discriminate between the /p/ in *pay* and the /s/ in *say*. The clinician speaks the two items and the student then indicates whether they are the *same* or *different*. The clinician attempts to speak with constant loudness and intonation. The next two objectives require students to discriminate between consonants that share place, but that differ on other signal parameters (Objectives 2 and 3 in Table 9–5).

Table 9–6 presents examples of consonant pairs and words pairs that might be used for achieving the first three consonant speechreading training objectives presented in Table 9–5.

Table 9–5. Consonant analytic speechreading training designed for young cochlear-implant users. These objectives also are appropriate for adults who have significant hearing loss.

The student:

---

1. Will discriminate consonant pairs that differ in place of production and share either voice or manner, for example, *tag* from *bag*.

2. Will discriminate consonant pairs that share similar place of production but differ in manner and voice, for example, *pan* from *man*.

3. Will discriminate consonant pairs that share place and manner and/or voice, for example, *park* from *bark*.

4. Will identify consonants that share manner of production, using a four-item and then a six-item response set; for example, *tag* from the response set of: *tag, bag, back*, and *gas*.

5. Will identify consonants from a four-item and then a six-item response set of voiced or voiceless consonants; for example, *pop* from the response set of: *pop, cop, cap*, and *top*.

6. Will identify consonants that share place of production, using a four-item and then a six-item response set: for example, *pan* from the response set of: *pan, man, bat*, and *mat*.

7. Will identify words from an open set of familiar vocabulary.

Source: Adapted from Tye-Murray, N. (1992c). Speechreading training. In N. Tye-Murray (Ed.), *Children with cochlear implants: A handbook for parents, teachers, and speech and hearing professionals* (pp. 115–136). Washington, DC: Alexander Graham Bell Association for the Deaf.

Table 9–6. Examples of consonant and word pairs that can be used in achieving the first three consonant speechreading training objectives listed in Table 9–5.

Objective 1: The student will discriminate consonant pairs that differ in place of production and share either voice or manner.

Consonant pairs:

/m/ versus /d, dʒ, g, j, l/

/p/ versus /d, tʃ, g, ʃ, h, s/

/b/ versus /t, dʒ, n, k, j, l/

/d/ versus /k, j, dʒ/

Word pairs:

meat/geese	pill/chill	top/chop
moose/goose	pot/hot	boat/coat
bit/knit	dog/jog	peal/heal
make/lake	tear/chair	pin/chin

Objective 2: The student will discriminate consonant pairs that share similar place of production but differ in manner and voice.

Consonant pairs:

/p/ versus /m, w/

/d/ versus /s/

/t/ versus /l, n/

/k/ versus /j, dʒ/

/g/ versus /ʃdʒ, tʃ/

Word pairs:

pan/man	tip/lip	geese/cheese
toe/low	day/say	deal/seal
dip/sip	pen/men	game/chain
tan/land	car/jar	tail/nail

Objective 3: The student will discriminate consonant pairs that share place and manner and/or voice.

Consonant pairs:

/b/ versus /m, p, w/

/d/ versus /n, t, l/

/v/ versus /f/

/t/ versus /s/

/k/ versus /g, ʃ, tʃ/

Word pairs:

bat/mat	keep/cheek	van/fan
dog/log	beak/week`	cap/gap
bun/one	tail/sail	doe/no
cat/gas	two/sue	curl/girl

After a student achieves the first three consonant speechreading training objectives, intermediate objectives in a speechreading curriculum (Objectives 4 and 5 in Table 9–5) might focus attention on identifying consonants that share manner and/or voice. The student will progress from performing a discrimination task, as in the first three speechreading training objectives, to performing a closed-set identification task. For example, individuals might identify the word *cat* from the response set of *cat*, *pat*, *pet*, and *kit*, words that all begin with voiceless consonants. Following a discrimination activity, they then may perform an identification activity, using a closed-set response format. For this kind of training activity, the clinician might set before the individual a set of six picture cards, such as the set shown in Figure 9–3. The clinician then speaks one of the items, and the student indicates which item was spoken. This kind of task is a precursor to open-set word recognition. Table 9–7 presents stimuli that might be appropriate when the goal is to identify words beginning with the /p/ and /b/ phonemes. (Figure 9–3 presents a corresponding picture set.)

Advanced objectives for consonant speechreading training (Objectives 6 and 7 in Table 9–5) often focus attention on identifying consonants that share place and manner, place and voice, or place, manner and voice in a closed-set and then an open-set format. For example, students may be asked to identify /p/ as in *pole* when one of the foils is *bowl*. The /p/ and /b/ sounds are visually and acoustically similar.

Synthetic Speechreading Training

In comparison with sentence-level auditory training objectives, sentence-level speechreading training objectives will begin with more challenging tasks (Figure 9–4). This is because most people can recognize more speech when they can both see and hear rather than only hear a talker. For example, if the student is a child, the first task in a speechreading training curriculum may be to practice recognizing simple directions. Such a task would occur much later in an auditory training curriculum.

Table 9–8 presents a sample hierarchy of synthetic speechreading training objectives. The first objective requires students to follow simple directions, in a closed-set format. Initially, the set should be small. For example, two crayons, blue and orange, might be placed before a young child. The clinician asks the child to draw a blue beach ball. As the youth advances,

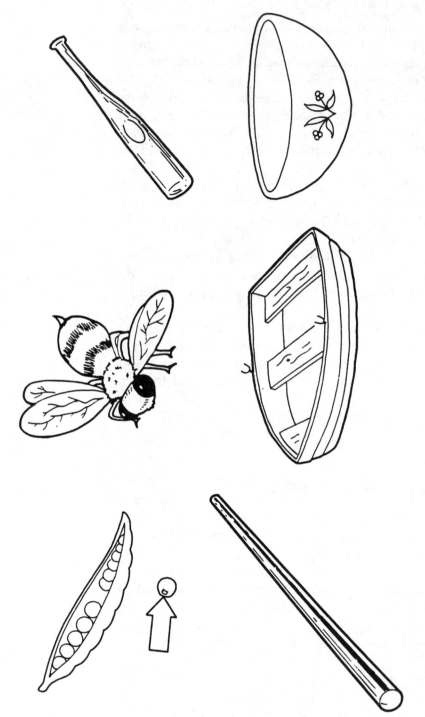

Figure 9-3. Illustrations that can be used with a closed-set identification task. (From *Communication Training for Hearing-impaired Children and Teenagers* (p. 18) by N. Tye-Murray, 1993. Austin, TX: Pro-Ed. Reprinted with permission.)

Table 9–7. Stimuli used for an identification activity when the target phonemes are /p/ and /b/ . A clinician might present each item five or more times during the training session. When the student can read and has fairly good listening skills, the target items can be more similar (i.e., they might rhyme), and the response choices can be presented orthographically.

That's the pole.

That's the boat.

That's the bowl.

That's the pea.

That's the bee.

That's the bat.

Source: Adapted from Tye-Murray, N. (1993b). *Communication training for hearing-impaired children and teenagers.* Austin, TX: Pro-Ed.

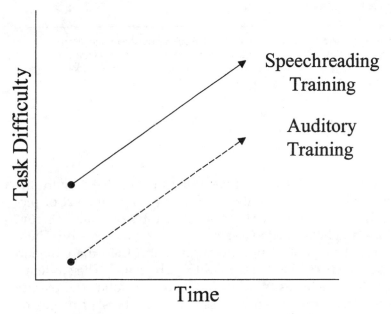

Figure 9–4. Initial synthetic speechreading tasks typically are more difficult than those for auditory training.

the set is enlarged, and the directions become more complex. In more advanced exercises, the clinician might present the following directions:

1. Color the ball orange.
2. Color the sand yellow.
3. Color the shovel purple.

Table 9–8. Synthetic speechreading training objectives designed for young cochlear-implant users . These objectives can be modified to meet the maturity and cognitive levels of adults who have significant hearing loss.

The student:

---

1. Will follow simple directions using a closed response set.

2. Will identify a sentence illustration from a set of four dissimilar pictures.

3. Will identify a sentence illustration from a set of four similar pictures.

4. Will listen to topic-related sentences, and repeat or paraphrase them.

5. Will listen to two related sentences, and then draw a picture about them or paraphrase them.

6. Will speechread a paragraph-long narrative and then answer questions about it.

Source: Adapted from Tye-Murray, N. (1992c). Speechreading training. In N. Tye-Murray (Ed.), *Children with cochlear implants: A handbook for parents teachers and speech and hearing professionals* (pp. 115–136). Washington, DC: Alexander Graham Bell Association for the Deaf.

4. Color the sky blue.
5. Color the water blue.

The second and third objectives listed in Table 9–8 require the individual to identify sentence illustrations from a set of pictures. The clinician might lay a set of pictures on a table (Figure 9–5) that might be used in a sentence recognition exercise. These are placed in front of the individual, and then the clinician speaks sentences that correspond to each picture. The student's task is to speechread the clinician, and then touch the picture that illustrates the sentence. Postcards, snapshots, or magazine pictures can be used to construct picture sets. Several sentences can be developed for each picture so that a single set can provide practice for speechreading a large number of sentences.

The fourth objective for synthetic level training requires the student to recognize topic-related sentences. These are sentences that concern a common theme. A set of topic-related sentences appears in Table 9–9 as an example.

The final objectives for formal synthetic speechreading training require students to speechread paragraphs. The clinician might present a picture that provides contextual cues for rec-

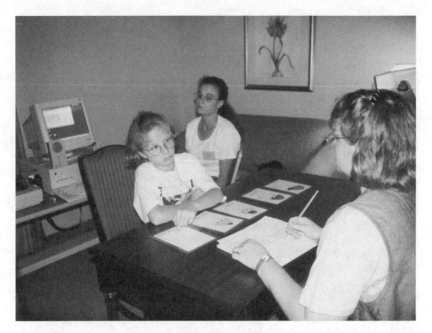

Figure 9-5. A clinician and child performing a sentence-recognition task using picture cards. By Kim Readmond, CID.

Table 9-9. Example of a set of topic-related sentences that can be utilized in achieving the fourth objective for synthetic speechreading training: The student will listen to topic-related sentences, and repeat or paraphrase them.

Sentences concerning cooking:

---

1. I added a cup of flour.
2. The bread is in the oven.
3. Will you hand me the measuring cup?
4. I need the box of sugar.
5. The mixer is in the cabinet.
6. The oven is set to 300 degrees.
7. Put the bowl in the sink, please.
8. The pan is filled with batter.
9. I will beat the eggs.
10. Please pour a cup of milk.

---

ognizing the passage. As in a continuous discourse tracking task (Chapter 3), the patient must repeat (or in this task, paraphrasing is also permitted) each sentence after speechreading the clinician speak sentences one at a time from a paragraph.

A **holistic** approach to speechreading incorporates several methods and includes the child in setting goals.

A Holistic Approach to Speechreading Training for Children

Yoshinaga-Itano (1988) describes a *holistic* approach that can be used to teach children speechreading. The training goals of this approach can be summarized as follows (Yoshinaga-Itano, 1988):

■ "Increase the child's knowledge of the speechreading process.
■ Increase the child's ability to generate strategies to facilitate more successful communication.
■ Increase the child's ability to generate strategies to facilitate more successful communication.
■ Increase the child's confidence in the efficacy of speechreading by providing situations that ensure a high probability of success.
■ Increase the child's tolerance for communicative situations that have a higher degree of frustration.
■ Increase the child's ability to generate personal goals for improving speechreading.
■ Increase the child's motivation to improve speechreading abilities" (p. 244).

In implementing a holistic approach, Yoshinaga-Itano suggests that children should participate in setting goals and should make a commitment to accomplish them. The holistic program should allow for both self-evaluation and clinician-evaluation, and speechreading practice should be provided in real-life versus drill situations.

EFFICACY OF SPEECHREADING TRAINING

Many researchers have considered whether speechreading skills can be developed through training and practice. At present, this issue has not been resolved clearly; some investigators report that training improves performance (e.g., Walden, Erdman, Montgomery, Schwartz, & Prosek, 1981; Walden, Prosek, Montgomery, Scherr, & Jones, 1977), whereas others report that speechreading training provides little measurable benefit (e.g., Heider & Heider, 1940; Lesner, Sandridge, & Kricos, 1987). When improvements do occur, they appear to be modest. For instance, investigators have demonstrated that adults with hearing impairment show only small improvement following training, typically improving by 10–15% in their ability to recognize speech stimuli (e.g., Alcantara, Cowan, Blamey, & Clark, 1990; Gagné, Dinon, & Parsons, 1991; Walden, Erdman, Montgomery, Schwartz, & Prosek, 1981).

Often, results are inconclusive or present contradictory findings. Some people may not show improvement in their performance on a test of audiovisual speech recognition. However, if you ask them whether they feel they benefited from speechreading training, they may provide an ardent testimonial in support of training (Binnie, 1977). Some individuals may become better test takers, so their speechreading skills only appear to improve, rather than actually improving. For instance, Gagné et al. (1991) evaluated the effectiveness of a computerized speechreading training program, in which participants received speechreading practice by using a modified continuous discourse tracking procedure. Changes in speechreading performance were determined by comparing scores on standard speech recognition tests obtained prior to the training program to scores obtained after training. The participants did not improve on most of the standard tests. However, they were able to repeat more words verbatim per minute during the continuous discourse tracking task post-training than pretraining. The researchers cautioned that the improved tracking rates might have resulted from 25–30 hours of practice with the tracking procedure during training, rather than from improved visual speech recognition skills.

Few investigators have examined the extent to which children improve following training. It is possible that they have more potential to benefit from this kind of training than do adults.

FINAL COMMENTS

At one time, many adults received aural rehabilitation that was comprised primarily of speechreading training. With the advent of sophisticated listening devices, and the increase of communication strategies training, few adults receive a great deal of speechreading training, and rarely is it provided in the absence of other aural rehabilitation services. Nonetheless, it is important for persons with hearing impairment to understand why speechreading is so difficult. The emphasis of speechreading training may be on ways to minimize the difficulty of the task, such as ways to manage the environment or ways to encourage appropriate speaking behaviors on the part of their communication partners.

KEY CHAPTER POINTS

✔ Speechreading training was very popular in the first half of the 20th century. The advent of more sophisticated listening devices, and questions about the benefits of training, have led to a reduced emphasis on speechreading training in an aural rehabilitation program.

✔ As with auditory training, a speechreading training program typically includes both analytic and synthetic training objectives.

✔ The logic underlying many speechreading curricula is gradually to increase students' reliance on the auditory signal for recognizing phonemic contrasts.

✔ Research suggests that speechreading training provides only modest if any benefit for adults. Little research has been performed with children.

PART III

---

*Aural Rehabilitation
for Adults*

10

Adults Who Have Hearing Loss

Topics

One of the major forces shaping American society at the onset of the third millennium is the aging of our population. As the baby boom generation matures, an increasing number of adults are seeking hearing-related services. In this chapter, we will be concerned with persons who are over the age of 16 years. Although much of what we review will be applicable to the entire adult population, Chapter 12 is devoted to special considerations for older adults, individuals who are over the age of 65 years.

It is important to develop a good sense of who the patient is and where the person is in terms of adjusting to hearing loss. We will consider first the "who" issue, and then the "where-in-terms-of-adjustment." Our guiding theme is as follows:

Any successful aural rehabilitation plan must be founded on a patient orientation.

A **patient orientation** to rehabilitation designs and delivers rehabilitation services based on the patient's background, current status, needs, and wants.

A **sales orientation** to rehabilitation emphasizes persuading the patient to pursue and procure services, interventions, and listening devices.

This is a simple idea that is the essence of a service practice. A *patient orientation* holds that the most successful aural rehabilitation program is one that best determines individuals' backgrounds, current status, needs, and wants and then accommodates them through the design and delivery of appropriate interventions. This is in contrast to a *sales orientation*, in which the emphasis is on telling or persuading people that they need certain aural rehabilitation services or listening devices and that your practice is better than the competition at providing them.

As we shall see, this philosophic orientation does not mean that we must begin with a blank slate with every new patient. Rather, certain aural rehabilitation offerings may be more appropriate for some persons than for others, and variable parameters of those services can be adjusted to meet a targeted individual need. A person who has minimal residual hearing may not receive auditory training, but rather, communication strategies and speechreading training. An individual with a mild hearing loss may receive only a hearing aid and counseling.

An important outcome of this philosophy is a high level of patient satisfaction with the aural rehabilitation plan. Individuals who receive services based on a patient orientation model usually report improved adjustment to hearing loss. They may remark, "The communication strategies program was great—I feel more in control of my hearing problems now," or, "My audiologist took the time to listen, and the hearing aid she gave me made a big difference in my ability to perform at work." Such satisfaction ensures continued compliance with the plan, as well as positive word-of-mouth publicity for your service. This, in turn, will allow you to attract and serve even more people.

HEARING LOSS AMONG ADULTS

Most adults lose their hearing gradually over time. The largest segment of the hard-of-hearing adult population has mild or moderate sensorineural hearing loss. Typically, thresholds for the mid and high frequencies are poorer than those for the lower frequencies, regardless of the patient's age. The magnitude of hearing loss tends to progress with advancing age.

Hard-of-hearing adults may perceive conversational speech as too soft and as sounding mumbled. The greater loss of sensitivity in the higher frequencies compared to the milder loss in the lower frequencies often results in reception of the low-pitched acoustic segments associated with vowel sounds but not the high-pitched segments associated with consonant sounds. Hence, a commonly heard complaint among hard-of-hearing adults is, "I can hear people talk but I can't understand what they say." The presence of background noise exacerbates this problem because it can further mask the high-pitched consonant sounds that are difficult to discriminate even in quiet. Similarly, females or children may be more difficult to understand than males, due to their characteristically high-pitched voices and softer speaking levels.

Although hard-of-hearing adults do not comprise a homogeneous group, trends have been identified in the demographic data. In terms of probability, the typical hearing-impaired adult is a white Caucasian male with a family income of less than $7,000 (in 1977 dollars) and an educational experience of less than 12 years. More males than females have hearing problems and those with less education and/or lower incomes are more likely to have hearing loss than those with more education and/or higher incomes. The incidence of hearing loss is greater among white Caucasians than African Americans. Age also is a factor. For instance, a 25-year-old man may have a pure-tone average of 5 dB, whereas a 65 year-old may have a loss of 22 dB (Ries, 1991).

WHO IS THIS PERSON?

In addressing the question, "Who is my patient?" you will consider a number of non-hearing-related variables, including a patient's stage of life, socioeconomic status, race and ethnicity, gender, life factors, and psychological adjustment (Figure 10–1).

Stage of Life

Jim Lawson and his 20-year-old son Kevin were in a car accident. Both received head trauma and, as a result, incurred irreversible bilateral hearing losses (Figure 10–2).

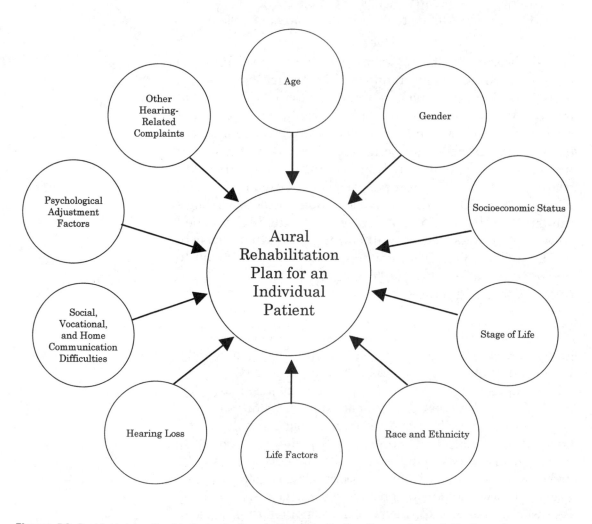

Figure 10–1. Variables that influence the design of a patient's aural rehabilitation plan.

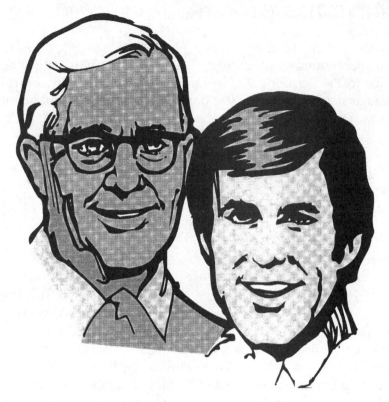

Figure 10–2. An aural rehabilitation plan may vary as a function of a patient's stage of life.

For both Lawsons, life with hearing loss will never be like it was before the accident. However, the impact differs somewhat because the two men are in different stages of life.

Jim Lawson owns a small advertising firm, which he started after college graduation. After many years of long hours and hard work, the firm is well-established and successful.

The accident has left Jim filled with bitterness. He believes life has dealt him a blow just when he was experiencing decreased responsibilities and more freedom to pursue leisure activities. He now contemplates early retirement because his hearing loss interferes with his ability to interact with clients, but also has misgivings because he had hoped to have a larger savings account before retiring. Jim no longer socializes at executive meetings and plays less tennis because he cannot converse easily with his friends on the court. He feels old and frequently is saddened by passing thoughts, such as the fact that he will never hear the voices of his grandchildren. Increasingly, he depends on his wife for communication with the outside world.

Jim's son is a junior in college with a major in public relations. Prior to the accident, Kevin Lawson participated in several extracurricular activities and dreamed of creating a public relations empire.

The hearing loss has left Kevin deflated. Because public relations entails communication, he wonders whether he should complete his college program. He feels embarrassed by the use of a professional notetaker in class, but fears that asking classmates to share notes might elicit pity. Kevin spends hours alone in the gym lifting weights, bedeviled by concerns for his future.

Life stages are ranges in which a hearing loss may have a different impact.

Table 10–1 summarizes *life stages* and indicates how hearing loss may have an impact (Van Hecke, 1994). Hard-of-hearing persons often experience similar emotions such as frustration and they experience common difficulties such as communication breakdown. However, as the example of the Lawson family illustrates, the impact of hearing loss relates to an individual's *stage of life*: that is, whether the individual is in young adulthood, in the 30s, 40s, 50s, or in the later years. Depending on their life stage, patients will confront different issues. By being sensitive to where they are in the life span, you will gain additional insight into their concerns and aural rehabilitation needs.

Life Factors

Life factors are conditions that help define one's life, such as relationships, family, and vocation.

By adulthood, most people have achieved what Kyle et al. (1987, following Rothschild [1981]) characterized as socialization. They have established relationships with others, embarked on a vocation, and developed a personality and a personal view of the world. *Life factors* are in place. These factors may be socially and culturally determined, controlled by the individual, fixed, determined by the environment, or influenced by other qualities of the individual and his or her life situation. As with demographic factors, life factors influence the ways in which people cope with the advent of hearing loss. For instance, an individual with a heart problem and an extended family may not be as concerned about a subsequent mild or moderate hearing loss than someone who has been

Table 10-1. Life stages and the impact of hearing loss (see Van Hecke, 1994).

Stage	Events Associated With Stage	Impact of Hearing Loss
Young adulthood	Develop intimate relationships with others	Begin to reassess dreams
	Develop a vision of one's future life and begin to pursue dreams	Experience self-doubt and concern about finding life partner
The thirties	Reassess life decisions (e.g., Is this the right job?)	Energy is not invested in reassessment
	Modify life structures or reverse decisions that now seem inappropriate	Hesitation about change arises
	Invest self in job, family, and friends	
Middle adulthood	Begin to consider own mortality	Upward mobility may cease
	Note clear signs of physical aging in self	Uncertainty about goals and ability to achieve them may increase
	May feel that this is last chance to make life changes	
The fifties	Children may have left home	May consider early retirement
	Career may be well-established	Fears of aging intensify
	Time is available to pursue leisure activities	Withdrawal from leisure activities may occur
Late adulthood	Deterioration occurs in health, physical attractiveness, and strength	Other problems related to aging are intensified (e.g., loneliness)
	Friends and family are lost through death or relocation as a result of retirement	Overall sense of loss is exacerbated
	One begins to review one's life and reflect on its meaning	

taking antidepressants and who has recently lost a job. Someone who holds prejudices about hearing loss beforehand may suffer from a negative self-image and self-stigmatization afterwards.

Socioeconomic Status

In addition to stage of life and life factors, one's socioeconomic status can affect the impact of hearing loss and the design of an aural rehabilitation plan. Social scientists have defined at least six socioeconomic classes in American society. One's classification within this schema is based on a consideration of income, occupation, educational level, and dwelling type. These six classes include:

■ high uppers
■ low uppers
■ high middles
■ low middles
■ high lowers
■ low lowers

Ways in which socioeconomic status may affect the management of hearing loss are illustrated in the following examples:

■ Financial status may relate to whether an individual can afford binaural hearing aids and/or assistive devices.
■ Educational history may determine how much background knowledge someone has about the anatomy of the ear and its possible disorders, and may dictate how the problem is discussed.
■ Work schedule and level of employment may determine whether someone is able to attend aural rehabilitation classes scheduled during a week day.

Race and Ethnicity

Race and ethnicity help define us. We are a nation of diversity (Figure 10–3), and this has become increasingly true with each passing year. About 30 years ago, the United States Bureau of the Census identified standardized categories for identifying race or ethnicity. These categories included:

■ White
■ African American

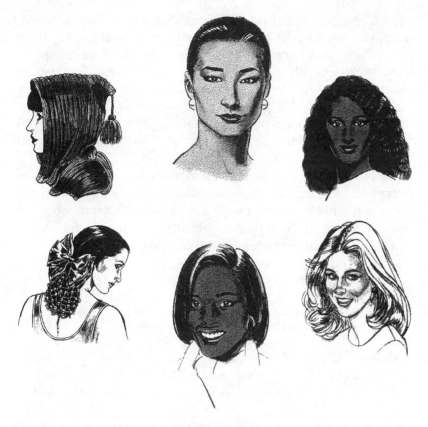

Figure 10–3. We are a nation of cultural and ethnic diversity. Speech and hearing professionals should try to be sensitive to this diversity, and tailor their aural rehabilitation plans accordingly.

☐ American Indian
■ Eskimo
☐ Aleut
☐ Asian-Pacific Islander
☐ Hispanic American

Almost as soon as they were described, these categories proved inadequate. For instance, within the Hispanic American category alone, there are at least four discrete subcultures:

☐ Puerto Rican
☐ Mexican
☐ Cuban
☐ Central American

Racial or ethnic groups often have distinctive customs, beliefs, and service preferences, and these must be considered when customizing an aural rehabilitation program. For example, hearing loss may have greater impact on self-concepts of masculinity and femininity within a subculture described as Mexican than within a subculture described as second-generation Japanese-American, so counseling may be different for the two groups. The content of a communication strategies training program may be appropriate for some groups but not for others. For instance, a member of an Aleut culture may feel uncomfortable in asking a conversational partner to repeat a message following a communication breakdown, as this may be interpreted as a sign of rudeness within his or her social milieu. Thus, it might be inappropriate for the hearing professional to encourage use of the repeat repair strategy during the course of a communication strategies training program.

Sensitivity to Cultural Issues

CalOptima is an HMO in Orange, California that provides training to health-care workers who provide services to Latino, Vietnamese, and Cambodian Patients. They offer these tips (Anders, 1997)

■ Seek eye contact with Latino patients.
■ Forgo eye contact with some Asian patients.
■ Avoid using patients' children as interpreters; family dynamics may make it difficult to get candid answers.
■ Address older patients in most nonwhite groups by surname and Mr. or Mrs. (p. B1).

Gender

Patients' gender may influence the content of their aural rehabilitation program (Figure 10–4). For example, in a traditional family structure, an adult female may fear that hearing loss decreases her ability to nurture her children, and she may experience a loss of self-esteem and sense of desirability. A hard-of-hearing male adult may worry that he has lost his means to provide financially for his offspring and believe that he has become less manly or less vigorous in the eyes of his friends. In these two examples, counseling will have to be tailored to suit the individual concerns.

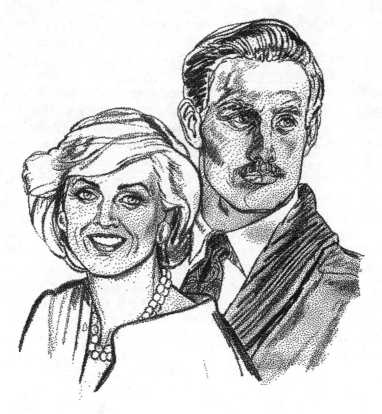

Figure 10-4. Gender may influence the design of an aural rehabilitation plan. Women and men may vary in their financial resources, their psychological responses to hearing loss, and their everyday listening demands.

As is the case with race and ethnicity, gender can be divided into subcategories. For instance, females can be divided into subsegments of "homemakers" and "workers." The latter group can be distinguished further as either clinical-technical or management professionals. As a function of their subsegment, individuals will require different aural rehabilitation interventions. For example, a homemaker may be interested in obtaining a baby-cry alerting assistive device, whereas a business executive may inquire about group amplification systems.

Psychological Factors

Psychological reactions that some hard-of-hearing individuals experience when learning of and adapting to a hearing loss may correspond to those experienced by terminally ill patients, although their emotions may be muted by comparison with sick persons. Where they are in terms of psychological adjustment will influence the kinds of aural rehabilitation services that are appropriate at any point in time.

Psychological responses to hearing loss may begin as shock and disbelief, followed by depression, then anger and guilt, and finally, acceptance (Van Hecke, 1994). Recently diagnosed hard-of-hearing patients first may experience *shock and disbelief.* Some feel numb or disorganized when the audiologist describes their test results. They then may deny a problem exists and may blame their listening problems on other factors.

Dissonance theory concerns situations in which one's self-perception does not coincide with reality.

A milder version of shock and disbelief relates to ***dissonance theory***. Most people do not want to receive messages that run counter to their own self-perception and self-image. They may object to audiological findings that do not fit well with their own cognitions. "Hey, I can't have a hearing loss," a young person may think, "I run marathons—my body is in great shape." Some individuals may attempt to reassert their views of the world either by searching for a disconfirmation of the diagnosis or by minimizing the importance of it. For instance, one woman made a point of telling a family member whenever she heard a noise in the next room, "See, I heard that! " Others may dismiss the hearing loss as being insignificant. "Yes," someone might say, "I miss some things, but most of what I miss isn't worth hearing anyway."

Depression often follows denial in reaching acceptance of a hearing loss.

Depression may follow denial, or a mourning for what has been lost (e.g., the loss of hearing, the loss of effortless conversation) and for what may lie ahead (e.g., a continued decrease in hearing, an increase in feelings of powerlessness). Persons may feel isolated from friends and family as they miss out on casual conversational exchanges. They may need to depend more on others for navigating communication with the outside world, and they may experience a concomitant decrease in self-esteem. An inability to hear environmental and body sounds, such as leaves rustling or their footsteps on the pavement, may intensify feelings of loss, as may a decreased ability to enjoy music. One woman reported, "For a while I felt tired and disinterested all the time. My daughter would ask me to go shopping and I'd say 'no.' Someone would say the sun was going to shine that day and I'd say 'so what?' I had a weight in my heart. I never felt elation and I never felt disappointment. It took me months to realize that I was depressed, and that the depression was related to my hearing loss."

Anger and guilt may bubble up after depression, as patients realize that their lives have been inalterably changed. "Why me?" they may ask, or "What did I do to deserve this?" There may be a perception of unfairness, and a person may protest, "But I am too young to be going deaf!"

Over time, *acceptance* of the hearing loss occurs. The intensity of feeling stemming from depression, anger, and anxiety cannot be maintained, and a sense of normalcy returns. The realization emerges that life goes on, albeit differently than before. As one man said, "I'm not too happy about my hearing, but I figure no one's going to take me out behind the barn and shoot me!"

Anger and **guilt** are stages that sometimes follow depression in adjusting to a hearing loss.

Acceptance: the final stage of adjustment to a hearing loss in which the patient realizes that life goes on, albeit differently.

WHERE IS THE PERSON IN TERMS OF ADJUSTMENT TO HEARING LOSS?

Now that we have considered the question of who is the patient, let us now address the question, *Where is the person in the adjustment process*? In this section, we will consider the time course of hearing loss, and where in the process the aural rehabilitation plan begins to be implemented. During your first interaction with an individual, you probably will ask questions about the progression of hearing loss. Questions may include the following:

■ **When do you think your hearing loss began?**
■ **How did you know you had a problem?**
■ **What brought you here today?**

In recent years, much research has focused on the time course of hearing loss in hard-of-hearing adults, and how the quality of life alters throughout. Familiarity with this research will prove helpful as you ask these kinds of questions, and as you consider the implications that the responses have for a person's aural rehabilitation plan.

The work of Jones, Kyle, and Wood (1987; Kyle, Jones, & Wood, 1985) provides a useful framework for considering adjustment to hearing loss. They identified four phases in the time course of acquired hearing loss. These four phases are summarized in Figure 10–5.

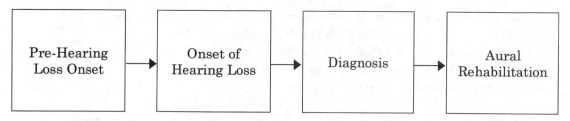

Figure 10–5. Four phases in the time course of acquired hearing loss.

Phase 1: Pre-Hearing Loss

As we have just learned, prior to incurring hearing loss, patients will have achieved a certain socioeconomic status, personality, and world view. Life factors are in place. With few exceptions, as in the case of adults who have a family history of hearing loss, few individuals ever anticipate they will suffer from hearing loss, especially while still younger than 65 years of age. Thus, when hearing loss begins, it usually takes a person by surprise.

Phase 2: Onset of Hearing Loss

Phase 2 is the time span stretching between the onset of hearing loss and diagnosis. Often, onset of hearing loss goes undetected. If asked when the loss began, a person may not know. As Hétu (1996) noted:

> It takes a rather striking invalidation of one's perceptual experience to start suspecting that one's sense organs no longer work properly. When hearing loss is progressive and symmetrical, there is no internal reference by which to measure the decrease in one's hearing capabilities. Furthermore, a comparison with others' hearing capabilities is very limited." (p. 17)

The advance from mild loss to awareness might last anywhere from a few days to many years. Situations that often alert people to a problem include having to turn up the television or radio volume, having to ask people to repeat their messages, not hearing a doorbell or someone calling their name, and missing out on conversations that occur in the home (Jones et al., 1987). One man, reflecting on this phase, noted ruefully, "For about two years, I was snapping at my wife for talking too soft. Then I begin to think that other people were mumbling too. It wasn't until my little grandson accused me of not paying attention that I thought to myself, maybe it's my hearing."

Other, less frequently cited indicants include complaining about bad telephone connections, believing that people mumble, and not knowing where sounds are coming from. Family members and others may remark about a patient's coping behaviors and rationalizations. In an initial interview, when a person may be exploring the possibility of hearing loss, the hearing professional might ask any of the following questions (based on Wayner & Abrahamson, 1996):

Do you frequently ask people to repeat?
Do you feel that most people mumble?
Do you sometimes hear sound, but can't understand what is being said?
Do you have to work hard to hear?
Are you tired after you have listened for a lengthy period of time?
Do people comment on the volume setting of your television programs?
Has someone said that you speak too loudly in conversation?
Has someone said that you missed what was said or did not react to speech?

When people begin to realize they have hearing loss, they often discuss the issue with family members before seeking formal diagnosis. However, they may not mention the problem at work. Many try not to disclose the presence of hearing loss to those outside the home, often for fear of stigmatization and discrimination.

Phase 3: Diagnosis

Phase 3 is a time when the hearing loss is identified by a professional and the extent of the problem is revealed. An individual may seek out the family doctor first, an otolaryngologist, or go directly to an audiologist. At this point, the individual might expect the hearing professional to provide a rapid solution, and he or she may expect a treatment and complete cure. Susan Jacobs was one such example. After her audiologist diagnosed a moderate bilateral sensorineural hearing loss, Susan responded, "My son had a hearing loss when he was 2 years old and the ear doctor gave him tubes. Now he's fine. You think surgery can help me?"

Upon realizing that hearing loss is here to stay, many people succumb to anxiety. They may worry about possible outcomes, such as decreased professional options, loss of independence, rejection by friends or family members, and altered social status. The magnitude of a person's anxiety may be mollified by what has occurred in Phase 2. For example, if someone has long suspected a hearing loss, then diagnosis may be less traumatic.

During the diagnostic process, the person's type and degree of hearing loss are determined, and the extent to which social, vocational, and educational activities are affected is explored. Typically, you will obtain a pure-tone audiogram and administer speech-recognition tests. You probably will administer a self-report survey or questionnaire aimed at assessing communication handicap and/or conduct an interview. The results will indicate how hearing loss interferes with everyday communication in the home, work, and social environments, and reveal related psychological difficulties. Answers to your questions will provide information about the need for amplification and assistive listening devices and the need for communication strategies training and psychological counseling.

The Interview

When asking about the home environment, you will want to gain an idea of with whom an individual communicates, what his or her specific communication problems are, and whether assistive listening devices might be appropriate. Example questions concerning the home environment include:

■ **Do you live alone? With a spouse? With children?**
■ **What are your communication demands in the home?**
■ **Do you watch television? Is hearing a problem?**
■ **Do you have difficulty in detecting or identifying warning signals (e.g., telephone ringing, doorbell, alarm clock, a baby's cry)?**

When exploring the work environment, questions are asked about the physical environment of the workplace, specific work tasks performed by the individual, and current hearing-related problems. This information will be important as you consider appropriate listening devices, the need for noise protection, and the need for employer/employee education. Example questions about the work environment include:

■ **Where do you work (e.g., a factory, an office, construction, in sales)?**

■ **What is your physical work environment like (e.g., noisy, open space, quiet, small office)?**
  Do you use or do you think you need protection for your ears against noise?
  Do you need to use the telephone? Is hearing a problem?
  Do you have to attend lectures or seminars?
  Do you need to recognize speech on a Dictaphone or a telephone answering machine?
  Does your employer know about the American with Disabilities Act?

As with any group of adults, persons with hearing loss vary greatly in their predilections for social activities. Some people engage only in quiet, one-on-one activities; others interact in groups and attend social events such as concerts or lectures. For those who are more reclusive, you may explore whether they avoid social activities because they do not enjoy them or because they experience so many communication difficulties that the activities are unsatisfying. If the latter is the case, then you have specific direction to target your aural rehabilitation efforts. Example questions concerning the social environment include:

  What do you do in your free time (e.g., go to movies, attend dinner parties, play bridge)?
  What kinds of social situations do you avoid because of your hearing loss?
  Have you ever used an assistive device in public?

Phase 4: Adjustment

In the final phase of adjustment to acquired hearing loss, Phase 4, individuals begin to adapt to hearing loss. During Phase 4, a person may receive any or all of the following rehabilitation services: Counseling, hearing aid(s), assistive devices, and formal speechreading, listening, and/or communication strategies training. Aural rehabilitation is focused on minimizing or solving the communication problems identified in Phase 3.

Costs

It is important to realize that the adjustment phase extracts numerous costs from patients, both monetary and non-monetary (Figure 10–6). For example, in the course of pursuing an audiological appointment, an individual may lay out

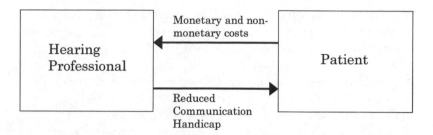

Figure 10–6. Monetary and nonmonetary costs associated with seeking aural rehabilitation services.

money for transportation, the appointment itself, lost wages for the time spent during the appointment, payment for a babysitter if he or she has young children, parking fees, hearing aid molds, hearing aids, and so forth.

Perhaps less obvious and often overlooked are the nonmonetary or *psychic costs* of seeking services and adjusting to hearing loss. Such costs for people may include any of the following:

Psychic costs are nonmonetary costs that relate to a person's psychological well-being.

■ **Acceptance** within themselves that they have a hearing problem.
■ **Anxiety** that they may be getting old.
■ **Awkwardness** for having to ask for time away from work and having to explain the reason for the request.
■ **Worry** that the hearing aid may cost too much or that the audiologist will take advantage of them.
■ **Fear** that nothing can be done to alleviate the communication difficulties.
■ **Embarrassment** for entering a hearing clinic.

Often, a primary goal of the experienced hearing professional is to maximize the benefits in exchange for real and perceived monetary and nonmonetary costs.

Apart from the costs associated with receiving services from a hearing professional, many adults discover that hearing loss extracts a toll both psychosocially and vocationally. It is important for you to be familiar with some of the psychosocial and vocational ramifications of hearing loss, and can express empathy.

Psychosocial Well-being

Hard-of-hearing adults may be more likely to suffer from feelings of loneliness than their normal-hearing counterparts and more likely to experience decreased self-esteem and other emotional difficulties, including embarrassment, shame, and uncertainty about one's social identity (Hétu, 1996; Jones et al., 1987). They may feel isolated both socially and emotionally. Outside the home, adults with hearing loss may be restricted in their ability to develop and sustain relationships and may feel disconnected from their community. As their hearing losses progress, they may begin to perceive that acquaintances avoid them. For instance, one person noticed that acquaintances gradually quit talking to her at the swimming pool and other community gathering places.

At home, individuals may believe that those closest to them do not understand the ramifications of hearing loss, nor do they adequately accommodate their listening needs (Lalonde, Lambert, & Riveria, 1988; Thomas & Herbst, 1980). Anger, frustration, and resentment directed toward one's spouse or children may be commonplace.

Vocational Status

Hard-of-hearing individuals may be more unhappy at work than the general population and have fewer vocational opportunities. Some people may experience a sense of being removed from the workplace mainstream, as they miss out on informal conversations and gossip. Professional growth and advancement also may be limited. For example, hard-of-hearing males between the ages of 45 and 61 years leave the work force in higher numbers than males who have normal hearing (Armstrong, 1991). Some workers may find themselves the subject of disparaging remarks by their colleagues. A hard-of-hearing secretary once walked into the office lounge and found a co-worker entertaining others with an impersonation of her. The man perched reading glasses on the end of his nose (worn in a similar fashion as the secretary), and repeatedly bellowed "Huh?" into an imaginary telephone receiver. The secretary reported to her audiologists that she had felt mortified and hurt, and thereafter she begin to eat lunch alone.

Adjustments by Family Members

Not only must patients adjust to hearing loss, but so too must their family members. Social and emotional issues that may

(continued)

arise include frustration over communication difficulties, impatience over the difficulties of communication (e.g., "Forget it, it's not worth repeating"), anger (e.g., "What am I supposed to do about your problem?"), guilt, and a sense of incompetence for not knowing how to minimize the listening problems for the hard-of-hearing person, pity, and anxiety (Wayner & Abrahamson, 1996).

We once posed the following question to a group of persons married to persons with significant hearing losses: "What are some of the most difficult aspects of living with a deaf family member?" Here are some of the responses:

Rhonda: "I'll list some of them: (1) Anger—communication is often difficult that he's 'not the same'; (2) concession—everyone has to change what it is he or she is doing or the way they do them (i.e., talking, listening to the TV); and (3) frustration—things have to be done his way to accommodate his hearing loss. It is just simply a whole new way of life. He has to deal with the fact that he is hearing impaired and being his family and loving him as we do, we deal (well or not) with all of the changes too. "

Gerald: "I cannot communicate with her by phone when she is alone. I once called a next-door neighbor to tell her of a tornado warning—she is so damn independent she was upset about my doing that."

Mike: "Communication with a hearing impaired family member requires patience and determination. I'm sure the frustration is equally disturbing to my wife. Tempers sometimes flare as one or both attempt communication and fail. Often times communication is abandoned by one or both parties, leaving both equally frustrated."

Jan: "We have a captioning device on the TV and the kids sometimes get mad when he wants to see the news captioned and they may go to another TV—poor kids, hah!"

Anna: "I have to move and make sure he can see my face when I speak to him. And we less and less enjoy 'small talk' together. Hearing aids have helped but we have finally reached the point where we cannot talk to each other without extra effort."

Pam: "Trying to do business and explain to him what's going on. Especially if someone else is around, he gets real rude and frustrated at me because he can't hear or understand."

TINNITUS—A RELATED PROBLEM

Now that we have considered the two questions posed at the beginning of the chapter, who is the patient and where the person is in terms of adjusting to a hearing loss, we will conclude with a consideration of two additional topics that are pertinent to the adult population: tinnitus, which we will consider in this section, and culturally Deaf adults, which we will address in the next section. *Tinnitus* is noise that is perceived in the ear and/or head and has no external physical source. The word is a derivative of the Latin word *tinnire*, which means to ring or tinkle (Jackson, 1983). Tinnitus often accompanies adult hearing loss, although individuals with normal hearing also experience it. The prevalence of tinnitus in the general population may be 35%, with 17% of the population reporting that it is continuously or frequently present. About 85% of those individuals who have ear problems report tinnitus (McFadden, 1982). Tinnitus is correlated with degree of hearing loss, with those who have greater hearing loss also having a greater subjective complaint of tinnitus. It is not correlated with age (Hazell, 1990).

Tinnitus is the sensation of noise in the head without an external cause.

Common descriptors of tinnitus include leaves rustling, the ocean roaring, crickets chirping, a radio playing off-station, a siren blasting, or a telephone ringing. The quality of sound might be crackling, pulsing, pounding, hissing, humming, musical, throbbing, whistling, popping, or whooshing. A person might perceive sound in the right ear, left ear, both ears, or inside or outside of the head.

As Table 10–2 indicates, etiologies of tinnitus relate to every level of the auditory system, although there is no clear understanding of the neuronal mechanisms that underlie it. Tinnitus can be triggered by factors associated with the external ear, middle ear, central nervous system, and especially, factors associated with the inner ear. Most tinnitus problems likely emerge from an interplay of peripheral and central factors. For instance, an abnormality at the level of the cochlea may lead to the generation of a weak neuronal signal. The signal may be detected on the conscious level as sound and, with continued occurrences, may become irritating to the patient and lead to a heightened cognitive awareness of the phantom signal. Subsequently, greater negative emotional reactions may result when the signal is detected, which may in turn lead to even greater awareness (Jastreboff, 1990).

Certain conditions or medications can exacerbate a tinnitus problem. For instance, some patients report that tinnitus worsens following stress or after taking aspirin. Table 10–2 presents a list of possible causes.

Table 10-2. Examples of causes of tinnitus.

Locus/Source	Cause
External ear	Impacted cerumen
Middle ear	Otitis media, otosclerosis, vascular anomalies, middle ear tumors
Inner ear	Ménières disease, presbycusis, ototoxicity, circulation problems, noise-induced hearing loss
Central nervous system	Migraine, acoustic neuroma, epilepsy, tumors
Other	Allergies, emotional or mental stress, medication, noise exposure, use of a hearing aid, physical work, lack of sleep

Source: Adapted from Stouffer, J. L., and Tyler, R. S. (1990). Characterization of tinnitus patients. *Journal of Speech and Hearing Disorders, 55,* 439–453.

For some people, tinnitus is a minor annoyance that is bothersome only in quiet situations, such as when trying to go to sleep. For a significant number, however, tinnitus is debilitating, the cause of frustration, depression, hopelessness, and even thoughts of suicide. Tinnitus can result in an inability to concentrate, increased difficulty in listening because it can mask the speech signal, and loss of sleep.

Because tinnitus cannot be measured objectively, it often is difficult to quantify its degree or to understand the magnitude of disability it presents. Some ways to obtain information include patient interviews and questionnaires. Some existing questionnaires include open-ended questions (Tyler & Baker, 1983). Some include quantifiable items concerning such as those listed below (e.g., Stouffer & Tyler, 1990), presented here with example kinds of questions :

■ **Location:** Is it in the left ear, right ear, or both ears?
■ **Pitch:** On a continuum corresponding to pitch, is it high pitched or low pitched?
■ **Constancy:** Is the tinnitus always present? Is it intermittent? Do you tend to notice it at a particular time of day?
■ **Composition:** Do you hear one sound or more than one sound?
■ **Fluctuations:** Does the tinnitus change from one sound to another? Does it change in pitch?

- **Loudness:** On a continuum corresponding to loudness, is it loud or soft?
- **Conditions that exacerbate the tinnitus**: What conditions exacerbate the tinnitus (e.g., drinking coffee, smoking)?
- **Annoyance**: On a continuum corresponding to annoyance, can the tinnitus be described as not at all annoying, extremely annoying, or somewhere in between?
- **Effects on concentration and sleep**: Does it have a slight effect? Extreme effect?
- **Depression:** Does it cause minimal depression? Extreme depression?

Unfortunately, many treatments for tinnitus have not been effective. Treatments include masking the tinnitus with an auditory signal, electrical stimulation, relaxation therapy and biofeedback, acupuncture, counseling, and pharmacological intervention. A relatively new approach to tinnitus management may hold promise. In this neurophysiological approach, patients listen to broadband white noise, for approximately 6 hours a day for 12 to 18 months, to habituate themselves to the phantom signal. Eventually, they do not attend to it, nor experience an emotional reaction, even though the tinnitus may still be present. There is some evidence that this treatment works for some patients (Jastreboff, Gray, & Gold, 1996).

Tinnitus Can Be Terrifying

Few people realize how debilitating tinnitus can be. Actor William Shatner, star of the Star Trek television series and movies, has experienced tinnitus for almost a decade. As the following excerpt demonstrates, he experienced desperate moments before finding some relief through a therapy offered by Dr. Pawel Jastreboff (Shatner, 1997):

> Over the years I tried herbal remedies. I tried eardrops. I bought masking devices to avoid the silence, and tapes and records of soothing sounds—Japanese music, running water. And inside my house is a little waterfall. The sound of the water is very soothing.
> Getting through the nights—that was always the worst. Sometimes I paced the halls. I often turned to writing and exercise, and fatigued myself to sleep. I'd have the tele-
>
> *(continued)*

vision on all night. It affected my marriage; if one person needs noise and the other person is sensitive to it, it can lead to separation . . . I could not sleep without sound. In my darkest moments I thought to myself, 'Will it be this way for the rest of my life, the way I am tormented by it now?' I began to think, 'What are the ways to take my life? How does one kill oneself?' I went so far as to start making plans. (p. 154–155)

Mr. Shatner's essay ended on a somber note. He related, "Recently I made a call to somebody in California who had promised Dr. Jasterboff money, and when I called, his wife answered and said he was dead. He had committed suicide because of tinnitus" (p. 155).

DEAF ADULTS

Heretofore, we have considered adults who are hard-of-hearing: adults who lost their hearing after acquiring speech and language. Now we will consider adults who acquired their losses before learning language and speech.

Deafness: Disability or Culture?

"Hearing people are always surprised to learn that deaf parents in neonatal wards cheer when they are told their babies cannot hear. Deaf Culture families see any effort to teach the deaf to speak as repugnant: The ASL sign for cochlear implant is a two-fingered stab to the back of the neck. 'Let me put it this way,' says Judith Coryell, head of Western Maryland's deaf education program and the mother of two deaf children. 'Say you were black. Do you think you'd be considering surgery to make yourself white?'" (Arana-Ward, 1997, p. 21).

Deaf Culture: a subculture that shares a common language (American Sign Language), beliefs, customs, arts, history, and folklore, primarily composed of individuals who have prelingual deafness.

Deaf Culture

Adult members of the *Deaf Culture* are individuals who lost their hearing early in life. They rely on sign language for face-to-face communication, and many believe they are culturally and linguistically distinct from hearing society. Members of the Deaf Culture use a capital D in the term "Deaf" to distinguish themselves from the audiologic condition of hearing loss. Membership in the Deaf Culture is not determined by one's degree of hearing loss, but rather, by one's identification with Deaf people. For example, two individuals may have identical severe bilateral hearing losses. One of them may use powerful hearing aids and feel a part of the hearing world whereas the other may socialize primarily with Deaf people (Giolas & Kaplan, 1997).

Deaf individuals become acculturated by means of educational experiences and social interactions. They usually have attended schools or classrooms for the Deaf and, as adults, they interact with Deaf groups, such as those centered around religious gatherings or sports. Most Deaf individuals marry a Deaf spouse.[1]

Recent History

Table 10–3 presents a chronology of significant events in the recent history of the Deaf Culture. The past few decades have brought about an increased visibility of the Deaf culture in today's world. Two landmark events in recent history are the appointment of I. King Jordan as president of Gallaudet College in 1988 and the approval of multichannel cochlear implants for use in children by the Food and Drug Administration in 1990. These two events signify two major forces affecting Deaf adults: the growth and expression of Deaf pride and advances in medical technology.

Unfortunately, these two forces often collide in purpose. Many Deaf adults reject the infirmity model of deafness implied by the use of cochlear implants (i.e., "there's a deficit here so let's fix it with surgery"). Some Deaf adults fear that use of cochlear implants may erase their culture, especially because post-implant rehabilitation for children often includes an emphasis on speech and listening skills and a de-emphasis on the use of American Sign Language (ASL). Deaf pride, personified by the protests at Gallaudet, leads to a celebration of cultural difference

[1]Not all Deaf individuals agree with the isolationist segment of the Deaf Culture. Some believe that deafness is a disability and that self-segregation is counterproductive. Although they still consider themselves to belong to Deaf society, these Deaf adults may not object to efforts to identify treatments, such as cochlear implants.

Table 10–3. Some significant events in the Deaf Culture movement since the 1960s.

1960s   Civil rights movement becomes visible in mainstream America; Deaf people became aware of their own ethnic possibilities.

The largest worldwide rubella epidemic in recorded history results in a great influx of deaf children into the public school systems from 1964 to 1965, while there is a concurrent decline in the number of children with normal hearing.

1970s   Congress passes Public Law 94-142, the Education for All Handicapped Children Act, in 1975, which mandates public education of children with handicaps within the public school system, and subsequently contributes to declining enrollments in public residential schools and increasing enrollments in public day classes.

A general consensus emerges among linguists that ASL is an official language.

Congress passes the Rehabilitation Act of 1973 (Section 504), which prohibits federally supported programs or activities from discriminating against qualified handicapped people.

1980s   A "Deaf Pride" movement grows rapidly among young deaf adults.

In 1988, I. King Jordan becomes the first deaf president of the country's oldest institute of higher learning for the deaf, Gallaudet University, after students stage a demonstration protesting the appointment of a hearing president.

Harlan Lane, a professor of psychology at Northeastern University in Boston, publishes *When the Mind Hears: A History of the Deaf*, a book condemning the history of oral communication in America.

1990s   Schools for Deaf children increasingly hire Deaf teachers and administrators.

The Food and Drug Administration (FDA) approves multichannel cochlear implants for use in children in 1990.

The Americans with Disabilities Act (ADA) (P.L. 101-336) is passed into law in 1990 and extends civil rights protection to people with disabilities in private and federal sectors.

The National Association of the Deaf presents a position paper, stating that "The NAD deplores the decision of the Food and Drug Administration (to permit cochlear implantation of children) which was unsound scientifically, procedurally, and ethically" (Broadcaster, 1991).

In 1994, some members of the Deaf Culture accuse Heather Whitestone, the country's first Deaf Miss America, of being an impostor because she primarily uses oral communication.

---

in which significant hearing loss is an entryway into a minority community with shared mores, language (ASL), art forms, and traditions (Lane, 1990).

Deaf and Hard-of-Hearing Adults

In some ways, members of the Deaf Culture have different problems than hard-of-hearing individuals. For instance, unlike many adventitiously hearing-impaired adults, many members of the Deaf Culture have limited or nonexistent speech production skills, and their voices may sound strained and harsh. They may be academically delayed (many Deaf individuals never achieve more than a fourth grade reading level), and they may gravitate towards certain professions that offer limited opportunity for professional growth. However, unlike hard-of-hearing adults, many Deaf adults do not experience being cut off from the life they have known as a result of hearing loss. They can communicate with fellow signers, they have comfortable companionship with their family and require no extraordinary patience or accommodation, and they are free of many of the anxieties associated with attempts to function in a hearing world (Giolas & Kaplan, 1997).

Psychological Profile

Some adults who incurred a significant hearing loss early in life present a shared psychological profile. They may be immature, and may demonstrate a lack of social judgment. Some may be less flexible than adults who have normal hearing, and they may be more likely to adhere to a set routine. Other tendencies include irresponsibility, impulsivity, passivity, overacceptance, and a failure to appreciate the feelings or opinions of others (Jackson, 1982). Of course, no general description such as this can characterize an entire group of people, and you must take the time and make the effort necessary to know the individual.

Professional Services for Deaf Adults

Deaf adults often do not solicit the kinds of services from hearing professionals that are sought by hard-of-hearing persons. For example, they may not seek hearing tests, they may not use hearing aids, and they may not be interested in communication training. Some of the professional services they may utilize include the following:

- Sign interpreting
- Notetaking
- Provision of assistive devices
- Academic and vocational counseling

Deaf persons who use speech may desire additional services as well. These include:

- **Speech and voice training:** Individuals may want to polish their speaking skills, especially if they have not received speech training for many years. They also may want an assessment of their speech, so they can better anticipate communication difficulties.
- **Communication strategies training:** Some individuals may desire training in the use of expressive and receptive communication strategies.

Professionals who interact with Deaf persons, even if only occasionally, should have some knowledge of sign language. In the best of circumstances, they should have enough skill in the use sign to allow functional communication interactions. Kinsella-Meier (1996) notes:

> If the language, cultural values, and beliefs held by Deaf persons are respected and understood by the clinician, then services can be provided more successfully . . . The Deaf person is likely to accommodate the hearing person by code switching to approximate English word order more closely if the hearing person is perceived to be willing to modify her own communication style. (pp. 9–10)

Sign Interpreters

Sign interpreter: a professional who translates the spoken signal into a form of signed English or ASL, or vice versa.

A *sign interpreter* is a professional who translates the spoken signal into a form of signed English or ASL, or vice versa. The interpreter does not participate in the dialogue, but simply conveys messages from one communication partner to the next. Examples of occasions in which a sign language interpreter might be utilized include one-on-one communication situations between a Deaf individual and an individual who does not know sign language, meetings, and lectures. Interpreters often accompany Deaf persons to medical, legal, and educational settings.

Professional interpreters may receive certification from the Registry of Interpreters for the Deaf (RID) or through other state-wide screening programs. They are expected to adhere to a set of professional guidelines established by the RID. Scheetz (1993) summarizes the RID code of ethics:

- Interpreters shall keep all assignment-related information strictly confidential.
- Interpreters shall render the message faithfully, always conveying the content of the message and the spirit of the speaker, using language most readily understood by the person(s) whom they serve.
- Interpreters shall not counsel or advise those whom they serve, or interject personal opinions.
- Interpreters shall accept assignments using discretion with regard to skill, setting, and the consumers involved.
- Interpreters shall request compensation for services in a professional and judicious manner. (p. 274)

FINAL REMARKS

Aural rehabilitation begins with a solid understanding of the patient population. In this chapter, we have considered how adults with hearing loss differ in their cultural orientation, their demographics, their reactions to hearing loss, their communication needs and problems, and many other factors. We also have considered the four phases of adjustment to hearing loss. This information lays the groundwork for providing aural rehabilitation services to adults. In the next chapter, we will consider the development of aural rehabilitation plans.

KEY CHAPTER POINTS

✔ A patient orientation holds that the most successful aural rehabilitation plan is one that best determines a patient's background, current status, needs, and wants and then accommodates these through the design and delivery of appropriate interventions.

✔ Most adults lose their hearing gradually over time. Typically, the loss is greatest in the high frequencies and least in the low frequencies.

✔ In following a patient orientation, you will determine "who the patient is." You will consider non-hearing-related variables such as stage of life, socioeconomic status, and psychological adjustment. These variables may affect the aural rehabilitation plan.

✔ Psychological responses to hearing loss may include the following stages: shock and disbelief, depression, anger and guilt, and, finally, acceptance. A milder form of shock and disbelief relates to dissonance theory ("this diagnosis runs counter to my self-image").

✔ There are four phases in an adult's adjustment to hearing loss: prehearing loss, onset of hearing loss, diagnosis, and adjustment. Aural rehabilitation often starts in the third phase. During this phase, you will want to identify a patient's particular communication problems at home, socially, and vocationally and begin to formulate solutions.

✔ Adjustment to hearing loss extracts both monetary and nonmonetary costs. Psychic costs include acceptance within one's self that there is a hearing problem and anxiety of aging.

✔ Hard-of-hearing people may have more psychosocial and vocational difficulties than normally-hearing adults. They may suffer from feelings of loneliness and decreased self-esteem. They may have a sense of being removed from the workplace mainstream.

✔ Tinnitus can be debilitating.

✔ Adult members of the Deaf Culture lost their hearing early in life. They rely primarily on ASL for communication.

Aural Rehabilitation Plans for Hard-of-Hearing Adults

Topics

- A Strategy for Plan Development
- Counseling
- Hearing Aids for Adults
- Assistive Listening Devices
- Follow-Up

- Case Study
- Final Remarks
- Key Chapter Points
- Key Resources

In the last chapter, we discussed demographics for the adult population, progression of hearing loss, and steps for evaluating the magnitude of hearing loss and communication difficulties. In previous chapters we have discussed services that might comprise an aural rehabilitation plan, such as provision of amplification, assistive devices, and communication training. In this chapter, we will bring these topics together and consider a systematic process for designing a patient-oriented aural rehabilitation plan for hard-of-hearing adults. This process usually requires the orchestration of a number of interventions, and these services often can be integrated in such a way as to achieve maximum benefit for the individual.

A STRATEGY FOR PLAN DEVELOPMENT

Figure 11–1 outlines the three component stages of developing a plan. These include:

1. *Evaluation:* First, the individual will be assessed, and his or her current status, wants, problems, and needs will be evaluated. This evaluation will allow the topics posed in Table 11–1 to be addressed. These topics pertain to patient demographics (e.g., Where is this person in terms of stage of life?), audiological and conversational needs (e.g., Is this person a candidate for a hearing aid?), and ecological concerns (e.g., Does the person work? If so, what are the communication demands associated with the workplace?). Topics to be evaluated also will include economics and psychosocial adjustment. For example, can the individual afford hearing aids? Is the person motivated to use them?

2. *Strategy:* The next stage will be to develop a broad strategy to guide your aural rehabilitation efforts. An aural rehabilitation strategy will be based on a consideration of an individual's needs, the availability of offerings within your particular practice, and the individual's ability and/or willingness to comply with the specifics of the plan. It is desirable to develop a strategy that can be communicated easily to the hard-of-hearing person. It should be one that is likely to meet with compliance and it should excite the individual because it offers the potential for benefit. The plan that is devised should not seem to be out of the realm of possibility in the eyes of the patient. For instance, the patient's immediate reaction on learning the specifics of a proposed plan should not be, "I would *never* wear a hearing aid!"

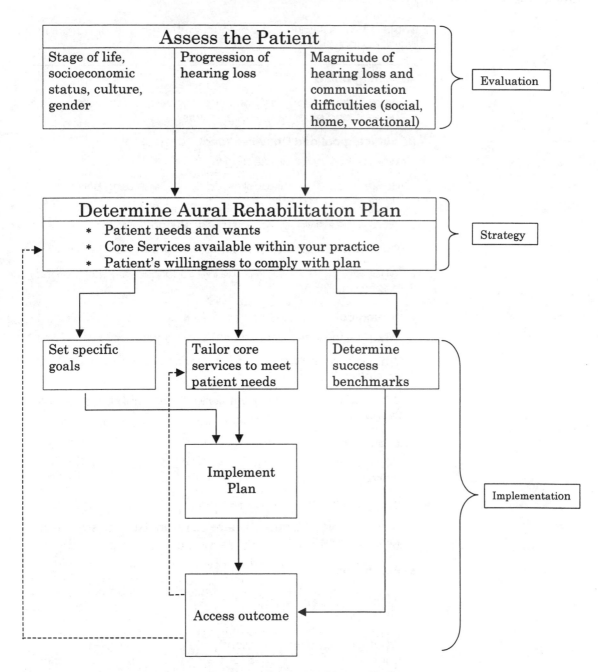

Figure 11-1. Stages in the design of an aural rehabilitation plan.

3. *Implementation:* The final stage in developing an aural rehabilitation plan is implementation. Specific goals (e.g., enhanced communication on the telephone) will be set, and existing services within the particular aural rehabilitation setting will be tailored to meet individual needs (e.g., the person may be invited to attend a communication-strate-

Table 11-1. Assessing the individual in the scheme of designing an aural rehabilitation plan.

A. Demographic

What is the individual's stage of life, socioeconomic status, culture, gender, and other relevant life factors?

B. Audiological and Conversational

What is the individual's hearing loss?

How well can the individual recognize speech using only audition? Using vision and audition?

What is the individual's communication handicap?

Does the individual use communication strategies effectively?

What listening devices does the individual currently use? Are they appropriate?

C. Ecological

What are the individual's communication demands in the home?

What are the individual's communication demands in the workplace?

What are the individual's communication demands in the social arena?

D. Economic

What are the financial resources available to support the individual's aural rehabilitation plan?

How does the individual make buying decisions?

How does the individual perceive aural rehabilitation services in terms of monetary costs and benefits?

E. Psychosocial

What are the psychosocial concerns related to the individual's hearing loss and communication difficulties, and how can they be addressed?

What are the nonmonetary costs related to seeking and receiving aural rehabilitation services for the individual, and how can they be minimized?

How motivated is the individual to receive services and to participate in aural rehabilitation interventions?

---

gies training program that includes other adults of similar age and hearing loss). The clinician will want to assess whether the plan is working. This will entail establishing success benchmarks and means for assessing them. The aural rehabilitation plan should be flexible. If new problems arise or the intervention proves unsuccessful, the plan should be adaptable.

Most aural rehabilitation services include counseling, dispensing of hearing aids and assistive devices, and provision of formal communication training classes. As aural rehabilitation specialists plan their strategy and implementation procedures, they consider how these services can be tailored to meet individual needs. For best results, patients should be involved in defining the plan and, together, clinician and patient should prioritize and update the key goals as circumstances change and evolve.

The typical progression of events involved in providing aural rehabilitation are represented in Figure 11–2. The hard-of-hearing person is evaluated and then receives counseling. Counseling can lead to discussions about psychological adjustment to hearing loss, receipt of hearing aid(s) and/or assistive listen-

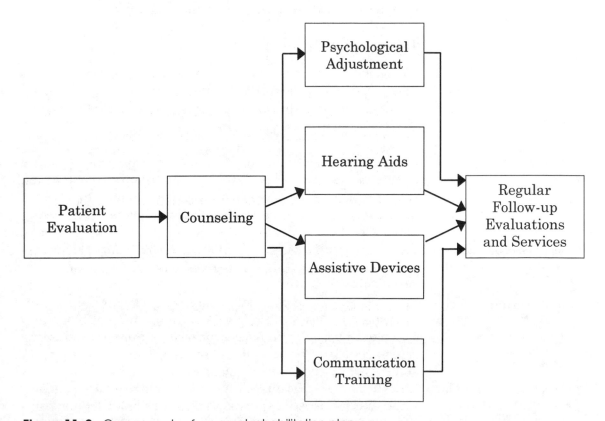

Figure 11–2. Components of an aural rehabilitation plan.

ing device(s), and participation in communication strategies training classes. Counseling is ongoing during these activities. Follow-up is provided regularly thereafter, often on an annual schedule.

COUNSELING

There are many reasons to include counseling in an aural rehabilitation plan. Counseling often provides patients with the following benefits (Erdman, 1993):

- Enhanced understanding of hearing loss and its effects on communication.
- Better self-disclosure and self-acceptance.
- Greater knowledge about how to manage communication difficulties.
- Reduced stress and discouragement.
- Increased satisfaction with aural rehabilitation services.
- Increased motivation to minimize listening problems.
- Stronger adherence/compliance with the aural rehabilitation plan, including use of amplification.

Types of Counseling

Clinicians often provide three kinds of counseling: informational, rational acceptance and adjustment, and emotional acceptance and adjustment (Alpiner & Garstecki, 1996; Wylde, 1982). These are summarized in Figure 11–3.

After a hearing test, an audiologist often explains the nature and degree of hearing loss to the patient, usually in conjunction with a review of the person's audiogram. There also may be a discussion of the benefits and limitations provided by a hearing aid and possibly a hands-on demonstration. In this interaction, the audiologist provides *informational counseling*. The professional instructs and guides and gives expert information.

Patients and their clinicians may discuss communication strategies and ways to improve communication at home and at school. During *rational acceptance and adjustment counseling*, clinicians focus on the permanence of the hearing loss and may introduce concrete means for managing communication difficulties. For instance, an audiologist might recommend specific assistive devices to use, such as a telephone amplifier.

Informational counseling includes imparting information about the hearing loss and the benefits and limitations of amplification.

Rational acceptance and adjustment counseling focuses on the permanency of the hearing loss and concrete means of managing communication problems.

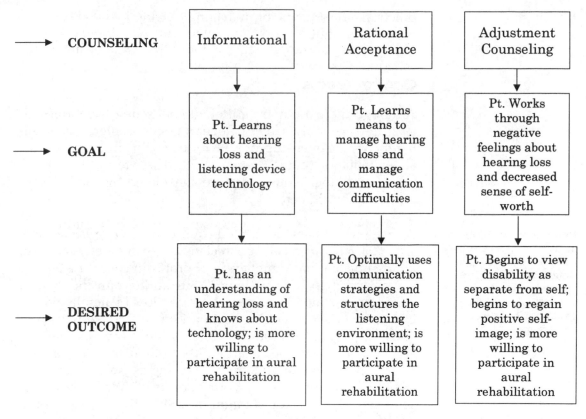

Figure 11-3. Three kinds of counseling provided in the aural rehabilitation setting (Pt. = patient).

Finally, clinicians may explore individuals' reactions to the loss of hearing. They talk about a person's feelings, ways in which social and vocational roles have changed, and whether and how self-image has been altered as a result of the loss. When persons' reactions are extreme, they may be referred to a mental health professional. Over time and with the help of *emotional acceptance and adjustment counseling,* patients usually attenuate their negative feelings about hearing loss and bolster their sense of self-identity and self-worth.

Emotional acceptance and adjustment counseling explores individuals reactions to loss of hearing.

Even though most clinicians are not trained counselors, providing informational, rational acceptance and adjustment, and emotional acceptance and adjustment counseling is an important component in their service arsenal. There is not always a clear boundary as to how far clinician should go when counseling and at what point referral to a professional counseling service should be made. A general rule of thumb is that counseling should center around the hearing loss. The clinician cannot resolve all problems that loom before the patient. Counseling is usually short term and focuses on solutions and practical adjustments for managing hearing loss and communication difficulties.

Central Tenets

Although there are many different counseling techniques, at least three central tenets of Roger's person-centered counseling theory are often appropriate for use with adults in the aural rehabilitation setting (Rogers, 1979). These tenets as they apply to audiologic counseling are considered by Clark (1994) and summarized here.

Congruence with self is the first tenet of person-centered counseling in which clinicians act as themselves in interactions with patients and do not assume a facade of professionalism.

A first tenet of person-centered counseling is *congruence with self*. This tenet means that clinicians act as themselves and do not assume an imposing facade of professionalism. Instead of saying to a first-time patient: "Your audiogram indicates a mild-to-moderate sensorineural hearing loss bilaterally with a conductive component," a pronouncement replete with professional jargon, an audiologist might instead say, "I know you are worried about your hearing. My tests seem to agree with your impression that you are not hearing as well as you used to hear. I'd like to answer your questions." With the former statement, the audiologist might inadvertently increase the patient's anxiety. With the latter approach, the audiologist has validated the patient's own opinions and allowed the patient to share the lead in discussing the test results.

In **unconditional positive regard**, the second tenet of person-centered counseling, clinicians assume that patients know best and assume that they have the inner resources to overcome their conversation difficulties.

A second tenet to follow when providing counseling is *unconditional positive regard*. The clinician assumes that patients know best and that they have the inner resources to overcome their communication difficulties. The professional accepts patients as human beings of stature, respects them regardless of their employment or social status, and brings appropriately placed empathy, sincerity, and caring to the interaction.

Empathetic understanding is the third tenet of person-centered counselng. The counselor listens to the patient's concerns and feelings about the hearing problem, reflects them back to the patient, and helps the patient identify solutions.

Roger's third tenet is *empathetic understanding*. The clinician listens carefully as patients perhaps rationalize and/or deny their hearing difficulties, as they talk about their concerns and feelings, and as they express their ideas and solutions. The professional establishes the patient's viewpoints, reflects them back, and then helps the patient to identify solutions. For example, a person might cite the soft presentation level as a reason for poor performance on a word discrimination test. In this instance, the audiologist would probably not say, "I presented the words at a normal conversational level, Mr. Smith. There is no doubt you have a word discrimination problem."

Instead, in order to show empathy and respect for the patient's feelings, the audiologist might respond, "I know the words were not very loud for you. Are there occasions during your typical day when speech seems too soft to hear?" With this remark, the patient's impressions are acknowledged, and the test results are related to situations that are relevant.

Targeting Counseling

As you develop your aural rehabilitation strategy and implement a plan, you will want to consider how best to target counseling for particular concerns. For example, one hard-of-hearing patient, Candice Brown, commented to her audiologist, "I worry that I can't be there for my 13-year-old daughter the way I want to be. It's too much of an effort for her to talk to me, she says. Lately, she just tunes me out." In this case, the aural rehabilitation plan might include the following counseling tactics:

■ **Provide informational counseling** by enrolling Candice and her daughter in a group communication strategies training program. Thus both Candice and her daughter will learn about difficult listening situations, appropriate speaking behaviors, and communication strategies.
■ **Provide rational acceptance and adjustment counseling**, and help Candice understand that communication between a teenage daughter and her parent is universally problematic, and not just an issue for a hearing-impaired mother. Encourage Candice in the optimal use of amplification and appropriate assistive devices such as telephone amplifiers.
■ **Provide emotional acceptance and adjustment counseling** by involving the daughter and Candice in aural rehabilitation group sessions, where both will have an opportunity to share their frustrations, feelings, and ideas for solutions.

HEARING AIDS FOR ADULTS

When determining whether to include provision of hearing aid(s) in an aural rehabilitation plan, an audiologist first must determine whether an individual is an appropriate candidate. If he or she meets the audiological criteria, the audiologist will perform a hearing-aid evaluation and provide a hearing-aid fitting and orientation session. Establishing an appropriate use-pattern will be a prominent goal in the aural rehabilitation plan.

You Want How Much?

Some people will demonstrate *consumer anxiety* when acquiring a hearing aid for the first time. This is a fear that they are being taken advantage of because they do not know much about hearing loss or hearing aids. Their concerns may include the following (Reiter, 1995):

■ How do I know I am being sold the proper hearing aid?
■ Why is the person down the street cheaper?
■ Why are hearing aids so expensive?
■ Do I really need two hearing aids?
■ How do I know this dispenser is really any good?
■ How do I know I am not being ripped off?
■ Why should I buy hearing aids when they really are not any good because my friend does not wear his any place but the chest of drawers? (p. 10).

Through good service, open communication, and mutual respect and goals, you can alleviate consumer anxiety. To this end, it is important that you provide adequate pre- and post-fitting counseling and follow-up aural rehabilitation services. As you establish satisfied consumers, they will begin to recommend you to others.

Candidacy

Who is a candidate for a hearing aid? The answer depends on the degree and the nature of hearing loss and on patient motivation.

Hearing aids are available to alleviate a wide range of hearing losses. A traditional view is that individuals with an average sensorineural hearing loss between 40 and 90 dB HL are most likely to benefit from conventional amplification. Those at the extremes of hearing acuity, with mild or profound loss, are least likely to benefit. In recent times, this view had changed. Even adults with mild high-frequency loss may experience difficulty in recognizing speech, and nowadays, may be fitted with a high-frequency emphasis hearing aid.

Whether a hearing loss is significant enough to warrant amplification relates at least in part to the individual's lifestyle and occupation. For example, a retired gardener and a school teacher may have similar hearing losses. The gardener may believe amplification is unnecessary for days spent weeding flower beds whereas the teacher may find it critical for hearing small voices emanating from the back of the classroom.

Motivation to use a hearing aid is an important but often overlooked issue when determining whether someone is an appropriate candidate. Many people who have hearing loss simply are not interested in obtaining a hearing aid. In fact, it has been suggested that only about 5.8 million of the 23.5 million persons (or 23%) in the United States who have hearing loss actually own hearing instruments (Kochkin, 1992). Factors that commonly influence persons to obtain a device include (Mueller & Bender, 1988):

■ Communication problems at home, on the job, or in social situations.
■ Encouragement of family members.
■ Direction from a medical professional, usually their audiologist or otolaryngologist.

Reasons why individuals may not be motivated include vanity, financial constraints, or fear of aging. Some persons fear a social stigmata associated with using a hearing aid and are concerned that they will be devalued by others. Some harbor a fear of operating a mechanical device or are not willing to commit time and effort to using an aid on a regular basis. Finally, many people believe their hearing loss is not problematic enough to warrant use of an aid.

In developing motivation in patients, you might implement the 10-step hierarchical model presented in Figure 11–4. These steps are based on a marketing model designed to change the behavior of a target audience (Kotler & Andreasen, 1996). The 10 steps are grouped into five sets of tasks for the clinician:

1. **Education.** To become successful hearing-aid users, individuals must have a clear understanding of the magnitude of their hearing loss and realize that the loss is not medically reversible. They also need to understand their options in managing their communication problems and understand the value and limitations of hearing aids.

Audiologist's Task	Step	Patient Stage
Educate	1.	Understands nature of his/her hearing loss.
	2.	Understands what a hearing aid can and cannot do.
Change Values	3.	Realizes hearing aids are not a sign of aging.
	4.	Considers using a hearing aid.
Change Attitudes	5.	Learns about appropriate hearing aid styles.
	6.	Perceives that the benefits accrued from using a hearing aid exceed monetary and non-monetary costs.
Motivate Patient To Act	7.	Understands steps for obtaining a hearing aid.
	8.	Acquires hearing aid.
Establish Use Pattern	9.	Completes trial period with hearing aid.
	10.	Continues appropriate usage.

Figure 11-4. A model for developing motivation in adults to use hearing aids for the first time.

2. **Value change:** Individuals must believe that hearing aids will not result in devaluation of them by others. Others will not see them as old or as damaged goods. Additionally, they must come to realize that hearing aids can reduce communication difficulties and that they are relevant to their own lives. This step may entail a discussion of current beliefs and values, and an eventual disregard for the influences of family, friends, or co-workers who may have negative views about hearing-aid use.

3. **Attitude change:** The audiologist may discuss appropriate hearing aid styles and ask patients about preferred styles. They may discuss the monetary and nonmonetary costs associated with obtaining a hearing aid. Ideally, the patient will come to believe that the benefits received from using a device outweigh the costs.
4. **Action:** The audiologist must describe the steps involved in obtaining a hearing aid. The person then undergoes a hearing aid evaluation and fitting.
5. **Establishment of use pattern:** Once an individual has obtained a hearing aid, the aural rehabilitation process is not over. In particular, the individual should continue using the hearing aid in appropriate communication interactions.

Hearing Aid Evaluation for Adults

Once motivation is established and candidacy is determined, the individual receives a hearing aid evaluation. The audiologist selects the appropriate electroacoustic properties for the hearing aid, commonly by means of a prescriptive procedure. The amount of gain is prescribed, usually so that more gain is provided for the poorer frequencies and less for the better frequencies. The maximum sound pressure level output (SSPL-90) is also determined, after measuring loudness discomfort levels (LDLs) (see Chapter 6).

During the hearing-aid evaluation, the audiologist and patient determine the style of hearing aid. This decision is based on a combined consideration of the magnitude of the individual's hearing loss and his or her personal preference. For instance, an audiologist might conclude that a BTE device is most appropriate for a person who has a severe sensorineural hearing loss. However, after discovering he is adamantly opposed to wearing a visible device, the audiologist may prudently recommends an ITE hearing aid. By following the patient's lead, the audiologist adverts certain nonuse of the hearing aid by the patient.

Other decisions that will be made during the hearing-aid fitting include whether the person will use one hearing aid (monaural amplification) or two (binaural amplification), the type of hearing aid microphone (e.g., omnidirectioanl versus directional), and whether various features are desired, such as a telephone switch or a remote control switch for adjusting volume.

Hearing-Aid Fitting and Orientation

Once a hearing aid has been selected, ordered, and received, the patient returns to the audiological clinic for a hearing aid fitting and orientation. This is a very important segment of the aural rehabilitation process. The person must become comfortable in handling the device and must feel confident that he or she can manage this new piece of technology.

Mail-In Daily Logs

A novel method to provide follow-up after the initial hearing-aid orientation is through the use of daily logs, similar to the procedure we considered in Chapter 3. The audiologist creates seven postcards, each addressed with the audiologist's business address and each with a stamp. On the other side of each card, a date is printed, with the seven cards having seven consecutive dates. Each day, the patient's task is to complete three items printed on the backside of that day's card: The time the hearing aid was put on, the time the hearing aid was taken off, and any additional comments. The patient mails a card every day, so the audiologist is assured that the cards were not completed on one occasion.

This daily log allows the audiologist to monitor the patient's progress during the initial period of adjustment. The audiologist can determine whether the patient is gradually increasing use time and whether the patient is experiencing any difficulties. For example, one patient commented that her hearing aid squealed, on three separate days. Any time a patient seems to be having difficulty in adjusting to the hearing aid (e.g., if the patient reports a problem on two or more days), the audiologist can call the patient and discuss the difficulties, and if necessary, schedule an appointment.

The hearing-aid is fitted to the patient's ear. Performance with the hearing aid is then evaluated, often first with real-ear measurements, in which a miniature microphone attached to a plastic tube is placed in the ear canal to measure loudness of sounds, both with and without the hearing aid. Speech recognition performance also is measured with and without the hearing aid. Finally, the new user is asked about sound quality. The clinician may ask such questions as the following:

- **Can you understand my voice? Does it sound natural? Am I too soft or too loud? Do I sound tinny?**
- **How does your own voice sound? Does it sound hollow? Do you feel like you are talking inside a cave or a barrel?**
- **How do environmental noises sound? Can you hear the telephone ring? How do your footsteps sound?**

Once the hearing aid is introduced, an overview of its operation and maintenance is presented. This overview includes a demonstration of how to clean it, how to troubleshoot problems, and how to turn it on and off. The new hearing-aid user might be given simple printed guidelines for maintaining the device, such as those presented in Table 11–2.

If the device has a telephone switch, the individual should practice turning on the switch, placing the telephone handset over the hearing aid, and then conversing on the clinic telephone. If the hearing aid does not have a telephone switch, the person might practice placing the telephone handset at a short distance from the hearing aid microphone. The patient should insert and remove the device several times and adjust the volume.

Individuals also practice putting the battery into the battery compartment and taking it out, and are shown the battery's negative and positive sides. They should receive information about where to purchase batteries, how much they might cost, and how long they should last. They also should receive printed materials concerning the proper disposal of batteries, because dead batteries pose a danger to children and pets.

Table 11–3 describes appropriate expectations for hearing aid use. The patient and the audiologist will probably review the benefits and limitations of hearing aids, even if they have done so already during a previous appointment. Other topics will include feedback (what it is, why it occurs, and how it can be minimized), adjustment (one must become accustomed to listening to amplified speech), and how to know when the aid is not functioning normally (what to try at home to fix it and when to return to the audiologist).

Printed information about the trial period and warranty are provided during the hearing-aid orientation. Usually, patients receive a 1-month trial period with a new hearing aid, and may return it for a full or partial refund if they are not satis-

Table 11–2. This handout can be provided to patients as a guide to maintaining their hearing aids.

Do's and Don'ts for Maintaining Your Hearing Aid

Do:

- Regularly remove earwax from the earmold or sound-outlet of the hearing aid, using a wax removal brush or a wax loop remover.
- Routinely wipe the hearing aid with a clean, dry tissue.
- Open the battery case every night.
- Store hearing aid in your carrying case with a dry-pack and place in a safe place.
- Ensure your hands are clean and dry and free of creams before handling the hearing aid.
- Keep the hearing aid away from moisture.
- Carry a spare fresh battery with you when you are out.
- Check your batteries and replace when necessary.
- Turn off the hearing aid before taking it out of your ear to prevent feedback.
- Keep hearing aid away from dogs and cats.
- Remove your hearing aid when you are perspiring, such as on a very hot day or during strenuous exercise.
- Clean the earmold and tubing on a weekly basis.

Don't:

- Leave a dead battery in the battery drawer.
- Apply hair spray or face powder when wearing a hearing aid.
- Bathe, shower, walk in the rain, or swim when wearing a hearing aid.
- Take your hearing aid out while standing on a hard surface such as a tile floor; hearing aids are fragile and may break if dropped.
- Wear your hearing aid when using a hair dryer.
- Discard batteries in a place that is accessible to children or pets.
- Force the battery compartment closed; if it won't close, recheck the battery position or try another battery.

Source: Adapted from *Hearing Aids: Who Needs Them?* by D. P. Pascoe, 1991. St. Louis, MO: Big Bend Books.

fied. Patients should be encouraged to have a hearing evaluation and a hearing-aid check on an annual basis. Some may return to the clinic more often because they are experiencing difficulties. For instance, the earmold may not fit properly. During this period of early use, the patient probably will be administered speech recognition tests to assess benefit of amplification and to validate performance. In addition, self-assessment questionnaires about the benefit of hearing aid use may also be completed. Common instruments used for this purpose include the Hearing Aid Review (Brooks, 1990), Profile of Hearing Aid Performance (Cox & Alexander, 1991), and

Table 11–3. Appropriate expectations for hearing-aid use.

1. Many hearing aids may make speech somewhat clearer because they are adjusted to amplify the sounds you have the most difficulty hearing.

2. Hearing aids not only amplify speech, but also noises in the background, so you will probably have difficulty understanding speech in noisy environments.

3. Hearing aids make soft sounds loud enough for you to hear, but are designed to keep strong sounds from being uncomfortably loud.

4. Even when wearing a hearing aid, you will probably experience problems understanding people who are talking from a different room and locating where sound is coming from.

5. Hearing aids may not be helpful in reverberent listening conditions, such as rooms that have hard walls and floors and no draperies or carpet.

6. Your voice and the voices of others may sound different; you might feel that your voice is emanating from inside of a barrel.

7. Hearing aids will let you hear some sounds that you have not heard for a while, such as your own breathing or clothes rustling.

8. You will still have difficulty understanding speech, even though you are wearing a hearing aid.

9. Your hearing aid should be comfortable to wear; if it is not, then contact your audiologist.

Source: Adapted from *Hearing Aids: Who Needs Them?* by D. P. Pascoe, 1991. St. Louis, MO: Big Bend Books.

the Hearing Aid Performance Inventory (Kricos, Lesner, Sandridge, & Yanke, 1987).

Establishing a Use Pattern

Research suggests that 18% of adults who own hearing aids do not utilize them. Forty-seven percent are dissatisfied with their devices (Kochkin, 1997). There are several possible reasons why people may not use their hearing aids. Some individuals find hearing aids uncomfortable to wear or difficult to handle. Some experience overwhelming problems when listening in the presence of background noise. Others may have had unre-

Hearing aid use pattern: the times, situations, and locations in which a hearing aid user wears the hearing aids.

alistic expectations about what a hearing aid can and cannot do, and they may receive less than expected benefit. For some, speech may sound "tinny" or loud. In some instances, patients may have wanted one kind of hearing aid (such as an in-the-ear aid) but the audiologist prescribed another, one that may be more appropriate for the hearing loss configuration (such as a behind-the-ear style). Research suggests that this state of affairs may lead to overall dissatisfaction (Mueller, Bryant, Brown, & Budinger, 1991). Prefitting counseling, allowing the patient to choose the hearing aid style, and ample postfitting follow-up can increase patient satisfaction and lead to greater hearing-aid use.

There are at least three identifiable patterns to describe the ways in which adults use hearing aids (Figure 11–5). Those who eventually become full-time users often increase the number of hours per day that they use the new hearing aid, so that after several days or weeks, it is used during almost all waking hours. Commonly, persons who reject their hearing aids, either return them to their audiologist or put them away in a drawer, trying them for only a brief trial period of a few days or weeks. Finally, some individuals never achieve full-time use nor do they reject the hearing aid(s). They may try wearing the hearing aid in a variety of situations initially, and then decide that they need it only for specific places. An intermittent use pattern is best established on the basis of experience, so the individual actually tries the device in a variety of situations before deciding when it is and is not helpful, rather than on assumptions made by either the patient or the audiologist. Intermittent use patterns are most common among those with a mild hearing loss.

ASSISTIVE LISTENING DEVICES AND OTHER ASSISTIVE DEVICES

Individuals may use assistive listening devices either in addition to or in lieu of a hearing aid. The need for various devices relates to a person's degree of hearing loss, his or her ability to recognize speech in quiet and noise, social and occupational demands, and motivation to use hearing aids and/or assistive devices. Probably the most common requests for assistive devices pertain to telephone amplification systems, and then television viewing. Although there are many exceptions, it is a general rule of thumb that the greater the hearing loss the greater the interest in and need for assistive listening devices. This is

Full-time Use Pattern

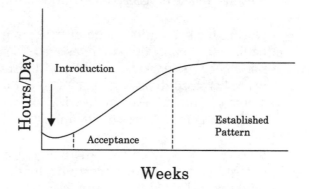

Rejection Pattern

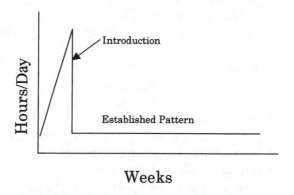

Intermittent Use Pattern

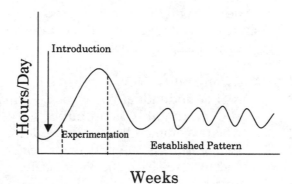

Figure 11-5. Patterns of use found in first-time hearing-aid users.

especially true for alerting devices, when individuals with severe and profound losses must rely on alerting stimuli to warn them of such conditions as fire or other emergencies, whether they are awake or asleep (and not wearing a hearing aid).

During the evaluation stage of designing a patient's aural rehabilitation plan, you will investigate the patient's capabilities, preferences, situational needs, and lifestyle as they pertain to his or her need for assistive devices. For instance, you may ask a person who has a severe hearing loss about interest in assisted listening for television viewing.

In assessing the need for assistive devices, the clinician might determine those communicative situations for which devices might be indicated. For example, Table 11–4 suggests those circumstances in which alerting, listening, and visual support systems might be appropriate for adults who have severe or profound hearing losses. In this framework, communicative interactions are classified as interactive or noninteractive, and warning needs are classified as basic or lifestyle-specific.

To obtain information about a person's need for and current use of assistive listening devices, some clinicians have employed written checklists like those presented in the Key Resources section at the end of this chapter. Preferably after a person has had an opportunity to gain experience with a hearing aid, the audiologist can review this checklist with him or her, and ask about situations that still are problematic. As problems are identified, the clinician can refer the individual to the checklist and then demonstrate systems that currently are not used, but that are appropriate for alleviating communication difficulties (Schum & Tye-Murray, 1995).

Issues that might be considered as the aural rehabilitation strategy is put together and recommendations for assistive devices are being formulated include (Compton, 1995):

■ **Affordability:** How expensive is the device? Especially if an individual has recently purchased a hearing aid, affordability is an important issue to consider when recommending assistive devices. It may be desirable to have the patient prioritize listening needs, and then to select the most useful/versatile assistive device(s) accordingly.
■ **Reliability and Durability:** Will the device work as promised, and will it hold up over repeated usage? Many manufacturers are now producing assistive de-

Table 11-4. Circumstances in which patients with profound or severe hearing losses may desire assistive listening devices.

I. Basic Warning Signals
   A. Smoke alarms
   B. Doorbell/knock
   C. Telephone ring
   D. Intruders

II. Lifestyle-specific Warning Signals
   A. Vehicle, such as sirens or horns
   B. Alarm clock
   C. Children/infants
   D. Household appliances, such as microwave or washer/dryer signals

III. Interactive Communication
   A. Face-to-face
   B. Telephone conversation
   C. Group
      1. home
      2. workplace
      3. social gatherings
      4. meetings
      5. classrooms

IV. Noninteractive Communication
   A. At home
      1. television
      2. radio
      3. stereo
   B. At work
   C. At public sites
      1. religious services
      2. movies
      3. concerts
      4. dramatic arts presentations
      5. lectures
      6. professional conferences
      7. sports events
      8. airport terminal

Source: Adapted from "Alerting and assistive systems: Counseling implications for cochlear implant users, by L. K. Schum and N. Tye-Murray, 1991. In R. S. Tyler and D. J. Schum (Eds.), *Assistive Devices for Persons with Hearing Impairment* (pp. 86–102). Needham Heights, MS: Allyn and Bacon.

vices, some of which vary in reliability, quality, and durability. When recommending an assistive device, you will want to balance the features of a particular device against its cost. Reliability may be of paramount consideration when safety is an issue, as in emergency alerting systems like fire detectors.

■ **Operability:** How does it work? The person must be able to manage the device. For instance, he or she should be able to replace the batteries, if applicable, and be able to operate the device. Sometimes formal instruction is necessary; therefore, the patient must have the time and the cognitive (and possibly financial) wherewithal to participate in a training session.

■ **Portability:** Can the device easily be transported from one locale to another? In some instances, portability is an issue. If someone travels frequently, for example, then the person will want a telephone amplifier that can easily be transported in a purse or coat pocket. A replacement handset amplifier would be inappropriate in this instance.

■ **Compatibility:** Can the device be used with a hearing aid? In many cases, patients wear their hearing aids at all times and will opt to wear the aid with any assistive listening device.

■ **Cosmetics:** What does it look like when in use? Some people may be self-conscious about using an assistive listening device. For example, pulling out a wireless FM listening device at a restaurant may be difficult. Counseling and opportunity for practice under the supervision of an audiologist may minimize cosmetic concerns.

In dispensing an assistive listening device, the following steps usually are followed (Sutherland, 1995):

■ Demonstrate how to use the device(s).
■ Review the advantages and disadvantages of the device and its capabilities and limitations.
■ Describe how the devices work and how to install them.
■ Demonstrate how to troubleshoot the devices.
■ Demonstrate the device to family members.
■ Answer any questions.
■ Review the Americans with Disabilities Act and talk about patients' legal rights.

FOLLOW-UP

Ideally, new hearing-aid users will participate in a group aural rehabilitation program following receipt of a hearing aid or other listening device. Information about the care and use of the device that was presented during the hearing-aid orientation may be reiterated, and provision made for supervised practice in handling the device and in using the telephone. Other class topics likely will include communication strategies, listening, and speechreading. The Key Resources section presents an example of a course syllabus for a 6-week adult aural rehabilitation group class.

For individuals who cannot or will not participate in a formal aural rehabilitation program, the clinician might provide written materials via the mail and occasionally write short letters inquiring about the patient's satisfaction and progress with amplification.

Apart from learning about their listening devices and communication strategies, patients also may learn about legislation concerning the rights of persons with hearing impairment. Several recent laws that are relevant to adults are presented in Table 11–5, along with a brief description of each one.

Individuals might be encouraged to join self-help organizations for hard-of-hearing adults. One such organization is Self Help for Hard of Hearing People, Inc. (SHHH), one of the largest in existence for hard-of-hearing adults. It is comprised of hundreds of local chapters and a national office that disseminates information about hearing loss and communication. The Key Resources section presents addresses for this group as well as other self-help organizations. In addition, it lists professional organizations that serve hard-of-hearing and Deaf adults.

You probably will want to follow up later on individual's progress with using any assistive devices, and evaluate whether the device is working for the person and meeting the targeted needs. In addition, you will want to ensure that the individual is using a device properly. If the person is embarrassed to use a device in public when appropriate, you might include assertiveness training in your formal aural rehabilitation classes (Compton, 1995).

Typically individuals should return to their audiologists on an annual basis for a hearing test and a hearing-aid check. During these visits, the audiologist can access whether hearing has worsened and whether the hearing aid is still functioning properly. Assessment usually includes an aided and unaided audiogram and word recognition testing. Sometimes, self-report scales are administered to access subjective hearing-aid benefit. Example scales are presented in Table 11–6.

CASE STUDY

Now let us consider a case study, as an example how the goals of the aural rehabilitation plan might be tailored to meet the individual needs of a specific patient.

Table 11–5. Legislation that hard-of-hearing and Deaf adults should be familiar with.

Legislation	Effect
Section 504 of the Rehabilitation Act of 1973	Prohibits discrimination against qualified disabled people in any federally supported program or activity
Hearing Aid Compatibility Act of 1988 (P.L. 394)	Mandates that all telephones manufactured for sale in the United States after August 16, 1989 (cordless phones by 1991) must be hearing-aid compatible
1988 Telecommunications Accessibility Enhancement Act (P.L. 100-542)	Requires that the General Services Administration make provision for telecommunications access to federal agencies, both for employees to be able to use the telephone and for deaf and speech-impaired individuals to have access to federal offices
Television Decoder Circuitry Act (Chip Bill) (P.L. 101-431)	As of July 1993, all television sets sold in the United States with screens 13 inches or larger must have built-in circuitry that can decode and display closed captions
The Americans With Disabilities Act (ADA) (P.L. 101-336)	Signed into law on July 17, 1990, this legislation extends civil rights protection for people with disabilities in private sector employment, public accommodations, state and local government services, transportation, and telecommunications relay services

Source: Adapted from "New perspectives in audiological rehabilitation, by C. A. Binnie, 1991. In G. A. Studebaker, F. H. Bess, and L. B. Beck (Eds.), *The Vanderbilt Hearing-aid Report II* (pp. 233–243). Parkton, MD: York Press.

Table 11–6. Self-assessment scales for measuring hearing-aid benefit.

Scale	Author(s)
Hearing Problem Inventory	Button (1980)
Hearing Aid Performance Inventory (HAPI)	Walden, Demorest, and Heper (1984)
Hearing Handicap Inventory for the Elderly (HHIE)	Newman and Weinstein (1988)

Mrs. Kerley is a mid-level manager in an investment brokerage house. She is 49 years old. She recently has experienced difficulty in talking on the telephone, which is why she is seeking aural rehabilititation. She does not report any other difficulties in her home or workplace. There is some evidence that Mrs. Kerley is reluctant to admit a hearing loss and may be underplaying the magnitude of her communication difficulties. For instance, she mentions that her teenage boys tend to mumble, but dismisses it as a "stage they are going through." Mrs. Kerley and her clinician identified the following aural rehabilitation goals:

■ **Assessment of hearing status.** Mrs. Kerley will receive a complete audiological evaluation, including speech recognition testing.
■ **Provision of counseling.** Counseling will be aimed at helping Mrs. Kerley accept and cope with her hearing loss.
■ **Consideration of a hearing aid with a telecoil.** In early discussions, she has indicated to her audiologist that she has mixed feelings about using a hearing aid, because she is afraid her employer may think her old. In turn, this may limit her career advancement. The audiologist will work with her to develop motivation to use a device.
■ **Receipt of a telephone amplifier.** Mrs. Kerley's work telephone will be fitted with a telephone amplifier.
■ **Practice in using communication strategies on the telephone.** Mrs. Kerley will receive one-on-one communication strategies training, with special emphasis placed on telephone use.

FINAL REMARKS

Technology has opened new vistas for the rehabilitation of individuals who have hearing loss. Sophisticated hearing aids, various assistive listening devices, and cochlear implants have made it much easier for clinicians to alleviate listening difficulties. Ironically, these very advances sometimes make us lose sight of the fact that many adults continue to have problems with communication even after receiving high-technology devices. They still need to receive aural rehabilitation follow-up services.

Many aspects of aural rehabilitation can be labor-intensive, expensive to provide, and time-consuming. Some services require much individualized attention for the patient, over the course of hours, weeks, and even months. As a professional, you may feel sometimes that you simply do not have enough time nor the financial resources to provide the high-quality aural rehabilitation you desire. However, many professionals are attempting to develop effective and efficient procedures that might alleviate these difficulties. Laser videodisc technology, VHS audiovideo tapes and home VHS players, personal computers with built-in audio stereo speakers, Compact Disc (CD)—ROM, and digital versatile disc (DVD) portend a broadened array of aural rehabilitation services for adults who have hearing loss. Moreover, the time spent in providing quality services will have a long-term payoff in patient satisfaction and in referrals to your practice.

KEY CHAPTER POINTS

- ✔ There are three stages involved in developing an aural rehabilitation plan: evaluation, strategy, and implementation. At each stage, the focus will be on customizing the plan for the individual.
- ✔ Counseling provides many benefits to the hard-of-hearing individual, including better self-acceptance and reduced stress and discouragement. A clinician might provide informational counseling, rational acceptance and adjustment counseling, and/or emotional acceptance and adjustment counseling.
- ✔ You may need to develop motivation in a patient to use a hearing aid. This may entail an education process, a change in the patient's value system and attitude, and establishment of a hearing-aid use pattern.
- ✔ Hearing aids are available to alleviate a wide range of hearing loss. Candidacy depend on degree of loss and also on a person's lifestyle, occupation, and motivation to use a hearing aid.
- ✔ A significant number of adults who receive hearing aids do not use them. There are several reasons for nonuse. For example, some people find the sound unacceptable, and others are disappointed that their hearing aids do not provide greater benefit.
- ✔ Issues to consider when recommending an assistive device include affordability, durability, operability, portability, compatibility, and cosmetics.

KEY RESOURCES

Alerting, Assistive, Listening, and Visual Support Systems Checklist

Date: _____

Instructions to the clinician: Place an (X) in the column that best describes client's use of, interest in, or need for, each listed system.

SYSTEM	CURRENTLY USES	USED TO USE	IS INTERESTED IN	DOES NOT NEED
Assistive Listening Systems				
Closed-caption decoder for TV	☐	☐	☐	☐
Telecommunication for the Deaf (TDD)	☐	☐	☐	☐
Direct audio input (to speech processor from battery-operated radio, tape-player, or portable stereo)	☐	☐	☐	☐
Telephone adapter	☐	☐	☐	☐
Telephone amplifier	☐	☐	☐	☐
Telephone answering machine	☐	☐	☐	☐
TDD Relay Message Service	☐	☐	☐	☐
Group System (FM, loop, hardwire, infrared)	☐	☐	☐	☐

(continued)

SYSTEM	CURRENTLY USES	USED TO USE	IS INTERESTED IN	DOES NOT NEED
Fax machine	☐	☐	☐	☐
Oral interpreter	☐	☐	☐	☐
Alerting Systems				
Telephone signaler	☐	☐	☐	☐
Doorbell signaler	☐	☐	☐	☐
Door Knock signaler	☐	☐	☐	☐
Smoke alarm signaler	☐	☐	☐	☐
Alarm clock signaler/vibrater	☐	☐	☐	☐
Baby cry signaler	☐	☐	☐	☐
Pet cat or pet dog	☐	☐	☐	☐
Trained hearing ear dog	☐	☐	☐	☐
Other (specify):	☐	☐	☐	☐

Comments: _____

_____

_____

Source: Adapted from "Alerting and assistive systems: Counseling implications for cochlear implant users," by L. K. Schum and N. Tye-Murray, 1995. In R. S. Tyler and D. J. Schum (eds.), *Assistive Devices for Persons with Hearing Impairment* (pp. 86–122). Needham Heights, MA: Allyn and Bacon.

Overview of a 6-Week Communication-Based Aural Rehabilitation Class for Hard-of-Hearing Adults[1]

Week 1

1. Introduction of class members
2. Pretraining assessment (self-assessment questionnaires, audio-visual, and vision-only speech recognition assessment)
3. Hearing loss and communication handicap
4. Hearing aids: Care, maintenance, and benefits
5. Discussion: How to be a good listener
6. Homework assignment
   a. Review listening strategies
   b. Identify difficult listening situations encountered during the week
   c. Review handout materials about assertive, aggressive and passive communication behaviors

Week 2

1. Discuss homework
2. Discuss handouts: What does assertive behavior have to do with hearing loss?
3. Assertive, aggressive, and passive communication behaviors exercises
4. Speechreading practice
5. Discuss second set of handouts: Factors that influence communication success
6. Topicon exercises (see Chapter 3, this text)
7. Homework
   a. Identify difficult communication situations encountered during the week
   b. Identify one situation in which you had a successful conversation, and describe factors that contributed to success

Week 3

1. Discuss homework
2. Group discussion: How to take control of the communication environment and optimize your residual hearing and speechreading skills
3. Environment exercises (with handouts)

[1]Modeled after a program offered at Central Institute for the Deaf (Mauźe & Frederick, 1995).

4. Speechreading practice
5. Group discussion: Communication is more than just hearing
6. Continuous discourse tracking exercises (see Chapter 4, this text)
7. Homework
   a. Use repair strategies during the following week, and be prepared to describe use to class
   b. Describe an incident in which you optimized the communication environment

Week 4

1. Discuss homework
2. Group discussion: Communication breakdowns and repair strategies
3. Speechreading practice
4. Group discussion: Communication is more than just hearing (continued from last week)
5. Role playing: Using repair strategies effectively
6. Homework: Construct examples of message-tailoring remarks (see Chapter 2, this text)

Week 5

1. Discuss homework
2. Group discussion: When hearing aids aren't enough: Assistive listening devices for the hard-of-hearing adult
3. Speechreading practice
4. Quest-Ar practice (see Chapter 3, this text)
6. Homework: Review handout materials concerning the communication environment

Week 6

1. Posttraining assessment
2. Group discussion: Putting it all together

Self-Help and Professional Organizations
That Serve Hard-of-Hearing and Deaf Adults

Alexander Graham Bell Association for the Deaf
3417 Volta Place, N.W.
Washington, DC 20007

American Deafness and Rehabilitation Association
P.O. Box 55369
Little Rock, AK 72225

American Athletic Association of the Deaf
2015 Wooded Way
Adelphi, MD 20783

American Hearing Research Foundation
55 E. Washington Street, Suite 2022
Chicago, IL 60602

American Tinnitus Association
P.O. Box 5
Portland, OR 97207-0005

Association of Late Deafened Adults (ALDA)
P.O. Box 641763
Chicago, IL, 60644-1763

Better Hearing Institute
P.O. Box 1840
Washington, DC 20013

Canadian Hard of Hearing Association (CHHA)
P.O. Box 3176, Station "D"
Ottawa, Ontario, Canada K1P 6H8

Canadian Association of the Deaf (CAD)
205-2435 Holly Lane
Ottawa, Ontario, Canada K1V 7P2

Ménière's Network
The Ear Foundation
2000 Church Street
Box 11
Nashville, TN 37236

National Association of the Deaf (NAD)
814 Thayer Avenue
Silver Spring, MD 20910

National Captioning Institute (NCI)
5203 Leesburg Pike, Suite 1500
Falls Church, VA 22041

National Center for Law and the Deaf
800 Florida Avenue, NE
Washington, DC 20002

National Center on Employment of the Deaf
National Technical Institute for the Deaf
Rochester Institute of Technology
1 Lomb Memorial Drive
Rochester, NY 14623

National Crisis Center for the Deaf
University of Virginia Medical Center
Box 484
Charlottesville, VA 22908

National Information Center on Deafness
Gallaudet University
800 Florida Avenue, NE
Washington, DC 2002-3625

Self-Help for Hard of Hearing People (SHHH)
7800 Wisconsin Avenue
Bethesda, MD 20814

12

Older Adults

Topics

- Presbycusis
- Speech Recognition
- Factors That Influence the Impact of Hearing Loss
- Aural Rehabilitation Plans for Older Persons
- Hearing Aids, Assistive Listening Devices, and Follow-up Aural Rehabilitation

- Aural Rehabilitation in the Institutional Setting
- Case Study
- Final Remarks
- Key Chapter Points

In this chapter, we consider the older members of our society. For our purposes, these are individuals who are 65 years of age and older. However, this age is a somewhat arbitrary benchmark, and people, agencies, and other concerns vary in how they define the term "older." Theaters, shops, and national parks confer the status of "senior citizen" to any individual over the age of 55 years. On the other hand, Congress has extended the mandatory age for retirement from 65 years to 70 years. Certainly, one reason for these ambiguous definitions relates to the heterogeneity of the population. For instance, one 65-year-old woman may be vibrant and healthy, and be a "youthful old," while another woman who is 60 years old may be sedentary and afflicted with illness.

It is very likely that, as a speech and hearing professional, you will at some point in your career work with older people (Figure 12–1). The elderly represent the fastest growing segment in American society. More than 30 million people in the United States are over the age of 65 years. This number is projected to rise to 39 million by the year 2010 (U.S. Census Bureau, 1986). In 1988, individuals 65 years and older comprised approximately 12% of the United States population. By the year 2020, this figure may swell to 13–18%

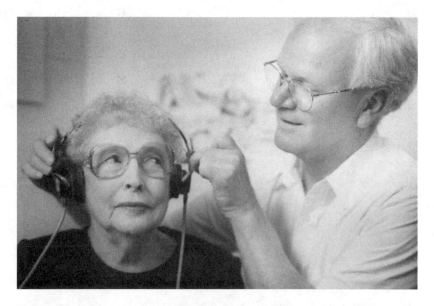

Figure 12–1. The number of elderly in the U.S. population is increasing. It is likely that they will comprise a significant segment of a speech and hearing professional's case load. (Photograph by Marcus Kosa, courtesy of Central Institute for the Deaf)

as the baby boom generation ages (Cunningham & Brookban, 1988). This group has the highest demand for medical care and social services than any other population group.

Victor

An audiologist and her family visit her husband's parents once a year. One year, the audiologist noticed that her father-in-law, Victor, seemed depressed as compared to the year before. He spent most of the pretty summer days sitting on an easy chair with his dog wedged beside him. When the family gathered in the family room to talk, Victor said little and often even read the newspaper. Victor refused to attend social functions, and had discontinued his daily walks with the dog. The audiologist noticed that Victor sometimes did not respond to his name being called from another room and often responded inappropriately to questions. For example, to the question, "Do you want peas or corn tonight?", he might grumble, "yes."

After several days of observing Victor, the audiologist began to suspect that he might have a hearing loss, and broached the possibility with Victor and her mother-in-law. With much coaxing, the audiologist convinced her father-in-law to have a hearing test while she was still in town. Victor was found to have a bilateral, moderate-to-severe sensorineural hearing loss. Driving home from the clinic that day, he turned to his daughter-in-law and confided, "Just between you and me, I was beginning to think I was losing my marbles. People were looking at me strange when I would try to join into a conversation, as if I said something peculiar, and I was thinking I was forgetting everything anyone told me. Maybe it is my hearing that's all that's wrong." Victor received a hearing aid shortly thereafter. The next summer, the audiologist found her father-in-law to be more his outgoing and gregarious self.

This narrative hints at several important points relevant to the older population:

■ **Hearing loss can be misinterpreted for other signs of aging, and might co-occur with depression.** In fact Williamson and Fried (1996) demonstrated that it is not uncommon for older adults to attribute hearing difficulties to old age instead of to a specific condition that can be alleviated with treatment.
■ **Hearing loss can decrease social engagement and increase social isolation.**
■ **Provision of aural rehabilitation services can have a positive effect on the quality of life for many older individuals.**

PRESBYCUSIS

Many older persons experience hearing loss. In fact, hearing loss is the third most common chronic condition afflicting the noninstitutionalized elderly (Hazard, Andrews, Bierman, & Blass, 1990). Although estimates vary, about 30% of individuals over the age of 65 years who dwell in the community have some degree of hearing impairment. Hearing impairment is more common among older men than women, and men are more likely to begin losing their hearing at a younger age (Gordon-Salant, 1987).

Presbycusis is age-related hearing loss.

Presbycusis is the global term used to refer to hearing loss associated with the aging process. The exact cause of presbycusis is not known. No doubt, age-related degeneration and one's genetic make-up are important factors. A lifetime of noise exposure in a modern society, in both recreational and occupational settings, also takes its toll in the later years. Disease and exposure to ototoxic agents can be contributing factors in some individuals.

Pure-Tone Thresholds and Auditory Processing

Figure 12–2 presents median thresholds for males for each decade of life between the ages of 20 and 80 years. As can be seen, hearing loss increases with age, and the audiogram displays evolve from a fairly straight line in youth, from 500 to 6000 Hz, to a precipice in the mid-years, with the fall-off frequency at about 2000 Hz. By the eighth decade, the display presents a falling slope, with the greatest loss occurring in the high frequencies. The decline in hearing thresholds accelerates over time, with the rate becoming more pronounced after individuals pass into their 40s. The hearing loss may become significant enough to seek audiological help only in the sixth or seventh decade, when the PTA might be 20 dB or greater than it was during young adulthood (Chessman, 1997).

In addition to sensorineural hearing loss, some older individuals experience changes in their auditory processing abilities. These changes are indexed by performance on psychophysical tests and on tests of altered speech or demanding listening tasks. For example, some older people have a reduced ability to discriminate two sounds that differ in pitch, intensity, and/or duration (Schneider, 1997). If you present a 60 dB tone and a 65 dB tone to an older listener, he or she may say that they are

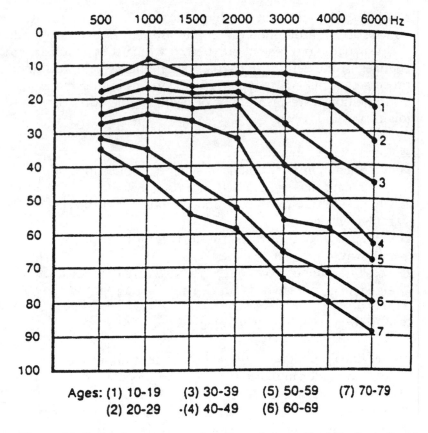

Figure 12-2. Audiograms as a function of decade of life. From *Aural Rehabilitation* (3rd ed.), by R. H. Hull, 1997, p. 300. San Diego: Singular Publishing Group. Reproduced with permission.

the same instead of different. Some persons have difficulty understanding time-compressed or frequency-filtered speech. Moreover, when a competing signal is presented to one ear, and the target speech signal to the other, many elderly adults experience greater difficulty in understanding the target signal than do younger listeners.

SPEECH RECOGNITION

A concomitant decline in speech recognition accompanies presbycusis. Beyond the age of 60 years, monosyllabic word recognition scores decline by 13% per decade in males and 6% per decade in females (Chessman, 1997). Speech recognition difficulties are exacerbated when an older person attempts to listen in a noisy environment, more so than is the case for younger listeners (Pederson, Rosenthal, & Moller, 1991; Plath, 1991).

Much research has been conducted to determine the extent to which speech recognition difficulties are caused by peripheral cochlear pathology and the extent to which they result from changes in the central nervous system and central auditory processing. This is a complex issue. We know that the aging brain demonstrates a number of changes, including the following (Willott, 1996):

■ A loss of neurons.
■ A reduction in the number of synaptic connections between neurons.
■ Changes in the excitatory and inhibitory neurotransmitter systems.
■ Changes in neural transmission along the auditory pathway.
■ Possibly, changes in cognitive processing of the acoustic signal (e.g., information processing, labeling, retrieval, and storage).
■ A decrement in long-term memory.

These global changes in brain functioning might have some effect on an older individual's ability to process rapid streams of speech information (Jerger, Chmiel, Wilson, & Luchi, 1995). They also may affect how well the individual comprehends the gist of a message.

Although these factors likely affect speech recognition, it appears that decreased word recognition is related primarily to changes in a person's hearing sensitivity at the cochlear level. Hearing sensitivity for the higher frequencies in particular relates to speech recognition performance. An older person's average hearing loss at the frequencies 1000, 2000, and 4000 Hz is the single best predictor of a variety of different speech recognition tests (Humes, 1996).

What Older Persons Have to Say About Hearing Loss

Sometimes you will hear comments that will clue you to the possibility of a hearing loss. Here are some remarks often made by older patients (Pichora-Fuller, 1997):

■ "I hear, but I have trouble understanding."
■ "Sounds seem all jumbled up."

- "It is difficult to tell where sounds are coming from."
- "I understand when it is quiet, but I have trouble when it is noisy."
- "I understand when I'm talking to one person, but I have trouble in a group."
- "In a group, if I know who is talking then I can follow the conversation, but I have trouble when someone else starts talking."
- "When someone else starts talking sometimes I have to look around to see who it is."
- "If I know the topic of conversation then I do pretty well, but I often get lost when the topic changes."
- "People seem to talk too fast; I need more time to make sense of what has been said."
- "It is not so much that I can't understand what is said but that it is tiring to listen."
- "I sometimes pretend to understand because it isn't worth it to ask the talker to repeat because I'm afraid that it would be an imposition and it could annoy or make the talker impatient."
- "I don't know for sure when I hear correctly and when I don't."
- "It's hard to get jokes; you have to get the punchline right away or it isn't funny."
- "When I'm with two or more people, they start talking to each other and leave me out."
- "I don't enjoy social events any more" (p. 125).

FACTORS THAT INFLUENCE THE IMPACT OF HEARING LOSS

Figure 12–3 indicates that a large number of factors influences the effect that hearing loss has on an older person's life. This figure provides a blueprint for compiling a profile of who the patient is and to develop an understanding of the impact of hearing loss. Impact will vary with an individual's economic circumstances, social circumstances, emotional status, and physical status. You will want to take into account these factors as you develop an aural rehabilitation plan for a particular patient and seek to minimize or eliminate specific communication problems.

Economic Circumstances

Longer lifespans and forced retirements have resulted in greater numbers of older persons living in poverty. Schulz

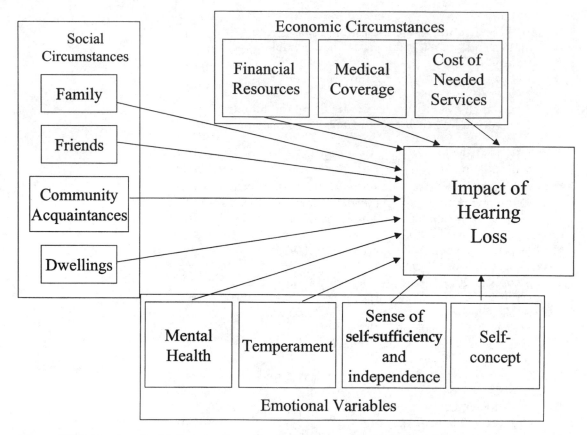

Figure 12-3. Factors that influence the effects of hearing loss for an older person.

(1992) suggested that the majority of elderly persons have only a modest income, and a significant minority live below the poverty level. However, the elderly as a group are not necessarily bereft financially as many stereotypes would suggest. In fact, their situation has actually improved since the 1960s and 1970s. Some individuals have prepared for retirement, and rely on Social Security incomes and/or work pensions. There are some older persons who do not have many expenses except those associated with health care, because their house is paid for, their children are grown, and other life expenses have been paid (Traynor, 1995).

Older woman tend to be economically disadvantaged as compared to their male counterparts. For example, twice as many women over the age of 85 years live in poverty than men (United States Census, 1984). Many women do not have independent resources to pay for hearing health care. This discrepancy in financial worth arises from such factors as wage discrimination and years of unpaid work in the home (Zones, Estes, & Binney, 1987). Largely because of social forces, many older women have not received higher education and technical training and have lived a life of financial dependence on a mate. The increase in divorce rate and the existence of no-fault divorce has undermined further the financial health of the nation's older females.

A patient's economic status may affect the impact of hearing loss and the aural rehabilitation plan, particularly if the individual does not have medical coverage. Decisions such as monaural versus binaural amplification or the selection of assistive listening devices may be influenced by a patient's financial resources, medical coverage, and cost of the devices and related services.

Social Circumstances

When examining the issue of social circumstances, we typically consider the people with whom patients interact and those individuals with whom they feel a connection. Social circumstances also include residency. For instance, does a patient live alone in a private home? In a private home with family members? In a nursing facility? Knowing the identities of a patient's communication partners and where the individual resides are important when designing an aural rehabilitation program.

A Family Affair

Sociologists and demographers tell us that most older persons have living children, and many older persons live within a 30-minute driving distance of at least one of their offspring. The majority of older persons see their children at least once a week, and three quarters of them talk to their children on the telephone on a weekly basis. As these data indicate, there typically is great potential to involve children in their parents' aural rehabilitation plan.

Social Contacts

The number of people a patient interacts with and the frequency of interaction influence the person's morbidity, mortality, and physical functioning (Strawbridge, Cohen, Shema, & Kaplan, 1996). Older people who have five or more contacts are less likely to suffer from loneliness and depression and more likely to have a higher quality of life than persons who have fewer social contacts. For example, a person who lives within a 30-mile radius of children and grandchildren and who works as a volunteer at the local zoo is more likely to have good mental health and be more interested in participating in an aural rehabilitation program than someone who has no family nearby and few interests outside of the home (Figure 12–4).

The extent to which an older individual maintains frequent and significant contacts with family, friends, and community acquaintances can ameliorate or exacerbate the impact of hearing loss. Social contacts allow an individual to feel more a part

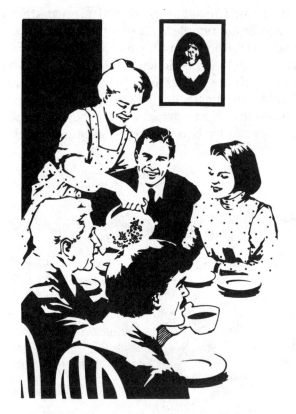

Figure 12–4. The number of social contacts and the frequency of contact can affect an older person's desire for aural rehabilitation. Persons who live near family members often are motivated to improve their communication effectiveness.

of life and more involved in the community and provide motivation to address a hearing loss. Individuals who do not have communication partners available often do not seek aural rehabilitation services (Figure 12–5).

Just as social relationships influence the impact of hearing loss, hearing loss can affect social relationships. It is not uncommon for a hearing loss to trigger a negative feedback loop like that illustrated in Figure 12–6. Lindblade and McDonald (1995) suggested that older persons may withdraw from social interactions because conversation becomes too effortful. In turn, family and friends may begin to perceive them as unsociable, preoccupied with health matters, forgetful, or paranoid (Figure 12–7). These perceptions may lead to an older individual mistakenly being labeled as demented, confused, hostile, or senile. For example, a son might find that his father frequently responds inappropriately to questions and suspect that he is experiencing cognitive decline. It may only be that the father has hearing loss, or has both hearing loss and mild confusion. As an older person withdraws, and appears to be less cooperative and/or less effective as a conversational partner, family and friends may begin to drift away and decrease contact. The older person may increasingly experience anger, frustration, apathy, and anxiety. This may lead to more withdrawal and more negative reactions from communication partners.

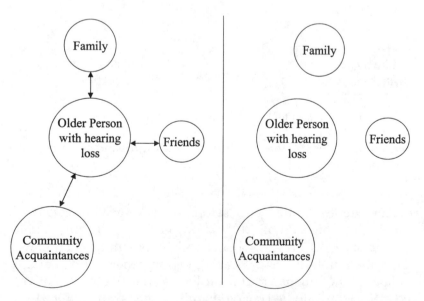

Figure 12–5. The number and frequency of social contacts influence a patient's motivation to seek aural rehabilitation services.

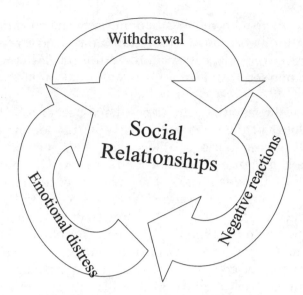

Figure 12-6. Hearing loss can trigger a negative feedback loop.

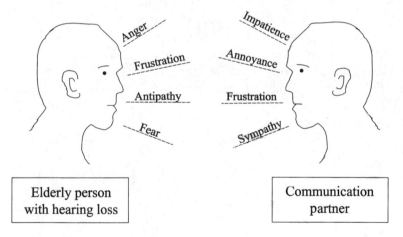

Figure 12-7. Hearing loss can create miscommunications between an older person and a frequent communication partner, and sometimes results in the older person withdrawing from social interactions.

To the extent possible, professionals working with an older individual should do all in their power to prevent this serial cascade of events. Provision of counseling for family and friends about the ramifications of hearing loss in general and characteristics of the patient's particular loss is crucial if this negative feedback loop is to be broken. Family, friends, and caretakers can learn how to counteract an older person's tendency to withdraw and avoid conversational interactions and encourage the individual to obtain aural rehabilitation services. In addition, they can actively participate in the aural rehabilitation program. They can learn how to use communication strategies effectively and/or learn how to help the older person handle a hearing aid or assistive listening device, or to handle the device for the person if necessary.

Residency

Most older persons live in private residencies, with only about 5% residing in nursing homes (Nussbaum et al., 1989). The majority of nursing home residents have hearing loss, and half of these have severe losses (Schow & Nerbonne, 1980; Voeks et al., 1990).

The residential-care population require special attention, as they are likely to have a multitude of impairments and health conditions, and their environments are likely to be more noisy than private home environments (Figure 12–8). Noisy environments can magnify communication handicap, and may result in

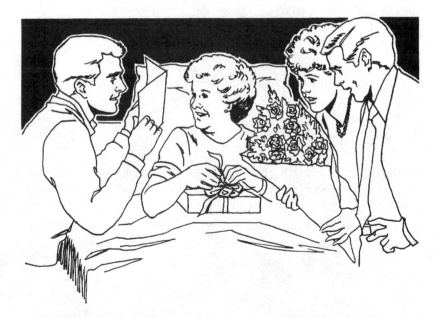

Figure 12-8. A patient's residence can have an impact on an aural rehabilitation plan. A person in a health-care facility or nursing home may have a particular need for assistive listening devices. In addition, health-care workers may need special instruction about how to communicate with an older person who has hearing loss; for example, making sure their mouth is clearly visible to the patient.

individuals withdrawing from communication interactions and social activities.

Emotional Variables

Now let's consider emotional variables, and how one's emotional state can influence the impact of hearing loss. A profile of a person's emotional state can be constructed by considering the following variables:

■ Mental health
■ Temperament
■ Sense of self-sufficiency and independence
■ Self-concept

Mental Health

A **mental health problem** is defined as psychopathology or clusters of other acute or chronic symptoms.

A person is said to have a *mental health problem* if he or she has psychopathology or clusters of other acute or chronic symptoms. As with any age group, older individuals vary widely in their mental health. However, it is not uncommon for an older person to suffer from depression. The following situations may trigger depression:

■ Loss of or separation from friends and loved ones.
■ Decreased ability to perform physical activities.
■ Retirement.
■ Empty-nest syndrome.
■ A decline in general health.

A hearing loss can magnify feelings of hopelessness, loneliness, and helplessness, and depression may decrease desire to seek hearing health care. Other mental conditions, such as anxiety, obsessive-compulsiveness, and neuroticism, also may increase the communication difficulties associated with a particular degree of hearing loss (Eriksson-Mangold & Carlsson, 1991).

Temperament

Temperament refers to stable personality traits.

Some people are, by temperament, more or less able to cope with hearing loss (Figure 12–9). *Temperament* refers to stable personality traits. Such traits as introversion versus extroversion, assertiveness versus passiveness, and optimism versus pessimism will relate to the impact of hearing loss (e.g., Knut-

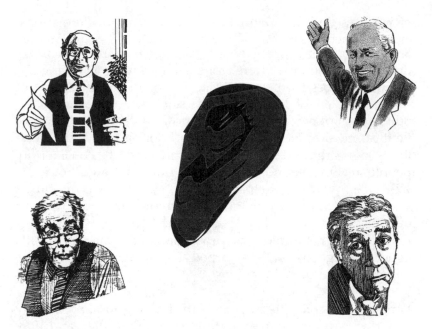

Figure 12–9. A person's temperament will affect how he or she copes with hearing loss.

son & Lansing, 1990). For instance, an older person might routinely be frustrated by minor irritations, such as getting stuck in traffic, breaking a pencil lead, or forgetting to set an alarm clock. This person may be more affected by hearing loss than someone who has a more easy-going temperament. He or she may be intolerant of talkers who are difficult to understand, and may over-react when a remark is missed or not recognized.

Sense of Self-Sufficiency and Independence

Self-sufficiency and independence relate to whether an individual can conduct day-to-day activities without undue reliance on others. Many older people feel increasingly dependent on others for daily activities. Some can no longer drive, some cannot do their own shopping, and some must have intermediaries accompany them to medical appointments. Hearing loss can be yet another signal of increased dependence, as an older person with hearing loss may have to rely on others to manage communication difficulties. One man complained, "My wife has to make all my telephone calls for me, and I hate it. It makes me feel like I'm 3 instead of 83!" One goal of the aural rehabilitation plan is to increase the older patient's sense of self-sufficiency and independence.

Self-sufficiency and independence relate to whether a person can conduct day-to-day activities without undue reliance on others.

Self-concept

Self-concept relates to how people view themselves; for example, does someone think of him- or herself as having a hearing impairment? Does the person think that he or she is capable of coping with a disability? Often one's self-concept does not match other people's perceptions, or an audiological report. One patient commented to her audiologist, "I don't feel old, and I certainly don't think of myself as a senior citizen. But the way people treat me reminds me I'm not young anymore. Someone will take my arm to help me up the stairs, or I go to buy a movie ticket, and they give me the senior citizen rate without even asking me if I'm eligible. It's weird." This woman was dismayed when her audiologist proceeded to describe the results of her hearing tests, and she learned she had a bilateral moderate hearing loss.

Persons' self-concepts interact with hearing loss. Some may experience difficulty in accepting aging altogether, and may refuse to wear a hearing aid. Conversely, another may accept hearing loss, and have no problem in maintaining a healthy self-concept.

Physical Variables

Physical variables as well as emotional variables influence the impact of hearing loss. Several physical changes occur as people age. Their skin wrinkles, age spots appear, hair may turn gray, joints stiffen, and muscles become weaker. Manual dexterity begins to decrease. The rate at which these changes occur varies among individuals, and some people are physically fit well into their 80s and even 90s. Physical fitness interacts with hearing loss to the extent that it may determine the kinds of communication interactions the individual engages in (e.g., Does the person attend parties? Still work?) and the kinds of listening devices that can be used (e.g., Is manual dexterity a problem if the patient desires an in-the-canal hearing aid?)

In addition to changes in physical fitness, many older persons experience chronic ailments, and these may influence the impact of hearing loss. About 40% of the elderly have some disabling and chronic condition (Atchley, 1993). The most common chronic ailments include (in order of frequency of occurrence, National Center for Health Statistics, 1987):

■ Arthritis
■ Cardiac disease

Hearing loss
Hypertension
Orthopedic problems
Cataracts

Three common physical conditions are especially relevant when we consider the impact of hearing loss for an older person. These are reduced vision, arthritis, and dementia.

Reduced Vision

Between about 30 and 40% of individuals over the age of 70 years have impaired vision (Castles, 1993; Vinding, 1989), and this percentage increases as a function of age. Unfortunately, the majority of individuals who have severe vision impairments also have significant hearing loss (Kirchner & Peterson, 1980). It is a sad twist of fate that, in the face of hearing loss, when someone could utilize the visual signal probably more so than at any other time in life for the purpose of speech recognition, this sense also begins to decline. Visual difficulties may relate to cataracts, glaucoma, diabetic retinopathy, or hemianopia, as well as other conditions.

In some cases, visual skills cannot be enhanced through the use of corrective lenses or ophthalmologic intervention. Reduced visual acuity has the following implications for the impact of hearing loss and the design of an aural rehabilitation plan:

Speechreading: The individual will not be able to utilize the visual signal maximally, so likely will experience more difficulty in day-to-day speech communication than a person who has similar hearing loss but normal vision.

Speech recognition training: Speechreading training may not be appropriate when vision is reduced, because the patient may not be able to adequately see lip movements and other facial gestures. Speech perception training might be aimed at helping the patient alert to auditory stimuli, and to utilize residual hearing to the fullest extent possible.

Communication environment: A patient who is less visually able will need optimal lighting in his or her communication environment, to maximize what clues are available from speechreading. Sometimes, the environment cannot be lit optimally for communication because bright lights cause the patient ocular discomfort.

■ **Hearing aids and assistive listening devices:** Reduced vision may mean that an individual is unable to manipulate the controls of a hearing aid. This consideration may influence the kind of listening devices you recommend, and you will want to be sure to instruct a family member or caregiver on how to check the batteries and handle the hearing aid. Any written materials should be reiterated with a different format. If a hearing aid is recommended, it is important to spend time with the patient so he or she learns to feel the parts of the hearing aid, and learns to adjust it by touch (Lindblade & McDonald, 1995).

Arthritis

Arthritis is a painful inflammation of the joints, and decreases an individual's ability to perform fine motor activities. For this reason, arthritis can decrease a patient's ability to use listening devices. For example, arthritis may pose the following difficulties for tasks related to using a hearing aid:

■ Putting the hearing aid on and taking it off.
■ Opening the battery compartment and inserting batteries.
■ Removing ear wax and performing other cleaning tasks.
■ Operating the controls.

Recommendations for listening devices will hinge on a patient's ability to handle them. In some cases, it might be more appropriate to recommend an assistive listening device that has large controls and is easy to manipulate than to recommend a hearing aid. It also may be appropriate to instruct family members or caregivers how to handle the listening devices.

Dementia

Another common physical problem among older persons is dementia. The symptoms of dementia include gradual memory loss, disorientation, decline in the ability to perform everyday tasks, and loss of language skills. *Alzheimer's disease* is a form of dementia. Approximately 10% of individuals over the age of 65 years has Alzheimer's disease. This percentage increases almost fivefold for persons over the age of 85 years. Seven out of every 10 afflicted people live at home and receive care from family or friends. Those who live in a nursing home may pay $25,000 to $35,000 annually (Jones, 1997).

Alzheimer's disease is a form of dementia that affects approximately 10% of people over the age of 65.

Hearing loss often co-occurs with dementia; in fact, older people with dementia are significantly more likely to have hearing loss than older people without dementia. If a hearing loss is present, it is more likely to be greater if the patient has dementia than if he or she does not.

Aural rehabilitation may be especially important for these people. Mulrow et al. (1990) demonstrated that use of hearing aids may improve cognitive functioning. Instruction for family caregivers also may improve communication functioning.

AURAL REHABILITATION PLANS FOR OLDER PERSONS

An aural rehabilitation plan for older patients will include assessment of hearing, communication handicap, and conversational fluency. It then may be appropriate to provide a hearing aid, a hearing aid orientation, assistive devices, speech perception training, and/or communication strategies training. In order to consider the special needs of a patient, and develop a good understanding of the relevant factors that have an impact on the patient's hearing status and communication, a hearing professional often begins with a case study and, sometimes, questionnaires.

Learning About the Patient

During the first interactions with an older person, you likely will take a case history and conduct an interview. As with younger adults, you will want to learn about the patient's current communication needs and conversational settings. You also might gather information from other sources, such as members of the family, or administer a questionnaire. Audiological testing will be performed to determine the presence of hearing loss and problems in speech recognition.

The Case History

The case history will provide information about the patient's subjective impression of communication difficulties and a description of listening problems. It also will furnish information about the patient's living arrangements, social interactions, vocational status, and hobbies. The case history also may include conversation with a family member or caregiver, during which you might ask about the patient's memory, emotional state, motivation to participate in an aural rehabilitation program, and the feasibility of doing so. It is important also to gather medical data about the following topics (Groher, 1989):

■ **Strokes, memory loss, vision problems, dizziness, and medications taken**, because they may have an effect on the patient's ability to participate in testing and subsequent aural rehabilitation.

■ **Arthritis and muscle weakness**, because, as we noted earlier, these conditions may interact with a patient's ability to handle a listening device.

■ **Ambulation, behavioral changes, and other pertinent conditions**, because they may affect the kinds of communication activities in which the patient may engage.

■ **Dementia and Alzheimer's disease**, as patients will require assistance from caregivers or family members to use hearing aids. There is some evidence that hearing loss can magnify cognitive dysfunction and accelerate dementia (Garahan, Waller, Houghtone, Tisdale, & Runge, 1992), so it is important that hearing-aid use be encouraged, when appropriate.

During the case history, it is wise to be alert for symptoms of dementia. For example, if someone cannot remember his or her birth date or seems confused by simple tasks, such as completing a questionnaire, the audiologist may want to alter the test procedures. Otherwise, performance may not reflect true hearing ability.

Communication Handicap and Conversational Fluency

As we have noted in previous chapters, communication handicap relates to the psychosocial effects of hearing loss. You might ask your patient to complete a questionnaire about perceived handicap, such as the Hearing Handicap Inventory for the Elderly (Ventry & Weinstein, 1982). Such instruments provide information about how the respondent perceives social and emotional consequences of hearing loss.

Conversational fluency, or the ease and effectiveness with which a patient can carry on a conversation with a communication partner, often is assessed informally when the patient is older. You might engage in conversation and note the frequency of communication breakdowns and the ways in which the patient attempts to repair them. You might question family members about how well the individual can engage in conversation.

Audiological Testing

In addition to learning about the patient and his or her communication handicap, it is important to quantify degree of hearing loss. Audiological testing for an older person typically includes collection of air- and bone-conduction thresholds for pure tones, speech reception thresholds, and speech recognition scores.

Traditional testing procedures may need to be adapted for the elderly. The audiologist will want to have ample time for patient instructions and may need to double-check to ensure that instructions are understood. If a patient is in the early stages of Alzheimer's disease, reinstruction may be necessary if the patient takes a short break because the person may forget the task. For someone in the later stages of dementia, testing may not be possible.

Other accommodations for the older patient that may be necessary include the following:

■ **During air- or bone-conduction testing, tone stimuli may need to be presented for a longer duration of time than for younger persons.** Some older persons have difficulty in grasping the concept of listening for a soft, brief tone.
■ **Stimuli for speech recognition testing may need to be presented live-voice rather than recorded voice, outside of the test booth, so that the patient and clinician can sit face-to-face (Hull, 1995).** Some older persons are disconcerted by listening to a disembodied, impersonal voice over headphones.
■ **Time for rest periods may need to be allocated, or testing spread over more than one day, as some individuals may suffer from fatigue.**

HEARING AIDS, ASSISTIVE DEVICES, AND FOLLOW-UP AURAL REHABILITATION

If audiological testing reveals a hearing loss, it may be appropriate to schedule the patient for a hearing-aid evaluation. However, many patients who receive an evaluation either opt not to purchase a hearing aid or do not use the device once it is acquired. In fact, only about 10–20% of older persons who have hearing impairment actually own a hearing aid (Weinstein, 1991) and, of these, only a fraction use them on a regular basis.

The audiologist will want to assess carefully motivation to use amplification before the fitting and then ensure that support systems for hearing-aid use are in place following fitting. Table 12–1 presents factors that affect a patient's motivation to use a hearing aid.

Many of the procedures we have reviewed for selecting hearing aids for adults (Chapter 11) are applicable for the elderly population When selecting the hearing aid, the audiologist might select one that has oversized touch-type volume controls and/or one that has easily manipulated battery compartments, especially if manual dexterity is problematic for the patient. Other factors that will influence the recommendation include finances (can the patient afford the device?), monaural versus binaural hearing aids, and whether assistive listening devices might be appropriate instead of, or as a supplement to, the hearing aid.

Sometimes the older patent will desire an assistive listening device in addition to or in lieu of a hearing aid. For instance, sometimes an elderly person is unable to handle a hearing aid or earmold because of arthritis, so may need a simple FM system instead. Kaplan (1996) suggested that, when arthritis or reduced tactile sensation is present, a simple hardwired system with earphones may be most appropriate. During conversation, a communication partner can talk into a microphone while the older person can wear earphones.

The same microphone-headphone system also can be used for viewing television or listening to the radio. The patient can

Table 12-1. Factors that may affect an older person's motivation to use a hearing aid.

- Degree of hearing loss
- Communication difficulties
- Self-concept
- Opinion of hearing-aid users (e.g., "Only really old people use hearing aids, and I'm not there yet.")
- Number and quality of conversational interactions in which a patient engages
- The availability of communication partners
- Physical health (such as manual dexterity and visual acuity)

simply place the microphone by the system's speaker. Alternatively, an older person may be interested in obtaining a listening system that plugs directly into the earphone jack of the television set or radio. For watching television, there is also the option of closed captioning.

When an elderly person lives alone, security is often an issue. It may be important to consider alerting devices to signal the doorbell and telephone ringing, and the smoke alarm.

One Versus Two?

Jerger et al. (1995) suggested that for some older adults, one hearing aid might be better than two:

> Conventional wisdom suggests that, because humans are normally two-eared listeners, two hearing aids (binaural amplification) ought to provide more benefit than only one (monaural amplification). This is indeed the case in most young people and in many older persons with hearing loss. It is not, however, a universal finding. Some older persons actually seem to do better with a monaural than with a binaural fitting. They report too much confusion of sounds when they wear two aids and that they do better when listening through only one. It is as if the second hearing aid interferes with the first to produce a confusion of sounds in which speech understanding suffers. (p. 934)

The importance of the hearing-aid orientation cannot be overemphasized, and whether the older person becomes a successful hearing-aid user may well hinge on the audiologist's willingness to take the time necessary to give a thorough orientation. There can be no shortcuts here. Ample time must be devoted to instructing the patient on how to insert and remove the earmold and how to handle the hearing aid. One patient, who stopped using his hearing aid shortly after purchasing it, was asked why he never developed a consistent use-pattern. He responded that he did not know how to work the wax removal device, that the battery door was too difficult to operate, and that it hurt his ear to remove the aid at night. This man's audiologist may or may not have provided information about these topics during the hearing-aid orientation. However, the audiologist obviously did not take enough time to ensure that the patient had an adequate understanding of how to handle the hearing aid and did not provide enough follow-up support to ensure successful use.

A component of a hearing-aid orientation may be instruction for family members, caregivers, and others involved in the patient's health care. They may learn about caring for the hearing aid, and also develop realistic expectations about what the hearing aid can and cannot do for the patient.

Many older people participate in group aural rehabilitation programs following receipt of a hearing aid, or even without obtaining one. The program may include such topics as the following (Lesner, 1995):

■ Hearing aids and their functions
■ Counseling about issues that are important to the participants
■ Hearing and hearing loss
■ Assistive listening device technology
■ Auditory and visual nature of speech
■ Communication strategies

Often, family members will participate in the aural rehabilitation program with their older relatives (Figure 12–10).

Research suggests that some older patients benefit from participating in formal aural rehabilitation programs. Information counseling and communication strategies may be especially helpful. For instance, research experiments suggest that many people may experience less perceived communication handicap following a counseling-based aural rehabilitation program, (Ventry & Weinstein, 1983). Some benefit from participating in a program that provides analytic auditory training coupled with communication strategies training, but not a program that provides only analytic auditory training (Kricos & Holmes, 1996). Perhaps the individuals who are most likely to benefit are those who have the greatest communication difficulties prior to the onset of training (Kricos & Holmes, 1996).

AURAL REHABILITATION IN THE INSTITUTIONAL SETTING

If you are designing an aural rehabilitation program for a patient in a nursing home setting, you may need to adjust the

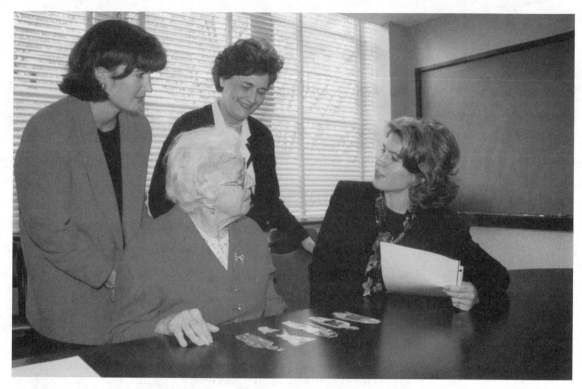

Figure 12–10. Family members and other close acquaintances might be encouraged to participate in the aural rehabilitation program for an older adult. (Photograph by Kim Readmond, Central Institute for the Deaf)

program for the institutionalized setting. Shultz and Mowry (1995) noted some of the problems associated with providing hearing health care to patients in a nursing home. These include:

■ **Managing the hearing loss when the patient may also have dementia or Alzheimer disease.** Often patients with dementia also have depression, which can decrease motivation to participate in an aural rehabilitation plan.

■ **Preventing hearing aids from being lost.** For instance, a patient may place the hearing aid in a bathrobe pocket, and the robe may end up in the laundry before the aid is removed.

■ **Involving the staff in the aural rehabilitation plan and providing inservice training.** Personnel should be aware of the communication difficulties associated with hearing loss. They should be familiarized with communication strategies and learn how to optimize the listening environment. Finally, they need to know how to handle hearing aids; for example, how to change batteries, how to clean earmolds, and how to insert and remove the devices from an older person's ear, as many residents will not be able to manage them alone.

■ **Dealing with the high turnover of facility personnel.** You may provide an inservice in August, only to discover that in December, half of the staff has been replaced.

CASE STUDY

The following example illustrates appropriate aural rehabilitation objectives that might be incorporated into a program for an older adult.

Mr. Gifford is a 70-year-old man who recently retired from his position at the post office. He is married and his daughter and her family live nearby. Mr. Gifford is concerned that his severe hearing loss may prevent him from giving tours to groups at the zoo. Although he is reluctant to admit this, he also feels that he is sometimes left out of the conversation at family gatherings, because he misses so much of what is said. Mr. Gifford tried using a hearing aid about 5 years ago, when he first noticed a hearing problem, but was dissatisfied with the sound quality. Besides, while delivering mail he found he rarely engaged in conversation with many people. Mr. Gifford's aural rehabilitation goals are to improve his ability to hear while working outside at the zoo and to improve his ability to participate in family conversations. Mr. Gifford is in fairly good health, although he does have arthritis in his hands.

Mr. Gifford and his clinician agreed that they were to establish goals for both his volunteer work and for his home setting. Aural rehabilitation goals included:

■ **Assessment and fitting of an appropriate hearing aid.** Mr. Gifford's ability to handle a hearing aid and work the controls also would be assessed. An instrument that he can handle, given his dexterity limitations, would be recommended.

■ **Provision of extensive follow-up-fitting support.** This would include establishing a use-schedule for the first few weeks of use, and a brief program of speechreading and listening training, to acclimate him to the amplified signal.

■ **Development of effective use of constructive facilitative communication strategies** (i.e., strategies aimed at structuring the environment for optimal communication by minimizing background noise and ensuring a favorable view of the talker, as discussed in Chapter 2). Instruction would be provided to maximize Mr. Gifford's listening potential in both indoor and outdoor environments.

■ **Development of effective use of other facilitative communication strategies and repair strategies to facilitate communication with family members and visitors to the zoo.**

■ **Involvement of family members in the aural rehabilitation plan.** Mrs. Gifford and her daughter would be encouraged to participate in a communication-strategies training program with Mr. Gifford, and to develop their use of communication strategies. Mrs. Gifford would also be invited to attend the hearing-aid fitting, and develop realistic expectations about what a hearing aid can do.

■ **Enrollment in a support group for hard-of-hearing individuals, such as Self-Help-for Hard-of-Hearing People (SHHH).** An attempt would be made to identify a group that has at least some other senior citizen members.

FINAL REMARKS

You may discover that working with older people provides some of your most rewarding professional experiences. One audiologist described how she tested an elderly woman who had terminal cancer. "Mrs. Kramer had a moderate, bilateral hearing loss," the audiologist related. "I knew by talking with her, and reviewing her medical records that she only had a few months to live. I suggested that she might not be interested in purchasing a hearing aid." Much to the audiologist's surprise, Mrs. Kramer not only wanted to buy a hearing aid, she wanted to buy two. She also wanted to borrow a VHF videotape that provides speechreading training. Mrs. Kramer's rationale was simple: "There is so much going on in my body that I can't control. It feels good to be able to actually do something positive about my hearing problem."

KEY CHAPTER POINTS

✔ The elderly represent the fastest growing segment of the U.S. population. Approximately 30% of the elderly population has hearing loss.

✔ Degree of hearing loss increases with age. Age-related hearing loss is called presbycusis.

✔ The impact of hearing loss on the older individuals may vary as a result of the person's economic status, social circumstances, social contacts, and emotional and physical health. Two persons may be of the same chronological age, yet vary greatly on these variables.

✔ Three physical conditions that may influence dramatically the design and success of an aural rehabilitation plan include reduced vision, arthritis, and dementia.

✔ Some changes may need to be made in the procedures for assessing hearing status, and for providing a hearing-aid orientation. In particular, more time usually must be scheduled to provide aural rehabilitation services for an older adult than for a younger adult.

Effects of Noise on Hearing and Communication

By William W. Clark

Topics

Few will debate the observation that we live in a noisy world. The clamor and din of modern society has increased in variety, if not prevalence and intensity, in the past decades. Whether it comes from air traffic overhead, from crowded urban areas replete with noisy traffic and public transportation vehicles, or from more personal sources, such as boom boxes, personal stereos, or noisy leaf blowers, noise is America's most widespread nuisance. But excessive noise is more than just a nuisance. Day and night, at home or at work or play, excessive noise exposure annoys individuals, produces stress, impairs the ability to communicate, interferes with work and play activities, and, in high enough doses, produces permanent damage to the auditory system that can lead to significant hearing loss.

This chapter will summarize the way we quantify sound and noise, describe how excessive noise exposure is measured and how it affects us, and provide suggestions concerning aural rehabilitation for those who must work or live or who choose to play in noisy environments.

A WORLD OF SOUND

What is sound? Acousticians define sound as "a particle disturbance in an elastic medium, which is propagated through the medium." In order for a sound to occur, a medium must have density and elasticity. Although sound can occur in any medium with these characteristics, including most solids, liquids, and gasses, we usually think about sound transmission in our medium, air. Air is composed of particles (air molecules) that have weight and elasticity. In fact, 1 cubic meter of air weighs about 1.3 kilograms (kg), and is quite elastic, that is, it can be compressed easily into a volume much smaller than 1 cubic meter. This is a useful fact for scuba divers who can carry one hour's worth of breathing air (about 1,500 liters) in a 20-liter tank.

The information provided above allows us to answer one of the questions we all were asked in elementary school: If a tree falls in the forest and no one is there to hear it, does it make a sound? The answer, from an acoustic point of view, is a resounding *yes*. But audiologists, speech-language-pathologists, teachers, and other professionals are concerned about the sense of hearing, that is, the perception of an acoustic event by a human listener. Adding a perceptual requirement to the definition then produces another definition: "Sound is a compression wave propagated through a medium that is capable of producing a sensation in the human ear" (Albers, 1970, p. 36). Now, when the tree question is asked again, the answer is *no*.

The discussion above highlights an important distinction between two different ways of considering sound. Engineers and scientists are concerned with sound as an energy that can be measured and quantified; no consideration usually is given to whether the sound can be perceived by humans. However, hearing health professionals usually are concerned about the *effects* of sound on humans: what and how we hear, what sounds please us, what sounds annoy us, what sounds interfere with our ability to communicate with each other, and what sounds can be damaging to our hearing. These definitions are necessarily more complex than simple quantitative descriptions of acoustic energy, and often are expressed in perceptual terms, like *loudness* or *pitch*.

> **Loudness** is the perception of the intensity of a sound.
> **Pitch** is the perception of the frequency of a sound.

MEASUREMENT OF SOUND

A general description of a sound should include a description of what the sound is, and how much of it is present. A *metathetic continuum* is used to describe the *what* quantity, and a *prothetic continuum* is used to describe the *how much* quantity. In acoustics and audiology, frequency of the sound is the metathetic variable, and the intensity or sound pressure level of the sound is the prothetic variable.

> A **metathetic continuum** is used to describe "what" quantity.
> A **prothetic continuum** is used to describe "how much" quantity.

First, let's consider frequency. *Frequency* is defined as the number of periodic repetitions of a sound in 1 second, that is, the number of cycles per second of that sound. By convention, the term *Hertz*, or *Hz*, is used to label the frequency of a sound. A sound of 1,000 Hz contains 1,000 cycles in 1 second. Similarly, a sound of 20 Hz repeats 20 times per second. As the frequency of a sound changes from low to high, the perception associated with frequency (known as the pitch) also changes from low to high. Note that the perceptual attribute, the pitch, does not get bigger as the frequency goes from low to high: it simply changes from one attribute, low pitch, to a different attribute, high pitch. This is what is meant by a metathetic continuum. The frequency of a sound is determined by the characteristics of the sound source. A tuba and a piccolo produce different frequencies of sounds because they differ in size.

> **Frequency** is the number of regularly repeated events in a given unit of time, usually measured in cycles per second and expressed in Hertz (Hz).

The second dimension is the "how much" dimension. By this, we are referring to the amount of energy present in the sound,

Intensity is the amount of energy present in a sound.

expressed commonly as its *intensity*. In acoustics, energy or intensity is defined as the acoustic power flowing through a unit of area, and the units of measurement are watts per meter squared (W/M²). In practice, engineers usually measure the pressure variations produced by the acoustic power, and the units are *Newtons* per meter squared (N/M²), or other equivalent measures expressed in *dynes* or *Pascals*. These funny-sounding units are metric equivalents to a unit more familiar to us: pounds per square inch. Therefore the energy, or intensity, continuum is a prothetic continuum; as intensity increases, the perceptual attribute, the loudness of a sound, also increases—it's not different, there's just more of it.

Newtons are a measure of the pressure variations produced by acoustic power, expressed as Newtons per square meter (N/M²).

Pascals (Pa): an alternative measure of pressure to the Newton. 1 Pa = 1`N/m².

Frequency and Period

As mentioned above, the frequency of a sound is the number of *periodic* oscillations per second, expressed in Hertz (Hz). The period of a sound is defined as the amount of time required to complete one cycle, and is the reciprocal of the frequency:

Period: the amount of time for a sound to complete one cycle of oscillation; the reciprocal of the frequency of the sound.

$$F = \frac{1}{P}, \text{ and } P = \frac{1}{F}$$

Therefore, the period of a 1,000 Hz tone is 1 millisecond (0.001 second), and the frequency of a tone with a period of 0.05 seconds is 20 Hz.

Speed of Sound

The **speed of sound** is dependent on the characteristics of the medium it travels through, i.e., its elasticity, density, and temperature.

Although the frequency of a sound is dependent on the characteristics of the source, the *speed of sound* is dependent on the characteristics of the medium, namely, the elasticity, density, and temperature of the medium. Sound travels faster in water than in air because water is more dense and less compressible than air. The speed of sound also is faster at higher temperatures. In air, sound travels at approximately 340 meters per second (1,125 feet per second) at a temperature of 72° Fahrenheit. We understand from common experience that some amount of time is required for sound to reach our ears. From the outfield bleachers, the crack of the bat is heard after the batter is observed hitting the ball. And, travelling at about ⅕ mile per second, we hear the sound of distant thunder some time after seeing the flash of lightning, the number of seconds telling us how far away the lightning struck (5 seconds = 1 mile).

Wavelength

Knowledge about the speed of sound allows us to calculate the other important variable of sound: its *wavelength*. Wavelength, abbreviated by the Greek symbol Lambda (λ), is the distance between two identical points on a periodic signal. It is equal to the speed divided by the frequency:

$$\lambda = C/F$$

At 340 meters per second, the wavelength of a 1,000 Hz tone is:

$$\frac{340 \text{ meters}}{1,000 \text{ Hz}} = 0.034 \text{ meters/cycle} = 13.4 \text{ inches/cycle}$$

Considering that a 1,000 Hz tone has a wavelength of about 1 foot, wavelengths of other frequencies commonly used in speech and hearing science can be estimated easily by remembering that doubling the frequency causes the wavelength to decrease by half and halving the frequency increases the wavelength by a factor of two. Using this rubric, Table 13–1 can be constructed.

> The **wavelength** of a sound is the distance between two identical points on a periodic signal; it is equal to the speed of sound divided by the frequency.

HEARING SENSITIVITY

Frequency Range

Humans cannot hear sounds of all frequencies. The range of human hearing extends from a low frequency limit of about 20 Hz to a high frequency limit of about 20 kilohertz (kHz) for ex-

Table 13-1. Relationship between frequency in Hertz and Wavelength in feet.

Frequency	Wavelength (approx) Feet
125 Hz	8 feet
250 Hz	4 feet
500 Hz	2 feet
1000 Hz	1 feet
2000 Hz	6 inches
4000 Hz	3 inches
8000 Hz	1½ inches

Infrasound: signals below the range of human hearing (less than 20 Hz).

Ultrasound: signals above the range of human hearing (more than 20 kHz).

cellent, young ears. Signals below 20 Hz are not perceived as sound, and sounds in this range are described as *infrasound*. Sounds with frequencies above 20 kHz also are not perceived, and these sounds are called *ultrasound*. Although ultrasonic signals are useful for cleaning jewelry, producing fetal images, and for motion detectors, they cannot be perceived and, therefore, are not sounds by Albers' definition.

Intensity or Sound Pressure

Intensity: the power or strength of sound, the power per unit area the source imposes on the medium.

The strength or power of a sound is described by its *intensity*, or the power per unit area the source imposes on the medium. A tuning fork, for example, does work as it vibrates and pushes air molecules back and forth. Each oscillation of the fork causes the air molecules next to it to be alternatively squeezed together and pulled apart. These local pressure disturbances then are propagated through the medium. Because it is much easier to measure pressure than intensity, sound level meters are designed to measure the atmospheric pressure variations caused by the sound, rather than the actual intensity of the sound.

The human ear is sensitive over a tremendous range of intensities. At threshold, a good, young, normal ear can detect an acoustic intensity of 10^{-12} watts/meter^2, a very small quantity indeed! That same young ear can be exposed to an intensity of 10^2 watts/meter^2 for a brief period without sustaining damage. The range from threshold to maximum tolerable level is called the dynamic range of the ear, and the ratio is 10^{14}:1, that is, 100 thousand billion to 1! The ratio of pressure variations (in air) for these intensities is 10^7 to 1.

These large pressure variations can best be understood by an analogy. Imagine a very large eardrum, which moves back and forth 1 foot at threshold. How far would that eardrum move at the maximum tolerable level? When asked that question, most elementary school children respond with guesses of 100 feet to 500 feet; a few adventuresome souls may hazard a 1 mile estimate. However, the answer is 1,894 miles! An eardrum in St. Louis would move back and forth 1 foot at threshold, and from St. Louis to San Francisco to New York to St. Louis for a very loud sound.

Because these large ratios were difficult to deal with, scientists and engineers invented a shorthand method to describe the strength of sound: the **decibel scale** (dB). A complete description of the derivation of the decibel scale is beyond the scope of this chapter. However, decibels commonly are used to express the sound pressure level of a given sound, and the ratio of intensities, or pressures, of two sounds to each other. Three characteristics of the decibel scale are relevant to the discussion. These are:

1. The scale is logarithmic.
2. It requires a stated reference value.
3. "0" dB does not mean there is no sound; rather it means the measured quantity is equivalent to the reference value.

In hearing science, the decibel scale is referenced to the threshold of human hearing (10^{-12} watts/meter^2 for intensity and the equivalent pressure of 2×10^{-5} Pascals), and the strength of sound is referred to as the *sound pressure level* (SPL) in decibels. The formulas for decibels are given below for informational purposes only.

$$\text{Intensity level: dB IL} = 10 \log (\text{I measured}/ \text{I reference}),$$
$$\text{where I reference} = 10^{-12} \text{ watts/meter}^2$$

$$\text{Sound pressure level} = 10 \log (\text{P measured})^2 /(\text{P reference})^2,$$
$$\text{where P reference} = 2 \times 10^{-5} \text{ Pascals}$$

In decibels, then, the range of human hearing extends from 0 dB SPL to about 140 dB SPL.

A further complication of the decibel scale is that the measures as stated above give no consideration to whether a sound is audible to a human listener. An ultrasonic jewelry cleaner may produce 140 dB SPL at 30 kilohertz (kHz), but it would be inaudible. Therefore, a filter network was added to approximate the human response to sound at moderate intensities. This network is called the *A-weighted filter network*, and sound pressure levels determined with the A-weighting network in place are noted as sound pressure level, dBA. Table 13–2 represents the typical maximum A-weighted levels of common household, transportation, recreational and hobby noises.

WHEN IS A SOUND A NOISE?

The definition of noise is actually rather complex. In acoustics, *noise* refers to any signal that is aperiodic. In engineering,

Decibel: a logarithmic unit of sound pressure used for expressing sound intensity; 1/10th of a Bel.

Sound pressure level (SPL): the magnitude of sound energy relative to a reference pressure of 0.0002 dynes/cm^2.

A-weighted scale: a filtering network used in a sound pressure meter weighted to approximate the human response to sound at moderate intensities, expressed in sound pressure level, dBA.

Noise is unwanted sound.

Table 13-2. Maximum sound pressure levels for common sources of nonoccupational noises.

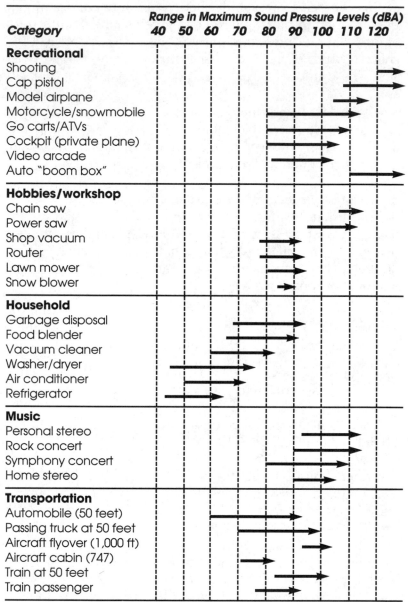

Category	Range in Maximum Sound Pressure Levels (dBA) 40 50 60 70 80 90 100 110 120
Recreational	
Shooting	
Cap pistol	
Model airplane	
Motorcycle/snowmobile	
Go carts/ATVs	
Cockpit (private plane)	
Video arcade	
Auto "boom box"	
Hobbies/workshop	
Chain saw	
Power saw	
Shop vacuum	
Router	
Lawn mower	
Snow blower	
Household	
Garbage disposal	
Food blender	
Vacuum cleaner	
Washer/dryer	
Air conditioner	
Refrigerator	
Music	
Personal stereo	
Rock concert	
Symphony concert	
Home stereo	
Transportation	
Automobile (50 feet)	
Passing truck at 50 feet	
Aircraft flyover (1,000 ft)	
Aircraft cabin (747)	
Train at 50 feet	
Train passenger	

Source: From "Hearing: Effects of noise," by W. W. Clark, 1992. *Otolaryngology—Head and Neck Surgery, 106,* 669–676. Reprinted with permission.

noise usually means a signal that interferes with the quality or detection of another signal. In psychoacoustics, noise usually is defined as unwanted sound. Although this definition is probably the most useful for our purposes, even it can be problematic. Is rock music noise? The answer depends on who is hearing it. Similarly, whereas a loud rattle coming from the engine of a car is most assuredly a noise to the owner, it may carry useful information to the mechanic whose job it is to repair the engine, and would not be considered noise.

Noise also differs in the way it affects people. In low doses, noise can be soothing and can be wanted sound. Patrons of libraries are less distracted by footsteps or page-turning when an air conditioner or ventilator produces a soft sound that masks the irregular noises. In moderate doses, noise annoys us. It makes communication difficult, affects task performance, increases blood pressure, and causes stress. In high doses, noise can cause permanent hearing loss.

Perhaps the most general, and most useful, definition of noise is the one proposed by Kryter (1996): Noise is an "acoustic signal which can negatively affect the physiological or psychological well-being of an individual" (p. 35). This definition covers all of the effects listed above. In this chapter, we will limit our discussion to one aspect of annoyance caused by noise, interference with speech communication, and more generally to the risk of permanent hearing loss posed by excessive exposure to occupational or recreational noise.

SPEECH COMMUNICATION IN NOISE

Background noise affects the ability to communicate orally. Figure 13–1 shows the relationship between background noise level, talker-to-listener distance, and vocal effort required for effective speech communication.

In Figure 13–1, the vertical axis is the A-weighted sound level of background noise measured in decibels. The horizontal axis is the distance between the talker and listener in feet. The regions below the contours are those combinations of distance, background noise levels, and vocal outputs wherein speech communication is practical between young adults who speak similar dialects of American English. The line labeled *expected voice level* reflects the fact that the usual talker unconsciously raises his voice level when he is surrounded by noise.

Consider a situation in which the background level is 50 dBA. Normal speech communication can occur at talker-to-listener

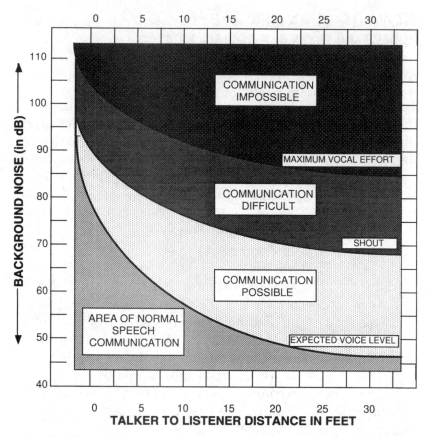

Figure 13–1. Speech communication. (Adapted from "Effects of Noise on People," EPA Report No. NTID 300.7, 50. United States Environmental Protection Agency.)

distances of about 20 feet; at distances greater than 20 feet, communication is still possible, but it is necessary to raise one's voice level. In a background level of 60 dBA, the normal communication range is reduced to about 8 feet. At greater distances, communication is possible, but only with increased vocal effort. For higher background levels, for example, 80 dBA, it is necessary to shout at distances greater than 5 feet, and communication is difficult. In many industrial settings, the background noise level is at or above 80 dBA; in these settings communication is difficult for distances greater than 5 feet without shouting and, for levels above 90 dBA, communication is impossible at distances greater than 10–15 feet. Clearly, speech communication is difficult or impossible for individuals who must work, or choose to play, in environments where the background noise levels are above 80 dBA.

HOW DOES EXCESSIVE NOISE AFFECT HEARING?

Mechanisms of Noise-induced Hearing Loss

The ear is injured by noise in two very different ways, depending on the level of the exposure. If the ear is exposed to a very high level, short duration exposure in which the peak sound pressure level exceeds 140 dB SPL, the acoustic energy in the signal can stretch the delicate inner ear tissues beyond their elastic limits, and rip or tear them apart. This type of damage is called *acoustic trauma*; it occurs instantaneously and results in an immediate hearing loss that is usually permanent. The organ of Corti becomes detached from the basilar membrane, deteriorates, and is replaced by a single layer of scar tissue that re-establishes the integrity of the fluid compartments of the inner ear. The hearing loss often is accompanied by tinnitus, a sensation of ringing in the ears, that usually (but not always) subsides within a few hours or days after the exposure.

Acoustic trauma results from exposure to very high level, short duration sounds (greater than 140 dB), resulting in immediate hearing loss that is usually permanent.

Because the ear is damaged mechanically by impulsive sounds, it matters little what the duration of the signal is; the important variable is the peak sound pressure level. Noises in the environment capable of producing acoustic trauma usually come from explosive events: a firecracker detonating near the head (170 dB SPL), a toy cap gun fired near the ear (155 dB SPL), or the report of a pistol, high-powered rifle, or shotgun (160–170 dB SPL).

Exposure to noise between 90 and 140 dBA damages the cochlea metabolically rather than mechanically. In this case, the potential for damage and hearing loss depends on the level and the duration of exposure. This type of injury is called *noise-induced hearing loss (NIHL)* and, in contrast to acoustic trauma, it is cumulative and insidious, growing slowly over years of exposure. Noise-induced hearing loss, commonly associated with workplace noise but in reality caused by any exposure that exceeds a daily average of 90 dBA regularly over a period of years, proceeds in three stages.

Noise-induced hearing loss (NIHL): sensorineural hearing loss that is the result of exposure to excessive levels of sound; auditory trauma caused by loud sound and resulting in permanent hearing loss.

In the first stage, sensory cells are killed by excessive exposure to noise. The cells do not regenerate, but are replaced by scar tissue. The losses are cumulative and insidious, and do not elevate thresholds for pure-tone signals. In fact, up to 50% of the outer hair cells in the apical turn of the cochlea can be killed without elevating thresholds for low-frequency pure tones.

In the second stage, which starts after a few weeks to a few years of exposure, depending on the level, beginning hearing losses can be detected audiometrically. However, these losses occur in the frequency region around 4 kHz. Because these losses do not affect speech understanding significantly, they seldom are detected unless the hearing is tested for some other reason (e.g., annual audiometry in a hearing conservation program).

Finally, with continued exposure for decades, losses continue to accumulate at 4 kHz, although at a slower rate than in the first decade, and they spread to the lower frequencies, which are important for speech understanding. It is at this point that the patient becomes aware of a problem that has been progressing for decades. If the diagnosis is noise-induced hearing loss, the recommendation made by the physician or audiologist is to avoid excessive exposure to noise and to wear *hearing protection* around necessary exposures. Of course, by the time this recommendation is made, much of the damage has already been done.

Hearing protection: devices designed to minimize the risk of noise-induced hearing loss.

HOW MUCH NOISE IS TOO MUCH?

If the ear of an individual is exposed to noise of sufficient strength, and/or of sufficient duration, a sensorineural hearing loss can occur. As stated, the hazard associated with a particular noise exposure depends not only on the strength or level of the sound, but also its spectral characteristics, temporal pattern, number or repetitions, and the duration of the exposure. Further complicating the attempt to provide a simple descriptor for hearing hazard is the fact that individuals vary widely in their susceptibility to noise exposure; it is not possible to specify an exposure limit that is guaranteed to protect everyone. An additional complication is that, because the effects of noise often go unnoticed by the patient, precise exposure histories are nearly impossible to obtain.

MEASUREMENT OF NOISE EXPOSURE

For centuries, noise exposure associated with the workplace has been known to produce hearing loss. In fact, *boilermakers' deafness* was the term coined to describe the now-familiar bilateral sensorineural hearing loss associated with excessive exposure to occupational noise. Largely on the basis of knowledge gained through field studies of hearing loss in industrial workers and military personnel, the U.S. Department of Labor promulgated regulations in the 1970s and 1980s designed to protect the hearing of employees who work in noisy environments. U.S. occupational noise exposure regulations specify that employees be protected against the hazardous effects of noise when daily sound levels exceed those listed in Table 13–3.

The levels stated in Table 13–3 represent the maximum allowable daily noise exposure, or the *permissible exposure limit* (PEL), as specified by OSHA and other federal agencies. The PEL for an 8-hour exposure is referred to as the *criterion*; it reflects the sound level in dBA that reaches the PEL after 8 hours of exposure. Note that for exposures that differ from 8 hours, the allowable daily exposure level is increased or decreased by 5 decibels for each halving or doubling of exposure duration. Ninety decibels is allowed for 8 hours daily, 95 decibels for 4 hours daily, etc. Each of the exposures listed in the table represent an equivalent *time-weighted average* (TWA) exposure of 90 dBA for 8 hours. By definition, an 8-hour TWA of 90 decibels represents 100% of the allowable dose.

Permissible noise exposure limit (PEL): a maximum allowable daily noise exposure specified by OSHA, expressed in dBA per 8-hour exposure.

Criterion: the maximum sound level in dBA that reaches the PEL after 8 hours of exposure.

When the daily noise exposure is composed of two or more periods of noise exposure of different levels, their effects are combined by the following rule:

Table 13–3. OSHA maximum daily noise exposure limit.

Duration per day (in hours)	Sound level (dBA)
16	85
8	90
6	92
4	95
3	97
2	100
1.5	102
1	105
½	110
¼ or less	115

Source: Adapted from Table G-16a of CFR 29 1910.95.

$$C1/T1 + C2/T2 + ...Cn/Tn,$$

where C = exposure duration at a given level and
T = allowable duration at that level.

Percent allowable dose then is calculated by multiplying the result by 100 percent. That is,

$$D = 100 * (C1/T1 + C2/T2 + ... Cn/Tn)$$

All exposures between 80 and 130 dBA are required to be integrated into the dose calculation. Exposures below the so-called "threshold" are not counted in the calculation of daily exposure; threshold values range from 80 dBA to 90 dBA among various regulations.

For example, consider the daily noise exposure for a sheet metal worker depicted in Table 13–4.

The employee's exposure, as shown in Table 13-4, would not exceed OSHA's PEL. The dose also could be expressed as a TWA level in decibels by calculating the 8-hour exposure level that would result in the same dose:

$$TWA = 16.61 \log_{10} (Dose/100) + 90,$$

or 87.8 dBA. It is important to remember that *dose* and *TWA* really refer to the same measurement: the 8-hour equivalent exposure for any measured duration or combination of levels and durations, expressed in percentages or decibels.

As amended in 1983, the current U.S. occupational noise exposure standard identifies a TWA of 85 dBA, or 50% dose, as an

Table 13–4. Calculation of daily noise exposure.

Activity	Level	Duration	C/T	Dose (%)
grinding	92 dBA	2.0 hrs	2/6	33
buffing	85 dBA	2.5 hrs	2.5/16	16
cutting	100 dBA	0.5 hrs	0.5/2	25
packaging	75 dBA	2.0 hrs	2/ infinity	0
lunch, breaks	79 dBA	1.0 hrs	1/ infinity	0
TOTAL			0.74	74%

action level. Workers covered by the standard who are exposed above the action level must be provided with an effective hearing conservation program, including annual audiometric evaluations, personal hearing protection if desired, and education programs. With a daily noise exposure of 74%, or a TWA above 85 dBA, the sheet metal worker described above should be in a company hearing conservation program.

The exposure limits set by OSHA were determined empirically from epidemiological and laboratory data concerning hearing damage from noise exposure and were designed to protect employees against sustaining a material impairment in hearing after a working lifetime. They were derived by subtracting the percentage of workers sustaining a material impairment in hearing as a function of exposure level from a control population without occupational exposure. The resultant percentage is the *percent risk* or *percent additional risk* of a material impairment in hearing after, say, 40 years of exposure, above that expected from presbycusis and sociocusis alone. Estimates of percent risk vary depending on which criteria and databases are used; on the basis of evaluation of all of the data, it can be concluded that the PEL of 90 dBA, with the 85 dBA action level, if enforced, would protect virtually the entire working population from occupational noise-induced hearing loss.

The OSHA noise standards are useful to the physician in arriving at a diagnosis, and for the audiologist in determining whether a recommendation about hearing protection should be made. First, because workers exposed to excessive occupational noise should be in a hearing conservation program, evidence of exposure history and prior company-obtained audiograms may be available for consideration. If the worker is not in a hearing conservation program, he or she may not work in significant occupational noise. Unfortunately, because not all workers are covered by OSHA standards and because enforcement has been weak, lack of participation in a hearing conservation program by a worker does not guarantee that he or she has not been exposed to excessive occupational noise. However, in evaluating a patient, if it is determined that exposure to occupational noise did not exceed a TWA of 85 dBA, or a dose of 50%, then exposure to occupational noise should be ruled out as the etiology.

Exposure Assessment

Two general types of exposure assessment commonly are used in industry: area noise surveys, and personal noise *dosimetry*.

Dosimetry: a method of calculating daily noise exposure in different workplaces.

Area surveys are used to identify job locations in which the TWA exposure may exceed 85 dBA; they are conducted by placing a sound level meter in a specific location and sampling the noise field. Exposures then are calculated based on the amount of time an employee works in that specific location. Area surveys also are useful in determining the sources of exposure in an industrial environment and for planning noise control engineering strategies for reducing exposure.

Occupational exposures can be measured directly by using personal noise dosimeters. These devices are small, computerized, integrating sound level meters that can record the minute-by-minute sound exposure throughout the workday. They are worn on a belt or in a pocket, and the microphone is positioned on the shoulder, approximately 5 inches lateral to the ear. Technological advances in microprocessor design, incorporating low-power consumption and component miniaturization, have led to sophisticated, small, lightweight dosimeters that can be worn. A distinct advantage to using dosimetry over other methods is that the measurement instrument travels with the worker and, therefore, can provide a more accurate assessment of exposure as he or she moves among different noise environments during the workday.

Exposure assessment using dosimetry does have some disadvantages. Because the instrument is mounted on the shoulder, reflection of sound off the body adds about 2 dB to the exposure assessment. In addition, it is nearly impossible to prevent bumping or touching the surface of the microphone during a normal workday. Contact with the microphone, even with a windscreen in place, will always increase the dose measure and, for short duration, high level impacts, the exposure can be inflated dramatically. Finally, because the dosimeter travels with the worker rather than staying under the control of the professional assessing the exposure, errors of commission and omission can occur. For example, a dosimeter attached to a jacket that then is deposited in a locker before the workshift begins will record the exposure of the jacket, rather than that of the worker.

TYPES OF OCCUPATIONAL NOISE EXPOSURE

According to a report published by the EPA in 1981, there are more than 9 million Americans exposed to daily average noise levels above 85 dBA. The breakdown is shown in Table 13–5.

Table 13–5. Workers exposed to average daily noise levels in excess of 85 dBA by employment area:

Agriculture	323,000
Mining	400,000
Construction	513,000
Manufacturing and utilities	5,124,000
Transportation	1,934,000
Military	976,000
TOTAL	9,270,000

Source: Adapted from *Noise in America*, EPA Report No. 550/9-81-101.

These numbers undoubtedly are outdated, but no more recent estimates are available. Although improvements in hearing conservation programs, advances in noise control engineering technology, and downsizing in major industries undoubtedly have reduced the number of individuals exposed to excessive noise, it still is safe to conclude that occupational noise exposure is a factor in causing hearing loss for millions of American workers.

It is impossible to specify precisely all particular job descriptions for which excessive exposure is a risk. However, as shown in Table 13–6, the textile industry, processing lumber and wood products, the food industry, and metal manufacturing industries employ large numbers of workers, a large percentage of whom work in noisy environments.

TYPES OF NONOCCUPATIONAL NOISE EXPOSURE

As effective as the federal regulations may be, if enforced, at protecting hearing in the workplace, they fail to consider hearing loss produced by noise exposure outside the workplace, and recent evidence suggests that these exposures are potentially hazardous for millions of Americans.

There are numerous sources of noise in the environment that have the potential to produce noise-induced hearing loss. The types of exposure sources span the recreational preferences of Americans. Evidence has been mounting over the past two

Table13-6. Estimate of production workers exposed to a TWA of 85 dB and above.

Industry	1000s of Workers Exposed to over 85 dBA	% of Workers Exposed to over 85 dBA
Food and Kindred Products	820	70%
Tobacco Manufacturers	48	76%
Textile Mill Products	855	95%
Apparel & Related Products	12	1%
Lumber & Wood Products	542	100%
Furniture & Fixtures	236.6	55%
Paper & Allied Products	395	71%
Printing & Publishing	132	20%
Chemicals & Allied Products	137	23%
Petroleum & Coal Products	58	50%
Rubber & Plastics Products	266	50%
Leather & Leather Products	3	1%
Stone, Clay & Glass Products	416	75%
Primary Metals		
Primary Steel	325	67%
Foundries	189	70%
Primary Nonferrous	63	27%
Fabricated Metal Products	786	70%
Machinery—Except Electric	956	70%
Electrical Machinery	959	70%
Transportation Equipment	880	65%
Utilities	445	71%
Total	6,524	59.3%

Source: Adapted from BBN Report #2671: Impact of Noise at the Workplace. U.S. Dept. of Labor, 11-30-73. Bolt, Beranek and Newman, Inc., 50 Moulton, Cambridge, MA 02138.

decades that there are sources of noise exposure outside the workplace that are potentially damaging. Precisely what the effects of these exposures are on an eventual noise-induced hearing loss has been the topic of many studies. Obviously, implicit in the assessment of the role of nonoccupational or recreational noise on NIHL is a determination not only of the level of exposure possible, but also some information about the typical exposure levels and patterns for groups of listeners.

A partial list of significant sources and maximum levels of nonoccupational noise was given in Table 13–1, which was used to demonstrate typical sound levels. If one considers a reading of >90 dBA as the borderline between safe and dangerous noise exposures, it is seen that nearly everything on the list, with the exception of household items such as refrigerators, falls in the dangerous category. Information about maximum levels does not, in and of itself, indicate a dangerous noise exposure (unless the continuous level exceeds 140 dB SPL): the hazards from exposure to noise from any device listed depend on the level and the duration of exposure for a typical consumer of that noise.

This report will be limited to an assessment of the effects of the two major sources of noise in the leisure environment: the discharge of firearms during hunting and target-shooting activities, and listening to music, either at concerts or through personal stereos.

Hunting and Target-Shooting

It is well known that individuals exposed to gunfire may sustain hearing loss associated with these exposures. Reported peak sound levels from rifles and shotguns have ranged from 132 dBA for .22 caliber rifles to more than 172 dBA for high-powered rifles and shotguns. Clinical reports documenting hearing loss after exposure to shooting can be found in the literature since the 1800s.

Numerous studies have attempted to assess the prevalence of hunting or target-shooting in the general population. On the basis of these surveys it is estimated that more than 50% of men in the American industrial workforce fire guns at least occasionally. The National Rifle Association estimates that 70 million Americans own guns, and 20 million purchase hunting licenses each year. The severity of injury produced by impulsive noise exposure and the prevalence of shooting by Americans make gun noise America's most serious nonoccupational noise hazard.

Because of the logarithmic nature of the decibel scale, it is difficult to grasp how much acoustic energy is in a single gunshot. Consider the following example: An individual is exposed to a single report of a high-powered rifle at 165 dB SPL and a duration of 0.003 seconds. How long would that individual have to work in an occupational noise environment in which the sound level was 90 dBA until the acoustic energy received was equal to the gunshot? The answer is almost a full work week of 8-hour workdays. In other words, one bullet equals 1 week of hazardous occupational noise exposure. Because shells often are packaged in boxes of 50, shooting one box of shells is equivalent to working in a 90 dBA environment for a full year! An avid target shooter can produce an entire year's worth of hazardous occupational exposure in just a few minutes on the target range.

One method of determining the role of shooting in hearing loss is to compare audiometric data in groups of individuals who engage in shooting with a matched group who do not. Variations of such an approach have been reported in a number of studies (e.g., Taylor & Williams, 1965). Virtually all of them show significant effects on hearing produced by gunfire noise, with the ear contralateral to the firearm exhibiting thresholds worse than the ipsilateral ear by about 15 dB for high-frequency (3–8 kHz) stimuli, and up to 30 dB for avid shooters.

Because shooting is so prevalent in our culture, it is the most important source of excessive noise outside the workplace. However, there are other significant nonoccupational sources of excessive noise exposure.

Listening to amplified music

Rock Concerts

There is a large body of research published within the past two decades that details exposure to individuals attending rock concerts and noisy discotheques. An analysis of all of the data indicated the geometric mean of all published sound levels from rock concerts was 103.4 dBA (Clark, 1991). In general, it is reasonable to conclude that attendees at rock concerts or noisy discotheques are exposed routinely to sound levels above 100 dBA. Studies of *temporary threshold shift (TTS)* after exposure to rock music most often have considered only the hearing levels of performers; a few studies have shown TTSs in listeners attending rock concerts. Generally, these studies show that most listeners sustain moderate TTSs (up to 30 dB at 4 kHz), which recover within a few hours to a few days after the exposure. The risk of sustaining a permanent hearing loss from attending rock concerts is small, and is limited to those who frequently attend such events. However, attendance at rock concerts remains an important contributor to cumulative noise dose for many Americans.

Temporary threshold shift (TTS): transient hearing loss following exposure to excessive noise.

Personal Stereos

Increased use and availability of personal listening devices, such as the Sony Walkman, have led to general concern about potentially hazardous exposures, particularly for younger listeners. The question of whether listening to music through headphones may cause hearing loss depends on, among other things, the volume level selected by the listener, the amount of time spent listening, the pattern of listening behavior, the susceptibility of the individual's ear to noise damage, and other noisy activities that will contribute to the individual's lifetime dose of noise (Clark, 1991).

Although several studies have suggested that personal stereos are capable of producing exposures above 120 dBA, analysis of listening habits suggests that most users of personal stereos listen at volume levels that do not pose a risk of hearing loss. Fewer than 5% of users select volume levels and listen frequently enough to risk any hearing loss whatsoever.

THE KEYS TO PREVENTION AND MANAGEMENT

With so many diverse sources of excessive noise exposure in our work and play environments, identifying strategies to prevent hazardous exposures, protect the hearing of individuals who must or choose to be exposed, and offer methods of rehabilitation for those who must communicate in a noisy environment or cope with a noise-induced hearing loss is a daunting task. However, it should be remembered that, unlike other diseases or injuries, noise-induced hearing loss is preventable. It can be avoided by reducing excessive exposure, or by protecting our ears during exposure.

If it's that easy, then why do so many people have noise-induced hearing loss? The answer lies in the insidious way in which noise-induced hearing loss creeps up on its victims. By the time enough damage has accumulated to produce a functional impairment, it is far too late to prevent the loss. Add to that the fact that protecting hearing generally is not considered a "macho" thing to do and that exposure to some loud noises can be exciting, and one has all the ingredients for a noise-induced hearing loss. It has been stated that prevention of excessive noise exposure would be accomplished more easily if the ear would bleed after a rock concert or an afternoon of shooting. What is needed is an approach that informs the patient about the potential for noise to cause a hearing loss before it is too late.

Key 1: Education

Whether in the workplace or at home, the key to prevention is education. Several national professional associations have been working to provide educational curricula about hazardous noise for elementary and secondary school children. These curricula are designed for use by science or health teachers to train healthy hearing habits for young ears, before the damage begins to accrue. Axelsson and Clark (1995) have suggested that schools invite hearing professionals to augment the curriculum with real-life experiences to help get the message across to children. Of course, professionals involved in aural rehabilitation would be ideal candidates for such a position.

Federal law requires that regular education programs be provided for employees exposed to potentially hazardous noise. However, these programs are only required to consider workplace noise, and they are often only given to employees in high noise environments. However, because the ear doesn't know the difference between an occupational and a recreational exposure to hazardous noise, education programs should be provided to all employees, and the emphasis should be placed on global hearing health and not restricted to job-related exposures.

Key 2: Prevention of Exposure

The second key is to prevent excessive exposure to noise. In the workplace, emphasis on engineering control of noise emission has reduced occupational exposures for many kinds of jobs. For example, lightweight fiber materials have replaced sheet metal in several manufacturing operations, and glues are now used to bond airplane wings, rather than the noisy rivets used in prior decades.

Administrative controls also can reduce employee exposure. An example of an administrative control is to assign workers to noisy jobs for only part of the workday, and to quiet areas for the rest. By careful placing of individuals, exposures can be reduced, even though the noise in the plant remains constant.

Administrative and engineering controls also can be employed in the home. One can avoid excessive exposure to unwanted noise, and become a judicious consumer of wanted noise. Are rock concerts your fancy? By all means, enjoy them, but limit attendance to the special concerts you really like. And don't participate in other noisy activities on the day you attend the concert (mow the lawn another day).

Key 3: Wear Hearing Protection

In situations in which the noise cannot be eliminated, hearing protectors should be worn. The two most commonly used protectors are earplugs or muffs. Earplugs come in a variety of styles and sizes. Recommended are the foam-type plugs, which are squeezed gently between the thumb and forefinger, and inserted into the external ear canal. The foam then expands and forms a seal. Other types of earplugs are made of plastic or silicone, and some are custom-fit for the user. The advantages of earplugs are their small size, comfort, and the fact that they are disposable. However, some individuals find the plug and the resulting occlusion of the ear canal uncomfortable.

The other type of hearing protector is a muff that fits over the ear. The advantage of this type of protection is that it is heavier and often provides slightly greater attenuation than the smaller earplug. Muffs are also reusable and, when kept in good condition, can be considerably cheaper than disposable earplugs. In occupational environments, it is easier to see that a worker is wearing a muff than a plug. A disadvantage of the muff-type protector is that a seal must be made between the earmuff cushion and the side of the head; any break in the seal renders the muff useless. Individuals who wear eyeglasses have a difficult time wearing the muffs because the temple piece of the eyeglass interferes with the seal.

In home environments, it is recommended that individuals wear hearing protection anytime they are exposed to loud, unnecessary sound. The type of plug or muff selected is of secondary importance. There is an adage in hearing conservation that says: "The most effective hearing protective device is one that is worn." Comfort is of utmost importance. Most individuals will find the foam plugs the protector of choice. They are cheap, comfortable, disposable, and readily available at hardware and drug stores.

Noise reduction rating (NRR): the decibels of attenuation provided by a hearing protector in laboratory conditions.

All hearing protectors are sold with a listing of the *noise reduction rating,* or the NRR. This rating refers to the decibel attenuation of the protector observed under laboratory test conditions, and varies from about 15 to 35 among various plugs or muffs. Although the NRR is useful for comparing among hearing protectors, it does not describe the actual attenuation one would expect in practice. In fact, studies have shown that muffs or plugs with NRRs of 25–30 actually provide only about 10 dB of protection when fit by the workers in actual working environments. However, most industrial and many environmental noise sources are in the 85–95 dBA range. In these environments, it is necessary only to reduce the level to below 85 dBA to make the environment safe, even for a working lifetime. Therefore, hearing protectors with attenuations of greater than 10 dB are not needed and, if they are used, they present additional problems for the user.

An individual working or playing in a 90 dB environment and wearing a hearing protector that provides 25 dB of attenuation will have difficulty understanding speech while he is wearing the protectors. Many workers fear they will not hear warning shouts from co-workers if they wear hearing protection, and for the worker using a protector with more than the necessary attenuation, this is a valid concern. In this scenario, it is far better to recommend a hearing protector with a more modest attenuation rating, and speech understanding will be preserved.

Special types of hearing protectors have been developed for special situations. One type—the *musician's earplug*—is developed specially to provide a flat attenuation. Unlike the traditional plug, which makes speech or music sound muffled, the musician's plug provides a much more realistic sound to the user and, although they are expensive, are preferred by musicians and others who desire a more realistic quality to their auditory perception.

Another type of hearing protector has a microphone and amplifier incorporated into its design. Sometimes called the *hunter's earmuff*, these protectors attenuate high-level sounds, like the report of a shotgun, but amplify low-level sounds, like the snapping of a twig by prey. They are particularly useful in environments characterized by high-level, impulsive sounds.

Finally, the field of ***active noise cancellation (ANC)*** technology has reached the hearing protector market, and several protectors are now commercially available that incorporate ANC. First developed by the military for use in tanks, ANC utilizes a very fast computer that samples the noise and generates a mirror image of it, which is then played along with the source noise, thus canceling it. Although the field is still in its infancy, ANC is an effective means of canceling low-frequency noise, and hearing protectors using it generate an extra 5–10 dB of attenuation in the low frequencies, considerable reducing the masking of speech. Hearing protectors incorporating ANC are expensive (about $300), but look for the price to drop rapidly as the technology advances.

Active noise cancellation: a form of noise reduction now used in hearing protectors in which a mirror image of noise in the environment is played alongside it to cancel it.

FINAL REMARKS

Excessive noise is a major pollutant in America. At work and at play, we are exposed to sounds that annoy us, interfere with our ability to communicate, produce stress, and, in high enough doses, lead to sensorineural hearing loss. Although much is known about the effects of noise on people, too little attention is paid to reducing noise at the source, to protecting the hearing of individuals who work or play in noisy environments, and to promoting the importance of preserving the sense of hearing in old age. Noise-induced hearing loss progresses in a cumulative and insidious manner, and usually is not noticed by the patient until the damage to the delicate sensory tissues of the inner ear has already occurred. Because the damage is permanent and irreversible, by the time it is noticed, it is too late. The key strategy to preventing noise-induced hearing loss is education. When our patients understand the importance of hearing later in life, and the risk noise exposure poses to it, they will be better prepared to take steps we recommend to avoid or limit their exposures. It is our job as hearing health professionals to get the message to them before noise-induced hearing loss starts, rather than after it has occurred.

KEY CHAPTER POINTS

✔ Humans with normal hearing can hear sounds over a ten octave range and of intensities that vary by a factor of 100,000 billion to one.

✔ Excessive exposure to noise can affect one's quality of life by producing annoyance, masking, and interference with speech communication at moderate levels, and can produce permanent sensorineural hearing losses in large enough doses.

✔ Noise-induced hearing loss is cumulative, insidious, and often is not noticed by the patient until it is too late to prevent the damage.

✔ Individuals who work in noisy jobs and individuals who engage in noisy hobbies such at sport shooting are at risk of sustaining a permanent noise-induced hearing loss.

✔ The keys to prevention are education, reduction of noise at the source, and wearing effective hearing protection during noisy activities.

PART IV

*Aural Rehabilitation
for Children*

Hearing Loss in Children[1]

Topics

- Demographics
- Hearing and Speech Recognition Skills
- Amplification

- Final Remarks
- Key Chapter Points
- Key Resources

[1]Parts of Chapters 14, 15, and 16 were adapted from "The Child Who is Deaf" by N. Tye-Murray. In J. B. Tomblin, H. L. Morris, and D. C. Spriestersbach (Eds.), *Diagnosis in Speech-Language Pathology*, 1994 (pp. 425–444). San Diego, CA: Singular Publishing Group.

Parents react in many different ways when a hearing professional tells them that their baby has a severe or profound hearing impairment. One common reaction is for parents to say, "O.K. We'll get hearing aids for her, and she can learn to lipread us." They assume hearing aids and lipreading lessons can make the hearing loss inconsequential. Unless the parents know someone who has had a significant hearing impairment from birth, they may not realize initially that their child's speech development, language acquisition, conversational skills, and literacy likely will differ from what is common for children with normal hearing. Parents may become aware of these consequences only gradually, as they receive counseling from speech and hearing professionals and as they acquire many months and even years of firsthand experience in watching their child grow. They also will learn to appreciate the long-term commitments that will be required of them, the child, other members of their family, and the child's school system in order for the child to realize his or her full potential.

With this chapter, we begin our consideration of children who have hearing losses. First we will focus on demographic issues and then hearing measurement. In subsequent chapters, we will focus on intervention plans and speech, language, and conversational skills.

Prelingual: hearing loss incurred before the acquisition of spoken language.

In this chapter, we will be concerned primarily with children who have prelingual hearing loss. As was noted in Chapter 1, children who are *prelingually* hearing-impaired had their hearing losses when they were learning language and speech. They may have been born with hearing loss (in which case they have congenital hearing impairment) or they may have lost their hearing early in life, perhaps as a result of meningitis, high fever, or head trauma. An *intervention program* includes family counseling, hearing-aid fitting (or cochlear-implant fitting), selection of appropriate assistive listening devices and follow-up support, and speech perception training. It also encompasses other aspects of a child's educational and rehabilitation program, such as speech and language therapy, educational and classroom placement, and communication mode. The intervention program also may include instruction for the child's parents about how to nurture their child's language, listening, and conversational skills

An **intervention program** for children includes family counseling, hearing-aid fitting, selection of appropriate assistive listening devices, speech perception training, and other aspects of a child's educational and rehabilitation program.

DEMOGRAPHICS

Over 1 million children in the United States have a hearing loss (Figure 14–1). For every 1,000 children in this country, 83 have

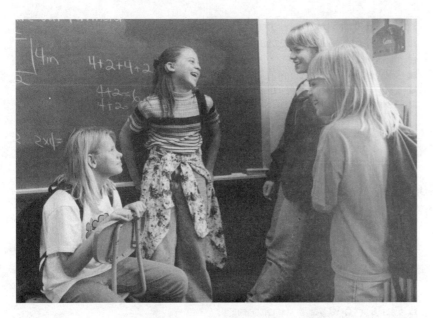

Figure 14-1. Over 1 million children in the United States have a profound hearing loss. By Patti Gabriel, courtesy of CID

what is termed an *educationally significant hearing loss* (U.S. Public Health Service, 1990). Severe and profound losses in infants have an incidence of 1 to 2 per 1,000 (Feinmesser, Tell, & Levi, 1982; Parving, 1985). Among school-age children, severe to profound hearing loss occurs in about 9 children of every 1,000 (Schien & Delk, 1974). If we consider children who have any degree of hearing loss, even a mild loss, then the incidence rises to as high as 1 in 25 (Teele, Klein, & Rosner, 1989).

Two important statistics to consider when reviewing the demographics of children who have significant hearing loss pertain to the occurrence of other disabilities and the hearing status of their parents.

Other Disabilities

Approximately 30% of hearing-impaired children have a disability in addition to hearing loss (Wolff & Harkins, 1986). Co-occurring conditions include mental retardation, significant visual impairment, learning disabilities, and attention deficit disorder. Emotional or behavioral problems, cerebral palsy, and orthopedic problems also may co-occur with hearing loss. Sometimes, the multiple disabilities stem from similar causes, such as trauma at birth or prematurity. Causes may also relate to ethnic background and heredity. Table 14–1 presents condi-

Table 14-1. Conditions that may co-occur with hearing loss.

■ Mental retardation
■ Behavior or psychiatric disorders
■ Learning disability, related to reading and/or writing
■ Nervous system ailments, such as seizures, vestibular disturbances, or spina bifida
■ Eye disease, including optic degeneration, ocular lens abnormalities, and retinitis pigmentosa
■ Renal disease
■ Musculoskelal abnormalities in the skull, oral cavity, face, outer and/or middle ear, limbs, or joints
■ Musculoskeletal disease, such as growth retardation or bone disease
■ Growth retardation
■ Skin disease, such as pigmentary disorder (e.g., albinism, white forelock, iris bicolor or heterochromia), keratosis, sun sensitivity, thick, coarse hair, and malformed fingernails and toenails
■ Metabolic disease such as diabetes, goiter, liver and spleen enlargement, or impaired metabolism or carbohydrates
■ Cardiac and vascular disease

Source: Adapted from "Speech impairment secondary to hearing loss," by S. R. Pratt and N. Tye-Murray, 1997. In M. McNeil (ed.), *The Clinical Management of Sensorimotor Speech Disorders*, (pp. 345–387). New York, NY: Thieme Medical Publishers, Inc.

tions that commonly co-occur with hearing loss. The relatively high frequency of co-occurring conditions suggests that the speech and hearing professional will need to take these into account when developing a child's intervention plan and aural rehabilitation strategy, and when working as a member of the child's multidisciplinary team.

Parent's Hearing Status

Ninety percent of children who have a severe or profound sensorineural hearing loss have parents who are normally hearing (Northern & Downs, 1991). This means that, prior to their child's birth, they may have been unfamiliar with the many ramifications of hearing loss. They probably will not know sign language. They also are unlikely to be members of the Deaf Culture (Chapter 10). Thus, they will have much to learn about hearing loss and aural rehabilitation, and they will need to make a decision as to whether to try and learn how to sign. They may also need to consider issues concerning the Deaf Culture. They may not (or may) be in agreement with the goal of enculturating their child into a culture that is different from their own.

HEARING AND SPEECH RECOGNITION SKILLS

Hearing loss that is severe or profound usually is sensorineural or mixed. Sensorineural hearing loss, in which the hearing loss is centered in the inner ear or auditory nerve, may stem from either environmental or genetic causes.

Environmental Causes of Sensorineural Hearing Loss

Environmental causes may be *prenatal* (occurring before birth), *perinatal* (occurring at birth) or *postnatal* (occurring shortly after birth). Prenatal factors that may affect a child's hearing status include the following:

Prenatal: before birth.
Perinatal: during birth
Postnatal: after birth

- Intrauterine infections, including rubella, cytomegalovirus, and herpes simplex virus
- Complications associated with the Rh factor (wherein maternal antibodies affect the Rh-positive blood cells of the baby)
- Prematurity
- Maternal diabetes
- Fetal alcohol syndrome resulting from mother's ingestion of alcohol during pregnancy
- Parental radiation
- Toxemia during pregnancy
- *Anoxia* (lack of oxygen)
- Syphilis

Anoxia: deficiency or absence of oxygen in the body tissues.

Hearing loss may be incurred during birth, in which case it stems from a perinatal cause. Perinatal causes of hearing loss include anoxia, which may be caused by a prolapse of the umbilical cord and a subsequent blockage of blood to the infant's brain. Although rare, the use of forceps during birth may cause damage to the cochlea, as might severe uterine contractions.

A postnatal loss often occurs because of meningitis or use of ototoxic drugs. A listing of ototoxic drugs appears in Table 14–2. Other postnatal environmental factors include measles, encephalitis, chicken pox, influenza, and mumps.

Table 14–2. Medications that may be ototoxic.

■ Aminoglycoside antibiotics, which are often used against gram-negative bacteria. Hearing loss is often bilateral and sensorineural. Some of the drugs may be more vestibulotoxic than cochleotoxic.

Amikacin
Dihydrostreptomycin
Garamycin
Gentamicin
Kanamycin
Neomycin
Netilmicin
Streptomycin
Tobramycin
Viomycin

■ Salicylates, used in large quantities for the treatment of arthritis and other connective tissue disorders. Their use may result in sensorineural hearing loss and tinnitus.

Acetylsalicylic acid
Aspirin

■ Loop diuretics, used to promote urine excretion. Their use may result in sensorineural hearing loss.

Ethacrynic acid
Furosemide
Lasix

■ Other drugs that may be ototoxic and that are used in chemotherapy regimens.

Cisplatin
Carboplatin
Nitrogen mustard

Source: Adapted from *Comprehensive Dictionary of Audiology,* by B. A. Stach, 1997. Baltimore, MD: Williams & Wilkins.

Genetic Causes of Sensorineural Hearing Loss

Genetic factors are thought to cause more than 50% of all incidents of congenital hearing loss in children (NIDCD, 1989). More than 400 kinds of genetic-based hearing losses have been described (see Gorlin, Torillo, & Cohen, 1995), and with increased activity in genetics research and the Human Genome Project, new types continually are being identified.

Chromosome pair: the basic units of genes; structures carrying the genes of a cell and made up of a single strand of DNA.

Important vocabulary for talking about genetics and hearing loss is defined in the Key Resources section at the end of the chapter. *Genes* provide the blueprints for development and function, and are arranged on the 23 pairs of *chromosome pairs,*

22 of which are *autosomes* and one of which is a pair of sex chromosomes. The different possible codes of a gene are called *alleles*. For example, an allele may specify blonde hair or red hair. If the same allele is inherited from both parents, then the resulting trait is *homozygous*. If the two are different, then the trait is *heterozygous*. Genetic hearing losses may be described as follows:

■ **Autosmal dominant trait:** One parent has a dominant allele for hearing loss which is passed on to the child, and typically, that parent has a hearing loss. The hearing loss is called *autosomal dominant* because a gene from only one parent is required for its manifestation. A child born to a parent with a dominant-trait hearing loss has a 50% probability of also having a hearing loss. If you examine the family history, you likely will find the reoccurrence of hearing loss in successive generations on one side of the family tree.

■ **Autosomal recessive trait:** A child may have parents who both carry a recessive gene for hearing loss, and yet both parents usually have normal hearing. The hearing loss is then related to an *autosomal recessive* trait. Approximately 80% of inherited hearing loss is of this type. The probability of a normally hearing couple's having a hearing-impaired baby, when both parents carry a recessive gene, is 25%. There may be no other family members who have hearing loss, and only a thorough examination of the family tree on either side of the family will reveal the rare occurrence of hearing loss. This is true only if both parents have normal hearing. If two deaf persons with the same recessive genes for deafness marry, all of their children also will be deaf.

■ **X-linked trait:** This rare kind of inherited hearing loss accounts for about 2% of genetic-based hearing losses. For a hearing loss to be related to an *X-linked trait*, the mother may have a recessive allele for hearing loss that is on the sex chromosome (labeled X on females and Y on males). When daughters inherit it, the trait is not shown, although they have a 50% chance of passing a hearing loss on to their sons. When males inherit the X-linked allele, they usually develop hearing loss.

Syndromes

Many hearing losses based in genetics are part of a *syndrome*, which in medicine means a number of conditions that occur

Autosomes: any of the 22 chromosome pairs that are not related to gender.

Alleles: the different possible codes of a gene.

Homozygous: having two identical alleles of the same gene; the same allele is inherited from both parents.

Heterozygous: having two different alleles of the same gene.

Autosomal dominant: one parent passes a dominant allele to the child; the probability of the trait being expressed in the child is 50%.

Autosomal recessive: both of a child's parents carry a recessive gene; the probability of the gene being expressed in the child is 25%.

X-linked: refers to the mother carrying a recessive allele for a trait on the sex chromosome, which is not expressed in female progeny but is passed to males.

A **syndrome** is a collection of conditions that co-occur as a result of a single cause and constitute a distinct clinical entity.

together and characterize a common disease. For example, Treacher-Collins is a syndrome that involves an autosomal dominant trait. In addition to hearing loss, which may range from mild to profound, the child with Treacher-Collins may manifest deficits in the oral cavity, nervous system, and pulmonary and renal systems. Another example of a syndrome that usually includes hearing loss is Goldenhar. In this syndrome, the afflicted child may have malformations in the mandible and outer ear, as well as a hearing loss that may range from mild to profound. Other systemic abnormalities associated with Goldenhar may manifest in the nervous system, eye, kidneys, and pulmonary and cardiovascular systems. This syndrome also involves an autosomal dominant trait. Examples of other syndromes that involve the auditory system appear in Table 14–3.

Table 14–3. Examples of syndromes that may include hearing loss.

Syndrome	Co-occuring Conditions
Richards-Rundle (autosomal recessive)	Ataxia, muscle wasting, hypogonadism, mental retardation, and progressive sensorineural hearing loss
Down syndrome (genetic abnormality)	Mental retardation, characteristic facial features, often accompanied by chronic otitis media, and associated conductive, mixed, and sensorineural hearing loss
Fetal alcohol syndrome (genetic abnormality caused by mother's abuse of alcohol during pregnancy)	Low birth weight, failure to thrive, mental retardation, wide-set eyes, recurrent otitis media, sensorineural hearing loss
Bjornstad syndrome (autosomal dominant disorder)	Congenital sensorineural hearing loss and pili torti
Mondini dysplasia	Congenital anomaly of the osseous and membranous labyrinths, severe loss of hearing and vestibular function
Latham-Munro	Myoclonus epilepsy, ataxia, and sensorineural hearing loss
Edwards (chromosomal abnormality)	Microcephaly, agenesis of bones, congenital heart disease, craniofacial abnormalities, mental retardation, and outer, middle, and inner ear anomalies
Alstrom (autosomal recessive)	Pigmentary retinopathy, diabetes mellitus, obesity, malformation of the brain, and progressive sensorineural hearing loss
Usher (autosomal recessive)	Congenital sensorineural hearing loss and progressive loss of vision
Epstein	Macrothrombocytopathia, nephritis, and sensorineural hearing loss
Lemieux-Neemeh	Nephritis, motor and neuropathy with sensorineural hearing loss
Formey	Joint fusion, mitral insufficiency, and conductive hearing loss
Robinson	Dominant onychodystrophy, coniform teeth, and sensorineural hearing loss

Table 14-3. *(continued)*

Syndrome	Co-occuring Conditions
Harboyan syndrome (autosomal dominant)	Characterized by progressive sensorineural hearing loss of delayed onset
Pendred (autosomal recessive)	Goiter and moderate-to-profound congenital sensorineural hearing loss
Jervell and Lange-Nielsen (autosomal recessive)	Electrocardiographic abnormalities, fainting spells, and sudden death accompanied by congenital bilateral profound sensorineural hearing loss
Alport (probably X-linked inheritance)	Nephritis and sensorineural hearing loss
Crouzon (autosomal dominant disorder)	Premature closure of sutures, hypertension, downward displacement of eyeballs due to shallow orbits, mild to moderate conductive hearing loss, may entail mixed loss; closure of external auditory canal
Pfeiffer	Premature closure of sutures, broad thumbs, broad great toes, short fingers and toes, hypertelorism, high arched palate, downward sloping eyes, absent external auditory canals, conductive hearing loss
Hunter (X-linked recessive disorder)	Sensorineural, conductive, or mixed hearing loss, growth deficiency, mental and neurological deterioration, coarse facial features
Stickler	Severe myopia, retinal detachment, flat facial profile, cleft palate, ocular anomalies, arthritis, sensorineural, conductive, or mixed hearing loss
Treacher Collins (autosomal dominant disorder)	Pinnae malformations, downslanting eyes, small chin, depressed cheek bones, large mouth, eyelid colobomar, conductive hearing loss related to atresia and ossicular malformation

Sources: Adapted from "Speech impairment secondary to hearing loss," by S. R. Pratt and N. Tye-Murray, 1991. In M. McNeil (Ed.), *The Clinical Management of Sensorimotor Speech Ddisorders* (pp. 345–387). New York, NY: Thieme Medical Publishers, Inc.; and *Comprehensive Dictionary of Audiology*, by B. A. Stach, 1997. Baltimore, MD: Williams & Wilkins.

Rapid Advances In Genealogical Research May Lead to Better Understanding of Deafness, and Even Prevention

In the past decade, our knowledge of genetic causes of deafness has increased by leaps and bounds. A major reason for this advancement is the Human Genome Project. This project may be summarized as follows (Allen, 1998):

(continued)

■ The Human Genome Project, is an ambitious and international scientific adventure—a kind of biological moonshot. The $20 billion project has been under way for about a decade.

■ The project first aims to decipher the genetic code hidden in our genes, the basic units of heredity.

■ Then it will help us understand how genes determine what we look like, the way babies develop and what diseases we get.

■ Finally, it will open new ways to diagnose, treat and even prevent disease, researchers say. Such revelations already have begun to occur. (p. 1)

These revelations about our genetic make-up have included the world of hearing and deafness. For instance Lynch, Lee, Morrow, Welcsh, Leon, and King (1997) traced the cause of deafness in a family in Costa Rica. *Nonsyndromic deafness* (meaning that deafness is the only symptom of the genetic defect) has occurred in generations of this family, since the 1700s. By mapping chromosomes on genes, in conjunction with performing traditional genealogy surveys with family members, the researchers were able to isolate a single gene that results in the affliction. This particular finding is important because this gene is thought to help determine how the hair cells in the cochlea respond to sound vibrations. By studying it, we may learn more about how the human auditory system operates, how deviations may occur, and what may trigger cell death.

Nonsyndromic deafness is deafness that is the only symptom of a genetic defect.

Mixed Hearing Loss

Some children have mixed hearing loss, which is a combination of both conductive and sensorineural components. Common causes of a conductive component of hearing loss (wherein sound cannot be transmitted normally through the outer or middle ear) include otitis media (fluid in the middle ear) and perforated tympanic membrane (eardrum). Mixed hearing loss is often a transient condition, so the child may have a conductive component only occasionally.

Speech Recognition Skills

Now let us turn our attention to the issue of listening skills in the child who has a severe or profound hearing loss. As Figure 14–2 illustrates, many different audiometric configurations fall

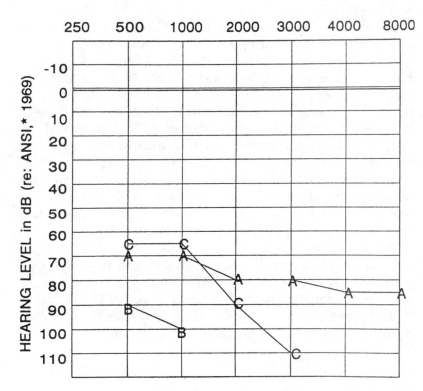

Figure 14–2. Audiometric configurations for three different types of hearing losses. Letters indicate the level at which a threshold was obtained. Child A has a severe hearing loss, Child B has a profound hearing loss, and Child C has a severe-to-profound impairment.

under the rubric of severe and profound hearing impairments. For instance, the child denoted by the letter A in Figure 14–2 has a severe hearing loss. He has some hearing across a wide range of frequencies (250 Hz to 8000 Hz). With appropriate amplification, Child A may recognize some speech with audition only and may speechread very well. This child also may hear many of his own speech sounds while talking, such as the vowel segments (which tend to be louder than consonants) and consonants that have high amplitude, such as the nasals /m/ and /n/. This child likely will hear the rhythm and prosody of his own speech.

Child B, also represented in Figure 14–2, has a profound hearing loss. Like many people with profound hearing loss, she is not completely deaf. She has some measurable hearing in the low frequencies (250 and 500 Hz). This child probably will not recognize any speech in an audition-only condition, nor recognize her own speech (although she may hear the rhythm of her intonation). She may or may not be a good speechreader.

Many children have a combined severe and profound hearing impairment. Their hearing typically is better in the low frequencies than the high frequencies. For example, Child C in Figure 14–2 has a sloping hearing loss. This child will hear some words using only audition. His listening skills will appear to be more inconsistent than those of Child A or B. Because he has some hearing in the low frequencies, he will often detect the presence of speech and recognize some words. However, because much of the acoustic information that distinguishes one word from another is contained in the mid and high frequencies, he often will not discriminate the words even though he seems to hear them. Thus, his family and teachers may sometimes accuse him of "not listening" or "not paying attention." Child C may have reasonably good speechreading skills and probably will hear the rhythm and prosody of his voice while speaking. He will not hear many of his own consonant productions, particularly sounds that have high-frequency information, such as /s/ and /t/. He may hear his own vowel productions but they may all sound similar to him.

Central Auditory Processing Disorders (CAPD)

Some hearing losses are due to *central* causes, which means that sound transmission between the brain stem and the cerebrum is disrupted, either as a result of damage or a malformation. Thus, the temporal cortex of the brain may receive incorrect information, or the information may not be processed correctly. These deficiencies in auditory processing skills sometimes are referred to as a central auditory processing disorder (CAPD).

Central hearing losses may result from head trauma, brain tumors, or neurologic vascular changes. Sometimes, a cause cannot be found. This is a difficult diagnosis to make. Children who have central hearing loss usually experience difficulty in discriminating sounds, associating meaning to sound, and listening in noise. They may have reduced auditory memory. Such problems sometimes are not implicit in the audiogram configuration (Bellis, 1996).

IDENTIFICATION AND QUANTIFICATION OF HEARING LOSS

At least two events may trigger a parent or caregiver to bring a child to an audiologist for a hearing test. The first is that the child may have failed a screening test. The second is that a parent may have noticed the child is not responding to sound in the same way as normally hearing children.

It is critical that hearing loss be detected as soon as possible, and that an intervention plan of appropriate services be developed. Hearing is essential during the first 3 years of life if a baby is to develop normal speech and language. In this section, we first will consider screening, and then more extensive audiological procedures.

Screening

When parents suspect a hearing loss, they often bring their child first to their family physician or pediatrician. The physician may perform an informal gross test, using some type of noise-maker. If the baby does not respond to the sound, a referral may be made for more extensive testing.

A hearing loss also may be detected during a screening program. If the child is a newborn, testing might be performed in the newborn nursery unit, especially if there is reason to suspect a hearing loss. High-risk registers include the following risk factors:

Low birth weight (less than 3.3 lbs)
Family history for hearing loss
In utero infections such as cytomegalovirus, rubella, or herpes
Ototoxic medications
Low *Apgar scores* (which reflect the normalcy of A = appearance, P = pulse, G = grimace, A = activity, and R = respiration at the time of birth)
Need for use of a ventilator for 5 days or longer
Cranial anomalies
Physical manifestations consistent with a syndrome

Apgar score: a numeric value between 1 and 10 assigned to newborns to describe their physical status at birth.

If the child is of school age (and hence, more likely to have a mild or moderate hearing loss), the loss might be identified during a school screening session. If a screening procedure indicates the possibility of hearing loss, the child is referred promptly for additional diagnostic audiologic testing.

A child's hearing may be tested in a variety of ways. The selection of a measurement technique is dependent on a number of variables, including the age of the child, and his or her ability to participate in the test procedures. Once a hearing loss has been identified, hearing should be tested twice per year for young children, and four times or more annually if other problems are present or if there is concern about the accuracy of the test results. Older children usually need to be evaluated only once a year.

Objective Tests

Two objective tests are used to determine the presence of hearing loss, auditory brainstem response (ABR) and otoacoustic emissions (OAE).

Auditory Brainstem Response Test

Auditory brainstem response (ABR): an auditory evoked potential that originates from the eighth cranial nerve and is generated by electrical stimulation of the cochlea via an electrode.

ABR testing often is used with babies between the ages of birth and 5 months. Electrodes are placed on the child's head, and brain wave activity elicited by the presentation of tone bursts or sound clicks is recorded. Usually, the child must be sedated for testing, as the patient must be very still in order to obtain accurate test results. ABR usually is used with individuals who cannot give behavioral responses or with individuals who provide inconsistent responses to sound stimuli.

ALGO: an automated ABR screening device used for screening newborns.

For screening purposes, a variation of ABR might be used: ALGO. *ALGO* is an automated ABR screening device, which compaires the baby's ABR response to a stored template of expected brain waveforms. The response is scored as either a pass or a failure.

Otoacoustic Emissions Testing

Otoacoustic emissions: low-level sound emitted spontaneously by the cochlea on presentation of an auditory stimulus.

OAEs are inaudible sounds that are the by-products of the mechanical actions of the outer hair cells in the cochlea. When sound stimulates the cochlea, the hair cells vibrate and initiate a signal in the eighth cranial nerve. Simultaneously, the vibration produces a sound that echoes back into the middle ear. The sound can be measured with a small probe inserted into the ear canal. Sound is presented, and the OAE is detected and traced. Persons who have normal hearing produce OAEs, whereas those who have hearing loss of 25–30 dB or greater do not. The procedure is used as a screening procedure. It is quick to administer and does not require the cooperation of the patient, other than to remain relatively still.

Behavioral Tests

Behavioral tests include the audiogram (Chapter 5). However, when a child is very young, it may not be possible to obtain one. Thus, to obtain information about the child's ability to detect a range of frequencies, the audiologist may utilize behavioral/observational audiometry (often referred to with the acronym BOA), visual reinforcement audiometry (VRA), or conditioned play audiometry.

Behavioral/Observational Audiometry

In *behavioral/observational audiometry*, the audiologist presents a sound stimulus and observes the child's behavior. Response to sound may be manifested by a change in sucking pattern, eye widening, cessation of activity, or a head turn.

Behavioral/observational audiometry (BOA): method of testing a child's hearing in which the tester presents a sound stimulus and observes the child's behavior for change.

Visual Reinforcement Audiometry

Visual reinforcement audiometry is used with children between the ages of 6 months and 2 ½ years. The child is tested in a sound-treated room. Sound is presented through an audiometer. When sound is presented initially, a box in the room lights up. Inside of the box is a toy that moves. For example, a box may light up to reveal a toy monkey clashing cymbals. The child is trained to look at the box when the sound is presented, and then testing is begun to determine the threshold for the frequencies of the audiogram.

Visual reinforcement audiometry (VRA): method of testing young children in which presentation of the sound is coupled to lighting of a toy for reinforcement of the child's response.

Conditioned Play Audiometry

Conditioned play audiometry is used to assess children, starting at about the age of 2 to 2 ½ years. Children may place a peg into a pegboard each time a sound is presented through the audiometer (Figure 14–3). He or she may drop a block into a jar. The child is trained to wait and listen for a sound, and then perform the response task when the sound is presented. Often, the child's parent may sit in the sound-treated room with the child during testing, while the audiologist may be in the adjacent room with the audiometer, watching through the win-

Conditioned play audiometry: method of testing children 2.5 years and older in which child is trained to perform a task in response to presentation of a sound.

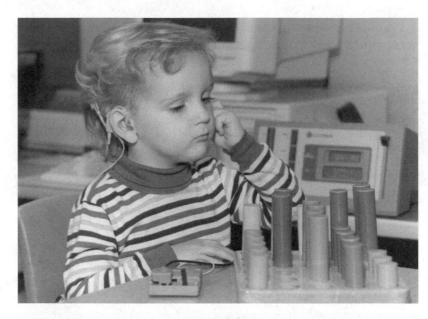

Figure 14–3. A young child is tested with conditioned play audiometry. He listens for a sound, and places a peg into the pegboard every time he hears one. (Photograph by Patti Gabriel, courtesy of Central Institute for the Deaf)

dow. The parent must be coached to sit quietly, and not provide cues about the presence or absence of sound to the child.

Coping With A Child's Diagnosis

Grief Reactions in Parents

The family must make many adjustments when they learn that one of their young members has a hearing loss. Carney and Moeller (1998) summarized some of the research that has examined the consequences of learning about the presence of hearing loss:

> It is common for parent to experience grief reactions and feelings of loss of control when a child is diagnosed with a hearing impairment (Luterman, 1979; Luterman & Ross, 1991). There is considerable evidence in the literature of negative consequences of such variable as high parental stress on child development. Quittner and Steck (1989) completed interviews with over 1000 mothers of hearing-

impaired children in Canada. They documented a high prevalence of maternal stress, with impact on family satisfaction and child development. Dunst (1985) reported that poorer feelings of well-being on the part of parents contributed to their lack of responsiveness to infant attention bids. Several researchers have found that parental language input can be seriously affected by the psychological state of the parents, which in turn can have far-reaching consequences for the child (Greenstein, 1975; Schlesinger & Acree, 1984; White, 1984). (pp. S64–S65).

This typically is a difficult period for families, and it is wise to be sensitive to the emotional turmoil that may be occurring.

After an audiologic appointment, the audiologist provides a written report to the child's parents as soon as possible. This provides a written documentation of what the audiologist has informed and counseled them about, and also recaps the audiologist's recommendations.

When you talk with many parents of children who have significant hearing loss, you may find a recurring theme: Many parents harbor hostility toward the medical profession. This hostility may derive from at least one of two sources. The first can be labeled as *anger because their concerns were dismissed*. Parents may tell you how they suspected a hearing loss in their baby, and took the baby to their family doctor or pediatrician. The doctor may have dismissed the parents' concerns, and thereby may have delayed diagnosis for several months or even years. As a result, the child was delayed in receiving amplification and intervention services. Often parents feel not only anger, but also guilt because they did not follow their instincts and pursue second and third opinions more promptly.

Another source of hostility may be labeled as *anger because the hearing loss may have been prevented*. These feelings often arise after a child has lost hearing because of meningitis. Kravitz and Selekman (1992) noted:

Many parents can identify the episode that resulted in their child's hearing loss; they blame it on improper medical care. In case after case, parents tell of their children being taken to hospitals because they had fever and appeared listless. The children were sent home with diagnoses of viral infection but within hours their conditions had worsened. The children spiked higher fevers, had seizures, and even arrested. The diagnosis was usually meningitis. While the children ultimately survived, they were left deaf and had other serious disabilities. Although years may have passed, these parents can vividly recall the harrowing details of their child's medical trauma. (p. 593)

In Chapter 10, it was noted that adults often pass through a series of emotional stages, just as most people who experience grief. These stages of emotional adjustment may include shock, denial, guilt, anger, and acceptance. Parents and family members may also pass through these stages when they learn of their child's hearing loss (Luterman, 1979; Luterman, 1991).

Shock, Denial, and Grief

Shock and denial are ways of protecting oneself from a crisis, and often result in parents focusing on minor details. An individual may deny that the hearing loss exists or may deny the enormity of its consequences. Grief then may occur, as parents realize that their ideal child has been lost.

Anger and Guilt

Anger and guilt may follow the denial stage, and often parents will become convinced that something they have done in the past may be responsible for the hearing loss. For example, one mother took anti-sea-sickness pills while on a cruise in the early weeks of her pregnancy. She experienced enormous guilt when her baby was diagnosed with profound hearing loss, because she was convinced that the medication had resulted in abnormal fetal development.

Acceptance

Finally, acceptance may set in, as parents begin to accept that their child's hearing loss is a reality. Ideally, the parents and family are willing to take constructive steps to deal with their child's hearing condition.

Many parents feel confused and overwhelmed during the early stages following diagnosis, and these feelings may be magnified as they interact with a variety of different professionals who may provide abundant, and perhaps conflicting, advice about how to handle the child's loss. They may feel inadequate when they realize how much time and effort will be required on their part to maximize their child's potential. An important role of the speech and hearing professional during this time is to provide support and reassurance that the parents can handle the new demands and to empower them to interact effectively with their child.

The stages just described are not necessarily like the rungs of a ladder, which parents climb up one step at a time, and never climb back down. Rather, parents may pass from one stage to another, return to an earlier stage, and then advance again. For example, when a child enters kindergarten, the child's parents may look at his classmates who have normal hearing and realize more fully what a significant hearing loss may mean in terms of their child's academic achievement. This may trigger new feelings of grief, even if they have come to terms with the permanency of the hearing loss.

Dealing With Feelings and Moving Forward

Kozak and Brooks (1995) suggested ways for parents to deal with their feelings. These practical nuts-and-bolts recommendations are as follows:

- **Accept your feelings:** The situation is difficult and it is understandable and appropriate to be upset. Accept that it hurts and try to find something you can do to help your child. This will allow you to feel something more positive too.
- **Talk to others:** Find a spouse, parent, friend or parent of another child with a challenge. Tell them what you are feeling and listen to them [talk about] their feelings. Get some support and see if you can give any . . .
- **Write in a journal:** If thinking and feeling are not enough to help but talking is too much for you right now or if you can't find the right listener, try writing some notes about your feelings in a journal, notebook or even a letter . . .
- **Find a group to support you:** You can find good listeners, help, support and encouragement in a group of parents whose children have any special challenges . . . Your local children's hospital, clinics and schools may be resources for finding such a group . . . Most parents of children with challenges say that other parents of

(continued)

these children provided the most important help they received in the early years. This type of support can help you learn and move forward while you cope with all your feelings.

■ **Other ways:** Some parents will look toward their ethical views or their religious values and comrades to help them find the way to feel better. Some people will delve into learning all they can about [hearing loss. Some may seek counseling] from a professional counselor or physician.

■ **Give yourself a break:** Don't demand too much of yourself. Pat yourself on the back for doing what you've already done to help your child. Ask someone who cares about you for some words of encouragement. Get a hug from your child . . . Cry if it feels better to do so. Do something good for you, even if it's only taking time to watch the quiet beauty of a sunrise or sunset. Be thankful for your child. Don't expect yourself to do every job perfectly. No one is perfect in our imperfect world.

AMPLIFICATION

Children usually receive amplification as soon as a hearing loss is identified, even if the child is only an infant. The earlier a child receives amplification, the more he or she is likely to develop auditory speech recognition skills. Support for this assertion comes from research about both animals and humans, and about vision and audition.

Support for Early Amplification

Research with vision suggests that young mammals have a more plastic nervous system than adult mammals. For example, kittens raised with goggles that expose one eye to vertical stripes and the other eye to horizontal stripes go on to develop abnormal binocular feature detectors (Hirsch & Spinelli, 1970). Children who have strabismus (crossed eyes) for several years may not develop stereopsis, even after corrective surgery (Kaufman, 1979).

Research with audition has shown that birds who do not hear their species' song patterns during a critical period of maturation never develop those patterns (Marler, 1989). Similarly, adults who have prelingual hearing loss receive minimal, if any, benefit from receiving a cochlear implant (Tong, Busby, & Clark, 1988). Children who are younger at age of implantation are more likely to develop better speech recognition skills than children who are older (Fryauf-Bertschy, Tyler, Kelsay, Gantz, & Woodworth, 1997).

These kinds of research findings underscore the importance of early identification of hearing loss, and the provision of amplification as soon as possible.

Selection of Hearing Aids

In Chapter 6, we considered the available styles of hearing aids. In this section, the selection of styles for children will be considered in more detail. Children who may benefit more from receiving a cochlear implant are considered in Chapter 18.

Traditionally, hearing aids for children included body aids, especially for children under age 3 years, because they are durable. More recently, body aids have become less popular, and most children receive behind-the-ear aids, no matter how young they are. Most behind-the-ear aids provide sufficient gain, even for profound hearing losses.

In-the-ear aids usually are not provided to young children, for a variety of reasons. These include the following:

■ The aid may not stay put in the ear.
■ The child's ear canal is still growing, so the aid must be recast frequently.
■ In-the-ear aids are difficult for parents to monitor. For example, parents may have a difficult time checking the position of the volume control.
■ These aids permit no direct auditory input.

An advantage offered by behind-the-ear aids is that they can be connected to many FM assistive listening devices. These systems include a wireless microphone worn by a talker and a receiver the child uses, connected to the hearing aid.

Once a hearing aid is fitted on a child, the audiologist provides instruction to the parents or caregivers about how to care for the device and how to perform a listening check (Figure 14–4).

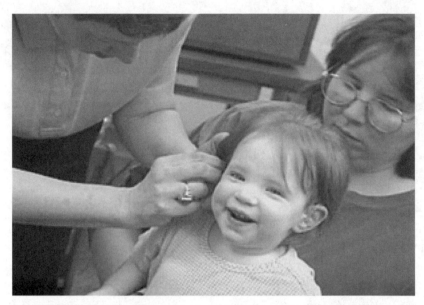

Figure 14–4. During the hearing-aid fitting, parents receive instructions about how to handle, maintain, and trouble-shoot the device. (From video footage by Rick Bernstein, courtesy of Central Institute for the Deaf)

Instruction may include how to wash an earmold, how to perform a listening check (i.e., how to monitor the child's ability to hear with the device), and how to troubleshoot the hearing aid (e.g., what to do if the hearing aid will not turn on, if the sound is weak or distorted, or if the hearing aid squeals).

Special Considerations for Children and Amplification

Special considerations for providing amplification to children include ensuring appropriate fit of earmolds. Ill-fitting earmolds can lead to irritation of the ear canal, as well as feedback. Because the ear canal is growing, infants and preschool children may need to receive a new earmold every 4–6 months. When children are between 4 and 9 years of age, new molds may be necessary only on an annual basis.

Another issue relevant to children is the adjustment period for establishing use of the device. Some children reject their devices or want to control when they do and do not use it. Some children react negatively to amplified sound, and some may view the listening device as a means of asserting independence or gaining control over parents. A speech and hearing professional can encourage parents to take responsibility and foster full-time use of the listening device at home and school. With a younger child, parents may provide reassurance and support to the child. Initially, the device can be worn for short time periods and then gradually increased over time. Routines of use should be established. Putting the listening device on in the morning should be part of getting dressed, and removing it should be part of getting undressed in the evening. For the older child, it is sometimes helpful to set a reinforcement system, in which some reward is received if the child wears the device for a specified amount of time every day.

FINAL REMARKS

In this chapter, we have focused on children who have severe and profound hearing losses. Children with lesser degrees of hearing loss also may experience listening difficulties. For instance, a child with a mild, high-frequency hearing loss may appear to have no problem in recognizing speech or responding to environmental sounds. However, the youth may not be performing optimally in the classroom setting, because he or she may have degraded listening performance in the presence of background noise. A child with a mild-to-moderate hearing loss may have decreased speech recognition and may be delayed in both speech and language development if appropriate amplification is not provided.

Children who have a lesser degree of hearing loss represent a fairly significant segment of school children in the United States. Ross (1990) suggested that 16 of every 1,000 school-age children have pure-tone-averages (PTAs, Chapter 5) between 26 and 70 dB HL. These children may need special accomodations in the classroom, as we will discuss at the end of Chapter 15, and may benefit from the use of special assistive listening devices, such as FM trainers (Chapter 5).

KEY CHAPTER POINTS

✔ About 30% of children who have significant hearing loss also have another disability.
✔ Hearing loss may arise from a variety of causes that may be prenatal, perinatal, or postnatal. The hearing loss may be due to environmental factors or genetic factors.

✔ Children with severe and profound hearing loss present a range of listening skills.

✔ A variety of audiologic procedures are available for identifying hearing loss and determining the magnitude of loss. Whereas most of the procedures rely on behavioral responses from the children, two procedures (ABR and OAE) are objective.

✔ Parents often have difficulty in accepting their children's hearing loss and may pass through a series of psychological stages before acceptance occurs. A primary role of the speech and hearing professional is to empower parents to interact effectively with their child and to make important decisions about their child's aural rehabilitation plan.

✔ Early and appropriate amplification is critical for normal speech and language development. Children often receive behind-the-ear hearing aids. In-the-ear aids usually are not prescribed, for a variety of reasons, including the fact that children's ears may still be growing, so aids must be frequently recast.

KEY RESOURCES

Important Terms to Know When Discussing Genetics[2]

Allele: one particular version of a gene.

Chromosome: structures bearing the genes of a cell and made of a single strand of DNA.

DNA: (deoxyribonucleic acid) nucleic acid polymer of which the genes are made.

Dominant allele: the allele whose properties are expressed as the phenotype.

Gene: a unit of genetic information contained within the chromosome that can be inherited.

Genotype: the total genetic make-up of an organism.

Heterozygous: having two different alleles of the same gene.

Homozygous: having two identical alleles of the same gene.

Mutation: an alteration in the genetic information carried by a gene.

Phenotype: the visible effect of the genotype.

Recessive allele: the allele for which properties are not observed because they are masked by the dominant allele.

Sex-linked: a gene is sex-linked when it is carried on one of the sex chromosomes.

[2]Definitions are from Clark & Russell, 1997, pp. 13–26.

Intervention Plans for Children

Topics

- The Multidisciplinary Team
- Roles of the Speech-Language Pathologist and Audiologist
- Decisions about the Intervention Program

- Factors That Influence Intervention Decisions
- Final Remarks
- Key Chapter Points

After the diagnosis of hearing loss is made and the child receives appropriate amplification, other rehabilitation services must be provided, including auditory training, language stimulation, and educational management. In this chapter, we will consider the multidisciplinary team and the intervention plan. The bulk of the chapter will be concerned primarily with children who have severe and profound hearing losses, At the end of the chapter, we will consider children with mild and moderate hearing losses.

The Beginnings of Deaf Education in the United States

The beginnings of deaf education in the New World follow two threads, manual communication and aural/oral communication (or oralism). Although there were sporadic attempts to educate deaf children in the United States before Alice Cogswell, many historians date the dawn of deaf education in this country to her birth in 1805. Alice was born into a well-to-do family in New England. At the age of 2 years, she contracted "spotted fever" and lost her hearing. Treatments of salt water poured into her ears, leeches, and special creams could not return what was lost. An ear trumpet bought by her distraught parents allowed her to hear a church bell, but not much more (Lane, 1984).

Alice's father, Dr. Mason Fitch Cogswell, a physician who performed some of the fist cataract surgeries in the United States, comissioned his young neighbor, Thomas Hopkins Gallaudet, to travel to Europe and learn instructional methods for the deaf. Gallaudet originally planned to visit the Braidwood family in England and Abbé Sicard in France, to gather instructional techniques in aural/oral communication and manual communication in the two countries, respectively. The Braidwood family proved to be secretive and unwilling to share their oral teaching methods. Thus, in 1816 Gallaudet left London for Paris, where he learned a manual communication system from Abbé Roch, Ambroise Sicard, and Laurent Clerc (himself deaf). Gallaudet returned to the United States, along with Clerc, and provided instruction to Alice. The two men went on to establish the American Asylum for the Education of the Deaf and Dumb (now the American School for the Deaf) in 1817, a school with a manual orientation. During the next 40 years, Clerc became one of the most influential educators of the deaf and the first (and one of the few) deaf teachers in the nineteenth century. Gallaudet's son, Edward Miner Gallaudet (1837–1917), became the president of the first college for the deaf in the new world, now named Gallaudet University (Lane, 1984; Moores, 1996).

The thread of oralism in the United States can be picked up several years later. This moment in time, too, was triggered when a young girl of a prominent family lost her hearing. Mabel Hubbard suffered scarlet fever in 1863 and, as a result, incurred an irreversible hearing loss. Her father, Gardiner Greene Hubbard, a lawyer in Massachusetts, helped to establish the Clarke School in Northampton, MA, in 1867, with the assistance of Samuel Howe, who also was the principal of the first school for the blind in the United States (Moores, 1996).

When Mabel Hubbard grew up, she married Alexander Graham Bell (Figure 15–1). In the latter half of the 19th century, Bell became an articulate and passionate advocate for oralism in the United States. In fact, an impetus for developing the telephone was a desire to develop an amplification device for his wife-to-be and for his mother, who also had a hearing loss. His counterpart who advocated an orientation that incorporated manual communication was Edward Gallaudet. In the late 1800s, these two men often were engaged in debate as to the merits of one method versus the other.

Throughout the 20th century, debates and controversies have flared on and off as to which of the two basic educational approaches, manual or aural/oral, is most appropriate for educating deaf children. The debate is likely to continue into the future.

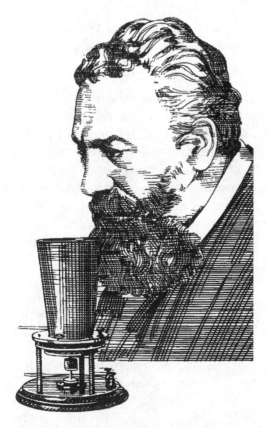

Figure 15–1. Alexander Graham Bell, advocate for oralism.

THE MULTIDISCIPLINARY TEAM

A **multidisciplinary team** is a group of professionals with different expertise who contribute to the assessment, intervention, and management of a particular individual.

An aural rehabilitation specialist usually works as a member of a *multidisciplinary team*. This team may include an audiologist, a speech-language pathologist, an educator, an otolaryngologist, and a psychologist. (In fact, the child's aural rehabilitation specialist may also be the child's audiologist or speech-language pathologist.) Depending on the situation, the team also may include a social worker or special education teacher. Each professional provides a different perspective of the child's abilities and needs. For instance, an audiologist collects information about the magnitude of hearing loss, a speech-language pathologist provides information about speech and language skills, and a psychologist and educator assesses cognitive skills, learning patterns, psychosocial adjustment, and academic performance. A multidimensional portrait of the child emerges and provides a foundation for making recommendations about the best course for intervention.

Team members share their information with one another, perhaps in the form of written reports, or as a group in a formal staff meeting. One person serves as a case manager and coordinates and integrates the various recommendations and services.

The team interacts with parents so that they can make wise decisions about a child's intervention plan. For preschool children, federal legislation, Public Law (PL) 99-457 (c.f. Roush & McWilliam, 1990), requires that a team of professionals focus on the family system and address issues specific to the particular family. PL 457 includes procedures for the identification of children with hearing loss (by means of at-risk criteria and audiologic screening methods), determination of extent of hearing loss, appropriate referral for medical and other services, provision of aural rehabilitation services such as auditory training, and determination of need for amplification and other listening devices.

The importance of early family-focused intervention cannot be overstated. Numerous studies suggest that families who receive counseling early, on a regular basis (such as weekly), who receive regular input from a teacher of the deaf, and who have an opportunity to interact with other families who have deaf children tend to have children who have better overall communication skills than families who do not receive this kind of support (Greenberg, Calderson, & Kusche, 1984; see also Clark,

1994; Greenberg, 1983; Greenstein, 1975; but also Musselman, Wilson, & Lindsey, 1988, for less definitive results).

The multidisciplinary team formulates an *Individualized Family Service Plan* (IFSP). It includes a description of child's current status and a report of the family and the expected outcomes of intervention. Specific details are included, such as the location and plan for service delivery, how long services will last, and how and when the child will be promoted into the public school systems (Roush & McWilliam, 1990).

Individualized Family Service Plan: a federally mandated plan for the education of preschool children, which emphasizes family involvement and is updated annually.

Federal law PL 94-142 concerns team management of children in the school setting. PL 94-142 (Education for All Handicapped Children Act of 1975) predates PL 99-452, and covers the identification of hearing loss in school-aged children, assessment of hearing loss, and the provision of aural rehabilitation activities, such as speech and language therapy, speech perception training, counseling, and determination of need for amplification. The key feature of PL 94-142 is that it stipulates a free and appropriate education for all children ages 5 through 21 years of age, in the least restrictive environment possible. Children who have disabilities should be *mainstreamed* whenever possible and appropriate, meaning that they are educated with children who do not have disabilities. The multidisciplinary team formulates an *Individualized Education Program* (IEP), which includes a description of the child's current levels of performance, a statement of annual goals (e.g., a listing of language structures that will be mastered), a recommendation for special education support with an indication of how support will be provided and to what extent, and finally, objective criteria for evaluating progress. An example segment of an IEP appears in Table 15–1.

Individualized Education Plan (IEP): a federally mandated plan for providing education to children with disabilities, which is updated annually.

ROLES OF THE AUDIOLOGIST AND SPEECH-LANGUAGE PATHOLOGIST

Because an audiologist or speech-language pathologist may serve as the aural rehabilitation specialist on a multidisciplinary team as well as a child's case manager, we briefly will consider their roles as team members. Exactly who does what is a gray area, as the roles of an audiologist and speech-language pathologist in the management of a hard-of-hearing or deaf child often overlap. What may be one person's responsibilities in one setting may belong to someone else in another location. In this section, we will consider what are often the responsibilities of each professional.

Table 15–1. Example segment of an Individual Education Program.

Domain	Status	Annual Goal	Short-term Objective
Audiologic	Can discriminate two utterances that differ in syllable length and intonation, such as *hello* from *how are you?*	To achieve closed-set identification of monosyllabic everyday words	Will correctly identify a spoken word when presented in the context of four then six alternatives with 80% accuracy
Language	Does not use bound morphemes, such as *-ed* or *-ing*	To establish consistent use of word endings in expressive and written communication	Will demonstrate use of past tense endings in 80% of written samples and 70% of spontaneous spoken language samples
Speech	Neutralizes vowels and omits final word consonants	To improve speech intelligibility	Will distinguish between /ɪ/, /a/, and /u/ in imitated speech tasks with 80% accuracy, and produce final consonants in at least 50% of words spoken during a spontaneous speech task
Psycho-social	Does not follow classroom rules	To demonstrate grade-appropriate classroom behavior	Will receive positive reinforcements for adhering to classroom regulations, and accumulate 100 points during a 3-month period
Educational	Reading is delayed by one grade level; can read aloud but has reduced comprehension	To improve reading comprehension	Will demonstrate comprehension on 85% of grade-appropriate reading samples

The Audiologist

An audiologist may perform any of the following duties:

- Evaluate hearing and speech recognition skills
- Select, fit, and help maintain appropriate listening devices, including hearing aids and FM trainers
- Provide speech perception training

■ Provide consultation to parents and other professionals on the multidisciplinary team

Audiologists identify and evaluate children's hearing capabilities and speech recognition skills. Although very young children may not be able to participate in word recognition testing, assessment of hearing thresholds can be performed with
almost all age groups. Following identification, the audiologist
may make any necessary referrals, such as to a physician or
other health-care professional. The audiologist also may initiate the formation of the multidisciplinary team and the case-
management process.

Audiologists also select and ensure proper use of listening devices. They will select and fit a hearing aid or make a recommendation for the child to receive a cochlear implant. They
likely will explore the child's home and school environments,
either through parent and teacher questionnaires or through
site visits to the home and school. For instance, the audiologist
may see that the child is in a noisy classroom and often misses
much of the teacher's speech. The audiologist then may recommend that the child and teacher use an FM auditory trainer
to reduce the effects of background noise. Follow-up maintenance and repair also will be provided.

Sometimes audiologists provide formal speech perception
training rather than, or in addition to, the speech-language
pathologist or classroom teacher. In some cases, they may
make recommendations to the person who provides training.

Finally, audiologists consult with parents and teachers about
the child's listening potential and difficulties and ways to encourage the development of listening skills.

The Speech-Language Pathologist

A speech-language pathologist may perform any of the following functions:

■ Evaluate speech and language performance
■ Provide speech and language therapy
■ Consult with parents, and classroom teachers
■ Provide instruction in sign language to child, class-
room teacher, and parents, if appropriate

- ■ Maintain bridges of communication between clinical setting, classroom and home, and ensure that therapy objectives are reinforced informally throughout a child's day
- ■ Advise audiologists about appropriate language levels for audiological tests
- ■ Provide speech perception training

A speech-language pathologist evaluates speech and language performance. If the child is 2 years old or younger, a speech and language evaluation may not be possible, simply because the child has so little speech and language to evaluate.

The speech-language pathologist also provides speech and language therapy. Test results are used to identify initial therapy objectives, and a hierarchy of steps to be followed over time is developed. Often, the objectives coincide with a curriculum that has been developed specifically for hard-of-hearing and deaf children.

A third role assumed by speech-language pathologists in the intervention plan is to provide consultation to parents, teachers, audiologists, and other members of the multidisciplinary team. Speech-language pathologists often provide general information. For instance, they may familiarize parents and teachers with their child's speech and language skills and how the child's skills compare to those of other children. They also can describe how speech and language skills progress in normally hearing children and children with hearing loss, and factors that may accelerate or impede progress. Such information helps those who know the child to develop appropriate expectations. It also may provide them with ideas about how best to nurture their child's development.

For families who use simultaneous communication or ASL, speech-language pathologists can help parents and teachers learn sign language. They may recommend printed or video resources that include sign dictionaries, and even provide direct instruction and practice.

Speech-language pathologists also can suggest ways for helping children to generalize what they learned in therapy to more real-world settings by informing parents and teachers about their child's current therapy objectives and suggesting practice materials. For example, a speech-language pathologist might observe a child in the classroom and then suggest ways in which the classroom teacher can integrate speech and language practice into the daily routine.

Speech-language pathologists may provide information about the child's language skills to audiologists and help them select appropriate audiological tests. For instance, if the speech-language evaluation reveals that a child has an extremely limited vocabulary, the audiologist may opt not to evaluate the child's speech recognition skills with recorded sentence lists.

In some cases, the speech-language pathologist provides formal speech perception training. The child's audiologist typically provides information about the child's listening performance, and this information is used to design training objectives. Again, the speech-language pathologist interacts with teachers and parents so that they can reinforce auditory and speech-reading training in everyday communication situations.

DECISIONS ABOUT THE INTERVENTION PROGRAM

Before an audiologist, speech-language pathologist, or educator begins to think about the specifics of an aural rehabilitation plan, such as auditory training objectives, four key decisions must be made about a child's intervention program. Typically, a child's parents or primary caregiver make them, although they receive information and recommendations from the multidisciplinary team before doing so. The decisions are summarized in Figure 15–2. All four decisions have an impact on how well a child de-

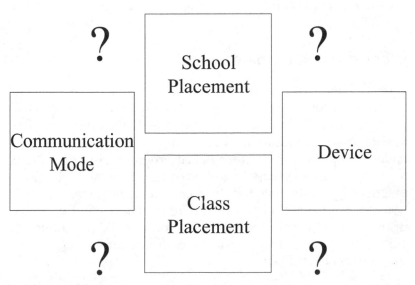

Figure 15-2. Decisions that must be made about a child's intervention program.

velops listening, speech, and language skills, and affect academic and psychosocial development. It is important to understand that no single route is appropriate for all children, and hence, each child must be considered on an individual basis.

One decision often affects or determines another. For instance, if a family opts for an aural/oral program, they also may opt for a private day school if an aural/oral program is not readily available in their local public school system. Decisions also may be revised many times during the course of the intervention program.

School Placement

One of the first decisions parents must make about their child's intervention plan relates to school placement. They must decide whether their child will receive services from a public or private institution and whether the child will attend a day or residential program. Since the passage of U.S. Public Law (PL) 94-142 (the Education for All Handicapped Children Act) in 1975, there has been a substantial increase in the number of children who remain in their home communities and receive a public education. Concomitantly, there has been a decrease in the number of children who attend residential and private day schools. Moores (1992) reported that enrollment in residential programs has declined by 6,945 students, whereas enrollment in public day classes has increased by 8,163 students since 1975. Enrollment in private residential and day schools has dropped from 6.0% of deaf children in 1974 to 1.5% in 1986.

Classroom Placement

A second decision relates to program placement. This decision is influenced by the age of a child at the time of diagnosis. For instance, if a child is a baby, than parents might consider either a center-based program or a home-based program, or a combination of the two. In a *center-based program*, children attend therapy for a designated number of hours each week. Their parents may participate too. In *home-based programs*, an early-intervention specialist visits the infant's home and provides instruction to the parents and child. Home-based programs occur in the home and emphasize one-on-one rather than group training (Scheetz, 1993).

In a **center-based program**, children attend therapy for a designated number of hours per week.

In a **home-based program**, an early interventionist visits the infant's home and provides instruction for the child and parents.

Beyond infancy and early preschool, two distinct classroom placement options, self-contained and mainstream, are available in many school districts and a third (a combination of the two), resource rooms, may also be available. *Self-contained classrooms* are contained within neighborhood or community schools and include only deaf and hard-of-hearing students (Figure 15–3), or may include children who have other disabilities, in which case it is classified as a *multicategorical self-contained* classroom. In *mainstream classrooms*, deaf and hard-of-hearing children attend classes together with children who have normal hearing. Sometimes children attend a self-contained classroom for part of the school day and a mainstream classroom for some subjects, such as art and physical education (Figure 15–4). When in a mainstream classroom, children often utilize support services, such as the use of a sign or oral interpreter and/or an FM trainer. Some children attend a mainstream classroom and also receive individualized instruction in a resource room. Children who attend *resource rooms* spend some part of their school day in a regular classroom, and receive instruction from an early intervention specialist for certain topics, such as language. An alternative or a supple-

Self-contained classrooms include only deaf or hard-of-hearing children.

In **mainstream classrooms**, deaf or hard-of-hearing children attend classes with their normally hearing peers.

Resource rooms provide instruction in particular areas for children who spend part of their day in regular classrooms.

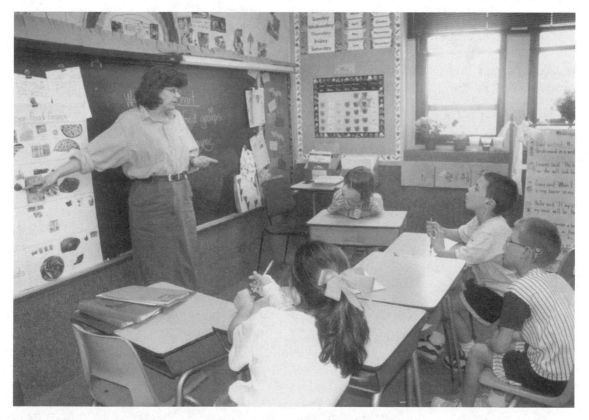

Figure 15–3. Self-contained classroom placement. Class sizes are usually small, and children sit in a circle around the teacher. (Photograph by Kim Readmond, Central Institute for the Deaf)

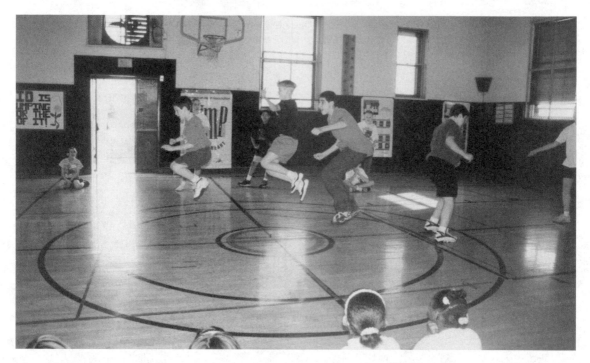

Figure 15–4. Partial mainstream classroom placement. Children may be mainstreamed for nonacademic subjects during the school day, such as physical education class. (Photograph by Kim Readmond, Central Institute for the Deaf)

Itinerant teachers work in several schools, providing support services to children who are deaf or hard-of-hearing and their teachers.

ment to a resource room is an *itinerant teacher*. The child attends school in a regular classroom, but receives support services from an itinerant teacher, who works in several schools and has expertise in issues related to deafness and the hard-of-hearing.

Figure 15–5, adapted from Deno (1970), illustrates one model for determining classroom placement. The goal is to move the child toward a regular mainstream classroom placement as expediently as appropriate. Only when necessary is a child placed outside of the mainstream classroom or taken out of the classroom to receive special support services. Not all speech and hearing professionals adhere to such a model. Sometimes a child is placed in a regular classroom at the onset of his or her educational program, so that the youth has normal classroom experiences from the onset and learns to identify with the hearing world. Alternatively, some children are educated in a self-contained classroom throughout their school years, with special emphasis on becoming enculturated into the Deaf community.

There is not a great deal of research data available to help parents make choices about classroom placement. Some evidence

Move this way as far as possible →

Self-Contained Classroom	Part-time Self-contained Classroom; Part-time Mainstream Classroom	Part-time Mainstream Classroom; Part-time Resource Room	Full-time Mainstream Classroom

← Return this way only as far as necessary

Figure 15-5. One model for determining classroom placement.

suggests children who attend mainstream classrooms have better speech and language skills than those who attend self-contained classrooms. However, the selection process determining classroom placement is often designed to place children with better skills in programs that provide fewer specialized services. As such, mainstreaming per se may not necessarily result in better communication skills. Northcott (1990) noted that children who are placed in mainstream classrooms usually have the following characteristics: "early fitting of hearing aids, early family oriented infant/preschool programming, auditory-oral approach to language learning, and . . . speech as the primary mode of communication." (p. 15)

Communication Mode

A third decision to be made about the intervention program relates to communication mode. Will the child use primarily speech to communicate? Manually coded English and speech? ASL? If a sign system is selected, the family also must learn the system as well as the child. Before we consider the decision process, let us first review the various communication modes.

The majority of persons with profound hearing impairments use one of three modes to communicate: *American Sign Lan-*

American Sign Language (ASL) is a manual system of communication used by members of the Deaf Culture in the United States.

guage (ASL), manually coded English, and spoken language. A relatively small minority use a system called Cued Speech.

American Sign Language

ASL is a manual system of communication. A person does not use ASL and speak at the same time. ASL has a different grammar than spoken English. One ASL sign might represent a concept that would require many English words to express. Facial expressions and body language can impart a variety of meanings to the signs. In both ASL and manually coded English, fingerspelling may be used if there is no sign for a particular word or concept. In fingerspelling, one handshape corresponds to each letter of the alphabet. The American manual alphabet appears in Figure 15–6.

Bilingual/bicultural model: teaching children with significant hearing loss ASL as their first language and then later English in school as they develop reading and writing skills.

A great deal of attention in recent years has been focused on the use of a ***bilingual/bicultural model*** for educating children with significant hearing loss. In this model, children use ASL as their first language for communication and then, later, learn English in school as they develop reading and writing skills (Mahshie, 1995; Paul & Quigley, 1994; Supalla, 1991). The premise is that, if children develop a language system for thought and expression first, basic skills will transfer to learning similar skills in a second language. The fact that deaf children of deaf parents (who use ASL) often have better language and literacy achievement than deaf children of hearing parents provides a primary rationale for this approach. A number of educational programs in the United States, Sweden, and Denmark have implemented this model, but definitive results of its success are not available (see Mahshie, 1995 for initial findings of support for a bilingual/bicultural approach).

Manually Coded English

Manually coded English is a form of communication in which manual signs correspond to English words.

As the name implies, ***manually coded English*** is comprised of manual signs corresponding to the words of English. It also has the same syntactic structures. Typically, a person who uses manually coded English speaks simultaneously while signing. For instance, as a boy says, "The cat is inside," he will sign the article *the*, and then one sign each for *cat, is,* and *inside.* The combined use of sign and speech as an educational philosophy is referred to as ***simultaneous communication***. The child uses every available means to receive a message, including sign, re-

Simultaneous communication: combined use of sign and speech.

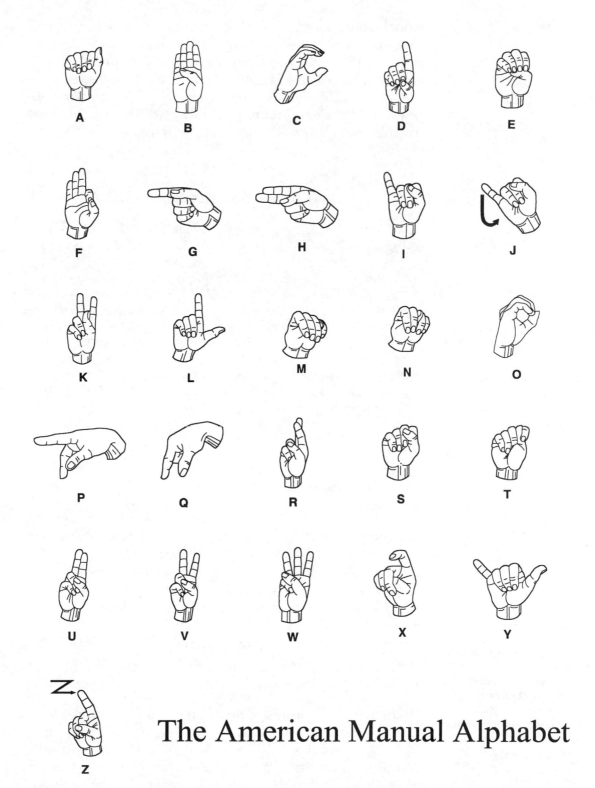

The American Manual Alphabet

Figure 15–6. The manual alphabet.

sidual hearing and lipreading. The majority of very young deaf and hard-of-hearing children use simultaneous communication. However, this could change in the future. The increased use of cochlear implants may mean that more children use an aural/oral mode. Conversely, the resurgence of Deaf pride and the Deaf Culture movement (which we considered in Chapter 10) may lead to more children using ASL.

More on Manually Coded English

There is no universally accepted English-based sign system. For example, under the rubric of manually coded English fall the systems of Signed English, Seeing Essential English (SEE I), Signing Exact English (SEE II), Linguistics of Visual English (L.O.V.E.), and the Rochester Method. People in one region of the country may sign a word one way whereas those in another region sign it in a different way.

Many teachers and children who use manually coded English actually sign a Contact form of English, omitting function words such as *the* and morphemes including those that mark past tense and plurality (Marmor & Pettito, 1979; Nix, 1983). Children who receive a Contact model of English may be at relatively high risk for developing deficits in language syntax.

Aural/Oral language

Aural/oral communication is the language used by persons with normal hearing.

Aural/oral language is the same language used by persons with normal hearing. The child with a hearing impairment who uses aural/oral language will speak messages and use speechreading to receive messages. Most children who use aural/oral language are educated with a multisensory approach, while a small number are educated with a unisensory approach. Children in a *multisensory approach* utilize both vision and hearing to recognize speech. In learning to talk, children rely on residual hearing, speechreading, and in some instances, touch.

Multisensory approach: use of both vision and hearing to recognize speech.

Unisensory approach: use of only residual hearing to receive spoken messages.

The **acoupedic approach** is a comprehensive habilitation program for infants and their families that emphasizes auditory training without formal lipreading instruction.

Children in a *unisensory approach* rely only on residual hearing to receive spoken messages. The classroom teacher may sometimes expect a child to recognize the signal auditorilly, even if the youngster has minimal residual hearing. This approach is sometimes referred to as an *acoupedic approach*, and is defined by Pollack (1970) as follows:

The term acoupedics refers to a comprehensive habilitation program for the hearing impaired infant and his family, which includes an emphasis upon auditory training without formal lipreading instruction. (p. 13)

Cued Speech

Cued Speech is a communication mode that is used by a handful of children with profound hearing loss. This communication system uses phonemically based hand gestures to supplement speechreading (Cornett, 1967). Thus, the talker speaks while simultaneously cueing the message. By themselves, the hand signals are uninterpretable. When coupled with the audiovisual signal, speech recognition increases because viseme members are distinguished from one another.

Cued Speech, a system for enhancing speechreading, uses phonemically based gestures to distinguish between similar visual speech patterns.

In the Cued Speech system, eight different handshapes are used to distinguish consonants and six locations on the face and neck are used to distinguish vowels. For instance, the consonants /p/ and /b/ resemble one another on the mouth. The consonant /p/ is distinguished by a 1 handshape and the consonant /b/ is shown by a 4 handshape. Thus, if talker said the word *pea*, he or she would hold a 1 handshape to the corner of the mouth, because a 1 handshape indicates the phoneme /p/ and a placement at the mouth corner indicates an /i/ vowel. If the talker instead said *bee*, he would hold a 4 handshape at the mouth corner. The word *boo* would be signaled by a 4 handshape at the throat. Figure 15–7 presents the Cued Speech system.

Selection of a Communication Mode

Much debate and controversy stems about the issue of communication mode, and many speech and hearing professionals take firm stands in favor of one mode versus another. Of all the decisions parents must make about their child's intervention plan, this decision can be the one they revisit most often.

Selection of communication mode is an area in which there are no clear answers to which is the best way to go, and it is likely that the best route is different for different children. With this said, there is some evidence that children educated with an aural/oral emphasis program achieve better speech and language performance and literacy development than children

Cued Speech Configuration

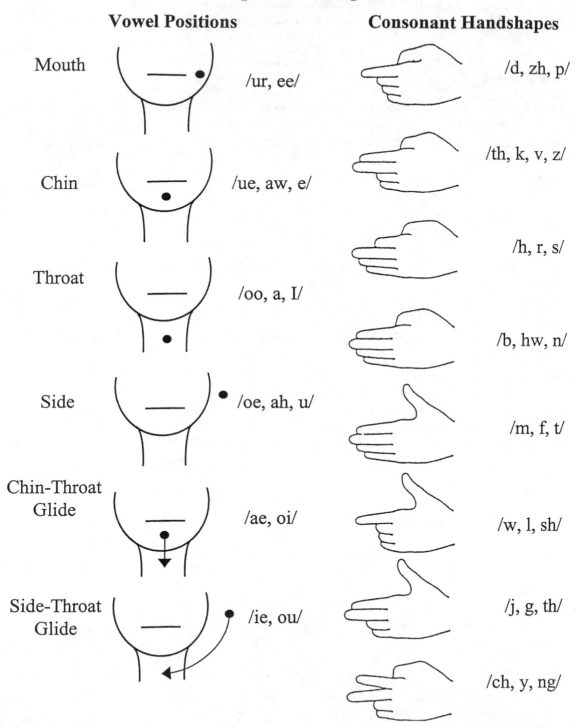

Vowel Positions		Consonant Handshapes
Mouth	/ur, ee/	/d, zh, p/
Chin	/ue, aw, e/	/th, k, v, z/
Throat	/oo, a, I/	/h, r, s/
Side	/oe, ah, u/	/b, hw, n/
Chin-Throat Glide	/ae, oi/	/m, f, t/
Side-Throat Glide	/ie, ou/	/w, l, sh/
		/j, g, th/
		/ch, y, ng/

Figure 15–7. Hand configurations and hand placement positions for Cued Speech. (Adapted from "Cued Speech: A Professional Point of View," by B. Scott-Williams and E. Kipila, 1987. In *Choices in Deafness: A Parent's Guide*, S. Schwartz, Ed. Copyright 1987 Woodbine House.).

who are educated in a program that uses sign language (Bench, 1992; Geers, Moog, & Schick, 1984; Quigley & Paul, 1984). For instance, Markides (1988) found that children from an aural/oral emphasis program were more likely to achieve better speech intelligibility than children from simultaneous communication programs, and their speech intelligibility was less likely to deteriorate over time.

Although such studies suggest that differences may exist between programs that implement different communication modes, most research investigations have provided relatively little control over other factors such as socioeconomic status or intellectual abilities. This is because there are many difficulties inherent in relating communication mode to outcome measures such as literacy or speech intelligibility. Complex interrelationships exist among demographic variables and the use of speech and sign. For example, children who use an aural/oral mode are more likely to have more hearing, to attend preschool, to come from higher-income families, and to use a hearing aid more often (Jensema & Trybus, 1978).

Some metrics have been developed for helping families choose communication modality. For example, Northern and Downs (1984) developed the Deafness Management Quotient (DMQ), a formula that factors in residual hearing, central intactness, intellectual factors, family constellation, and socioeconomic situation. Similarly, Geers and Moog (1987) developed the Spoken Language Predictor (SLP), which is a sum of five weighted predictor factors that include hearing capacity (which is determined by speech recognition performance), language competence, nonverbal intelligence, and family support. If a child achieves a certain score or better with one of these metrics, an aural/oral mode is recommended. If not, a modality that includes sign language is advised. More recently, a system has been devised that bases this decision both on family- and child-centered measures, as well as the progress a child makes during a 6-month period in a program conducted by speech and hearing professionals. This program, called Diagnostic Early Intervention Project (DEIP) (Moeller, Coufal, & Hixson, 1990), appears to be highly effective in determining optimal placement in an education program, and relatedly, optimal communication mode (Moeller et al., 1990).

Listening Device

In addition to deciding about school and classroom placement, and selecting a communication mode, a decision must be made about a listening device. The decision usually is made fairly soon after diagnosis of hearing impairment as to whether a child will be fitted with a hearing aid or a cochlear implant. Before receiving a cochlear implant, the child must have a trial period with a hearing aid (Chapter 17).

Parents have a plethora of information available to help them make a decision about a listening device. For instance, research suggests that children who use cochlear implants surpass hearing-aid users who have similar degrees of hearing impairment in their speech recognition (Tyler, 1993), speech production performance, and language and reading (see Chapter 16). Moreover, children who are younger when they receive a cochlear implant are more likely to perform better than children who are older.

In light of such experimental findings, it is likely that cochlear implant use will become more prevalent in the future. Indeed, there is potential for the cochlear implant to become the most commonly used listening device by young deaf children.

FACTORS THAT INFLUENCE INTERVENTION DECISIONS

Now that we have reviewed some of the decisions that must be made about a child's intervention program, let us consider the factors that often influence how these decisions are made. Figure 15–8 lists some factors that might influence a family's decisions. In many ways, the factors overlap.

Locale

Because urban and rural areas of the United States afford different educational opportunities, decisions about the intervention plan are to some extent, dependent on geographic location (Yoshinago-Itano & Ruberry, 1992). In large cities, parents often have a choice between intervention approaches. In rural areas, familial choice may be minimal. Because of limited resources,

Location	A. Urban B. Rural
Professional Counseling	A. Pediatrician B. Otolaryngologist C. Speech and Hearing Professional D. Educator E. Psychologist F. Other
Family Variables	A. Income B. Acceptance C. Education D. Expectations E. Participation F. Structure G. Familiarity with Deafness H. Other
Child Variables	A. Age B. Residual Hearing C. Age at hearing loss onset D. Vocalizations E. Behavior F. Language

Figure 15–8. Factors that influence the decision-making process.

many rural school districts historically have endorsed only one intervention option and offered few publicly supported education services. Thus, for children who do not live in urban areas, many decisions about intervention may be made at the district and state level, by persons other than the family.

Locale

Brackett (1990) describes how school factors can affect the design of an intervention program:

Some school districts, especially those in rural communities, do not have staff specifically trained or with appropriate credentials for working with hearing-impaired students. With no teacher of the hearing impaired to provide academic support, and with only one itinerant speech-language pathologist to cover a 150-mile area and visit schools twice weekly for the most severe cases, the question arises, "Is it possible to provide a quality program with the personnel who are available?" The answer may be "no" if caseloads are heavy and coordination time is difficult to arrange. Or the answer may be a resounding "yes." Many highly individualized programs have been implemented by support personnel who, with some in-service consultation, provide exactly what a child needs even though they do not possess the "correct" professional credentials.

The school district's attitude . . . can affect the service delivery model selected. A district may not want the bother of generating a local program, preferring instead to send the student to an already existing out-of-district program. Conversely, a small district may be able to hire that special teacher who can effectively design a suitable program for a specific child. Economics also affect the choice of a model for a particular child. It may be less expensive to initiate a program locally, rather than pay a large tuition to centralized special education services. However, it is difficult to effectively implement a quality program without sufficient resources." (p. 92)

Professional Counseling

Most families of recently diagnosed deaf and hard-of hearing children receive advice and counseling from a fleet of professionals. In addition to members of the multidisciplinary team, they also may receive advice from their family doctor and other professionals in their communities. The intent of professional counseling is to provide families with information, support, and opportunities for participation. Such counseling can be invaluable to families who are wrestling with issues that were unfamiliar to them before they had a hard-of-hearing or deaf child. Perhaps one of the most important roles you will play in a family's life will be to provide informational and emotional adjustment and acceptance counseling to families.

What Parents Say They Want From Professionals

Jackson Roush invited a group of parents to write about their experiences with speech and hearing professionals, and to describe what was helpful in their interactions. Roush (1994) summarized the responses in the passage below:

1. The early stages of identification are among the most stressful some parents will experience in their entire lives. Families want professionals to provide facts and information, but also to consider the affective domain. A sincere, caring attitude from professionals, even if they don't know all the answers, is noticed and appreciated. This is particularly important during the early stages of identification and intervention. Consideration of the parents' emotional state apart from the specific needs of the child, is especially appreciated.
2. Early on, many parents want the "right choices" presented to them; but eventually, most want to make their own decisions. They must depend on professionals, however, to provide honest, unbiased information, delivered at a level appropriate to their knowledge and experience. Most families seek professionals who will support and encourage them along the path of their own choosing.
3. Families want flexibility in methodology and placement decisions. What may be the "right decision" at a given point in time may change later on. Families want to be supported in the options they choose, and not made to feel "locked in" to these important decisions.
4. Families need to be praised and supported for what they are able to do, and not 'judged' for what they are unable to do.
5. Parents want and need the support of other parents. Many families report an emotional 'turning point' when they connected with a supportive group of other parents.
6. Professionals should consider the impact of hearing loss on the entire family. Parents are particularly appreciative when professionals seek creative ways to encourage the participation of all family members rather than designating a given individual, usually the mother, as the family expert and decision maker. (pp. 349–350)

Family Variables

In addition to locale and professional counseling, a third factor that influences decisions about the intervention plan is the family. Certainly home reinforcement and support is desirable no matter what program options are chosen.

Many family variables potentially affect the design of the intervention program. How these family variables interact and affect the decision-making process are no doubt complex. These variables include at least these, the family's:

■ Socioeconomic status, and availability of medical insurance.
■ Acceptance of the hearing loss.
■ Level of education and professional interests.
■ Expectations about who the child will become, and what he or she will achieve.
■ Willingness to participate in an intervention program.
■ Structure, including the number of siblings and whether both parents live in the household.
■ Familiarity with deafness.

The impact of these kinds of variables may be great. Let us consider four of them in more detail in order to demonstrate this point:

■ **Socioeconomic status:** A wealthy family may have the resources to afford extensive private speech-language therapy and hence opt to use an aural/oral mode of communication with their deaf child. They are more likely to have medical insurance and their insurance policies may provide coverage for cochlear implants. A family with little income and no insurance will not have these resources.
■ **Acceptance of hearing loss:** A family that has not accepted a child's deafness may not seek intervention services for several months or even years following diagnosis.
■ **Family structure:** A family headed by a young, single mother with several children may participate less in decisions made about her child's intervention program, or participate less in the implementation of the program. For example, one mother enrolled her 1-year-old daughter in a center-based program. She had two other young children and also worked the evening shift in a factory. She soon dropped out of the intervention program, unable to follow the program routine while coping with other life demands.

■ **Familiarity with deafness:** Families who are familiar with deafness, perhaps because of another relative's hearing loss, may be influenced by choices that are familiar to them. They also may be more accepting of the child's deafness and seek assistance quickly.

Child Variables

Not only general family-related variables influence intervention choices, so do characteristics of the individual child. These characteristics might include the presence of other disabilities, the child's intelligence, and/or degree of residual hearing. For example, if a child has mental retardation as well as significant hearing loss, an aural/oral communication mode likely will not be selected. On the other hand, if the child has residual hearing and receives good benefit from amplification, this option may be chosen. Less tangible child variables, such as whether the child is an introvert or an extrovert and whether the youngster is willing to accept challenges and competition, also will affect intervention decisions.

A child's progress and success also influence choices about intervention. For example, parents may enroll a child in one kind of program, but a lack of progress may lead them to enroll the child in a different program. A child's progress in developing receptive and expressive language, intelligible speech, and a positive self-concept impinge on whether and when a plan of intervention is modified.

A psychoeducational assessment usually is performed to obtain information about the child. The *psychoeducational assessment* usually includes an evaluation of the following child variables (Heller, 1990, p. 62):

  Intelligence, both *verbal* (cognitive abilities demonstrated via language-based performance) and *nonverbal* (cognitive abilities demonstrated by performance that is not language-based)
  Verbal function, written language, and reading
  Arithmetic skills
  Visual-motor skills
  Visual and auditory memory and multimodal integration
  Social and emotional function and problem solving
  Attention

The results of this assessment may be used to design a child's intervention plan, and also, to assess whether the child is progressing within his or her current program.

CHILDREN WHO HAVE MILD OR MODERATE HEARING LOSSES

Heretofore, we have focused on children who have severe and profound hearing loss. Children who have mild and moderate hearing losses also may need aural rehabilitation, although usually not to the same extent as children who have severe and profound hearing losses. Children with a mild hearing loss (hearing thresholds between 20 and 40 dB HL) may have some difficulty recognizing speech that is spoken quietly or at a distance. They usually have little problem when speaking on the telephone. It is not unusual for children with mild hearing losses to be diagnosed later in childhood, perhaps during an elementary school screening program, because they rarely seem to have significant problems in hearing or in developing speech and language.

Children with a moderate loss (thresholds between 40 and 70 dB HL) have difficulty understanding speech presented at a conversational level, and may have difficulty comprehending speech in a group setting. However, children with either a mild or moderate loss tend to receive a great deal of benefit from the use of hearing aids.

Children with mild or moderate hearing losses usually have an IEP developed. In particular, they should receive a speech-language evaluation to determine whether their speech and language acquisition is progressing according to age-level normally hearing peers. Sometimes, children will have mild misarticulation errors, such as errors in the production of fricatives and affricatives (Elfenbein, Hardin-Jones, & Davis, 1994). Children with moderate hearing losses may also have some delays in vocabulary development. Children with mild or moderate hearing losses may or may not need speech-language therapy, and may need to use a free-field FM assistive listening device system (Chapter 6). Often a child's classroom teacher will consult with a speech and hearing professional about how to adjust the classroom environment to accommodate the child with hearing loss. Information such as that summarized in Table 15–2 might be provided to the classroom teacher. Elfenbein (1994) provides a more in depth consideration of children who are hard-of-hearing.

Table 15–2. Guidelines for the classroom teacher.

The following suggestions should help _____'s teacher understand although he/she receives benefits from his/her hearing aid, it does not make speech clearer, only louder. What he hears might be called indistinct speech since there are individual sounds that are distorted or that she may not hear at all. Therefore anything that can be done to improve the listening conditions would be helpful.

1. **Let _____ sit as close to the teacher as possible. In this way he/she will be able to benefit from both the auditory and visual cues.** This seat should be far away from noisy distractions of hallways, radiators, or windows. Expect _____ to have more trouble listening and paying attention when the room is noisy than when it is quiet.

2. **Speak naturally to _____ in a good clear voice. The hearing aid is an amplifier therefore it is unnecessary to shout.**

3. **If _____ does not understand something that was said, the teacher can:**
   a. repeat-perhaps a little slower.
   b. rephrase.
   c. write the word or sentence on the board.

4. **In order to follow a group discussion, it would be helpful if _____ could sit where she could see most of the faces, and if the teacher or children could try to let her know who is talking and let her look before the speaker begins to talk.** It is also ideal if the teacher can repeat the most important things said.

5. **In order to understand what is said, it is usually helpful for _____ to see the speaker's face and lips.** This is called speechreading. For speechreading it is helpful if
   a. _____'s back is to the major light source.
   b. The speaker does not move around too much.
   c. The speaker speaks clearly and distinctly and faces _____ when talking.

6. **Sometimes the hearing-impaired child may miss the small words and misunderstand a sentence, especially if it is a long sentence and the room is noisy.** If _____ seems confused or gives a silly answer, repeat what was said and if he/she said something inappropriate let her in on the joke. _____ may not always tell the teacher if he/she has not understood, but she should be encouraged to do so. Hearing-impaired children are sometimes embarrassed to keep asking for repetitions.

7. **New vocabulary words may be difficult for _____, and he/she may require a little extra help in vocabulary development.**

8. **In some cases a notetaker can be a help to the hearing-impaired student. Sometimes a "buddy" in the class can be assigned to repeat directions to the hearing-impaired child without disrupting the classroom routine.**

Source: A handout from Central Institute for the Deaf Hearing, Language, and Speech Clinics, Reprinted with permission.

FINAL REMARKS

This chapter has presented an overview of children's intervention programs. We have considered the decisions that must be made and factors that influence them. A variety of organizations exists that provide information about hearing loss in children and information about intervention plans. Many of these organizations are state speech-language-hearing associations. In addition to providing information, many of these organizations are comprised of professionals who provide speech, language, and hearing-related services to children and their families. The Key Resourcers section provides a list of many organizations and their addresses.

In the next two chapters, we will consider the specifics of an aural rehabilitation plan. Unlike the situation with adults who have postlingual hearing loss (i.e., a hearing loss that was incurred after the acquisition of speech and language), the aural rehabilitation plan typically includes speech and language therapy as well as more traditional aural rehabilitation interventions.

KEY CHAPTER POINTS

✔ A multidisciplinary team is assembled to evaluate a child and to provide support and services to the child and his or her family. The team may include an audiologist, a speech-language pathologist, an otolaryngologist, an educator, and a psychologist. The audiologist or speech-language pathologist often serves as the aural rehabilitation specialist and the case manager. The team interacts with a child's family to formulate an IEP or an IFSP.

✔ Some of the decisions parents must make about their child's intervention program relate to school and classroom placement, communication mode, and listening device.

✔ Parents' decisions may be affected by several factors, such as their locale or their familiarity with deafness. You may play an important role in providing information and in making recommendations.

✔ Most children in the United States who have severe and profound hearing loss live at home and attend school in their home community. The majority of children use simultaneous communication.

✔ Most children with mild and moderate hearing losses can attend classrooms for normally-hearing children. Usually, they will receive an IEP, although they may or may not require specialized speech and hearing services.

KEY RESOURCES

Organizations that Provide Hearing-Related Services to Children and Their Families

Overseas Association of Communication Sciences
Argonner Elementary School
Unit 20235 APO,AE 09165

Alaska Speech-Language-Hearing Association
P.O. Box 944
Bethel, AK 99559

Arkansas Speech-Language-Hearing Association
P.O. Box 3835
Little Rock, AR 72203

Colorado Speech-Language-Hearing Association
1325 South Colorado Boulevard
Suite B401
Denver, CO 80222

Delaware Speech-Language-Hearing Association
P.O. Box 7383
Newark, DE 19714-7383

Florida Language, Speech and Hearing Association
335 Beard Street
Tallahassee, FL 32301

Hawaii Speech-Language-Hearing Association
1350 South King Street
Honolulu, HI 96814

Illinois Speech-Language-Hearing Association
435 North Michigan Avenue, Suite 1717
Chicago, IL 60611-4067

Iowa Speech-Language-Hearing Association
8305 University Boulevard, Suite F-1
Des Moines, IA 50325

Kentucky Speech-Language-Hearing Association
366 Waller Avenue
Lexington, KY 40504

Maine Speech-Language-Hearing Association
The Old Richardson Place
510 C Main Street
Gorham, ME 04038

Massachusetts Speech-Language-Hearing Association
518 North Main Street
Randolph, MA 02368

Speech and Hearing Association of Alabama
719 Franklin Street, SE
Huntsville, AL 35801

Arizona Speech-Language-Hearing Association
7622 North 48th Drive
Glendale, AZ 85301

California Speech-Language-Hearing Association
825 University Avenue
Sacramento, CA 95825

Connecticut Speech-Language-Hearing Association
213 Back Lane
Newington, CT 06111

District of Columbia Speech-Language Hearing Association
P.O. Box 91016
Washington, DC 20090-1016

Georgia Speech-Language-Hearing Association
P.O. Box 6708
Athens, GA 30604

Idaho Speech, Language and Hearing Association, Inc.
Box 8116 - Department SPA
Idaho State University
Pocatello, ID 83209

Indiana Speech-Language-Hearing Association
P.O. Box 984
Noblesville, IN 46060-0984

Kansas Speech-Language-Hearing Association
3900 17th Street
Great Bend, KS 67530

Louisiana Speech-Language-Hearing Association
8550 United Plaza Boulevard, Suite 1001
Baton Rouge, LA 70809

Maryland Speech-Language-Hearing Association
P.O. Box 539
Columbia, MD 21045

Michigan Speech-Language-Hearing Association
855 Grove Street
East Lansing, MI 48823

Minnesota Speech-Language-Hearing Association
3386 Brownlow Avenue
P.O. Box 26115
St. Louis Park, MN 55426

Missouri Speech-Language-Hearing Association
MSHA Central Office
713 PCA Road, P.O. Box 45
Warrensburg, MO 64093

Nebraska Speech-Language-Hearing Association
455 South 11th Street, Suite A
Lincoln, NE 68508

New Hampshire Speech-Language-Hearing Association
P.O. Box 3251
Nashua, NH 03061-3251

New Mexico Speech-Language-Hearing Association
P.O. Box 53580
Albuquerque, NM 87153

North Carolina Speech-Language-Hearing Association
P.O. Box 28359
Raleigh, NC 27611-8359

Ohio Speech and Hearing Association
P.O. Box 549
Miamisburg, OH 45343-0549

The Oregon Speech-Language-Hearing Association
Professional Administration Services
Salem, OR 97308

Organizacion Puertorriquena
P.O. Box 20147
Rio Piedras
Puerto Rico, PR 00928-0147

South Carolina Speech-Language-Hearing Association
3008 Millwood Avenue
Columbia, SC 29205

**Tennessee Association of Audiology
and Speech-Language Pathology**
530 Church Street, Suite 700
Nashville, TN 37219

**Utah Speech-Language-Hearing
Association**
P.O. Box 171363
Holladay, UT 84117-1363

**Speech-Language-Hearing Association
of Virginia**
P.O. Box 35653
Richmond, VA 23235

Mississippi Speech-Language-Hearing
3748 Highway 468
Pearl, MS 39209

**Montana Speech-Language-Hearing
Association**
P.O. Box 9627
Helena, MT 59604

**Nevada Speech-Language-Hearing
Association**
7235 Lingfield Drive
Reno, NV 68508

**New Jersey Speech-Language-Hearing
Association**
170 Township Line Road
Bellemead, NJ 08502

**New York State Speech-Language-
Hearing Association**
25 Chamberlain Street
P.O. Box 997
Glenmont, NY 12207-0997

**North Dakota Speech-Language-Hearing
Association**
P.O. Box 12775
Grand Forks, ND 58208-2775

**Oklahoma Speech-Language-Hearing
Association**
P.O. Box 53217
Oklahoma City, OK 73152-3217

**Pennsylvania Speech-Language-Hearing
Association**
100 High Tower Blvd., Suite 302
Pittsburgh, PA 15205-1134

**Rhode Island Speech-Language-Hearing
Association**
P.O. Box 9241
Providence, RI 02940

**South Dakota Speech-Language-Hearing
Association**
808 South Thompson
Sioux Falls, SD 57103

**Texas Speech-Language-Hearing
Association**
P.O. Box 140046
Austin, TX 78714-0046

**Vermont Speech-Language-Hearing
Association, Inc.**
4 Caroline Drive
Bennington, VT 05201

**Washington Speech and Hearing
Association**
2033 Sixth Avenue, N.E., Suite 804
Seattle, WA 98121

**West Virginia Speech-Language-Hearing
Association**
Hodges and Associates
109 Elizabeth Street
Charleston, WV 25301

**Wyoming Speech-Language-Hearing
Association**
P.O. Box 587
Thermopolis, WY 82443

American Speech-Language-Hearing Association
10801 Rockville Pike
Rockville, MD 20852

Autism Society of America
7910 Woodmont Avenue
Bethesda, MD 20814

Cleft Palate Foundation
1218 Grandview Avenue
Pittsburgh, PA 15211

Learning Disabilities Association of America
4156 Library Road
Pittsburgh, PA 15234

National Consumer Board for Stuttering
P.O. Box 8791
Grand Rapids, MI 49518

National Easter Seal Society
230 West Monroe, 18th Floor
Chicago, IL 60606

National Spasmodic Dysphonia Association, Inc.
P.O. Box 203
Atwood, CA 92601-0203

Orton Dyslexia Society
Chester Building, Suite 382
8600 LaSalle Road
Baltimore, MD 21286-2044

Stuttering Resource Foundation
1233 Oxford Road
New Rochelle, NY 10804

United Cerebral Palsy Association, Inc.
1660 L Street, NW, Suite 700
Washington, DC 20036

Wisconsin Speech-Language-Hearing Association, Inc.
P.O. Box 1109
Madison, WI 53701-1109

Alzheimer's Disease and Related Disorders Association
919 North Michigan Avenue, Suite 1000
Chicago, IL 60611-1676

The Arc
500 East Border Street, Suite 300
Arlington, TX 76010

Children with Attention Deficit Disorder
499 NW 70th Avenue, Suite 101
Plantation, FL 33317

International Association of Laryngectomees
c/o American Cancer Society
1599 Clifton Road, NE
Atlanta, GA 30329-4251

National Aphasia Association
P.O. Box 1887
Murray Hill Station
New York, NY 10156-0611

National Council on Stuttering
9242 Gross Point Road, #305
Skokie, IL 60077-1338

National Head Injury Foundation
1776 Massachusetts Avenue, N.W.
Suite 100
Washington, DC 20036-1904

National Stuttering Project
5100 E. La Palma Avenue, Suite 208
Anaheim Hills, CA 92807

The Selective Mutism Foundation
P.O. Box 450632
Sunrise, FL 33345-0632

TASH
29 W. Susquehanna Avenue, Suite 210
Baltimore, MD 21204

Alexander Graham Bell Association for the Deaf
3417 Volta Place, NW
Washington, DC 20007-2778

American Society for Deaf Children
2848 Arden Way, Suite 210
Sacramento, CA 95825-1373

Cochlear Implant Club International
P.O. Box 464
Buffalo, NY 14223

League for the Hard-of-Hearing
71 W. 23rd Street
New York, NY 10010

National Cued Speech Association
Speech-Language Pathology Department
Nazareth College of Rochester
4245 East Avenue
Rochester, NY 14618

Telecommunications for the Deaf
8719 Colesville Road, Suite 300
Silver Spring, MD 20920-3919

Association of Auditory-Verbal International
2121 Eisenhower Avenue, Suite 402
Alexandria, VA 22314

International Federation of Hard-of-Hearing People
Telderssatraat 7
NL-8265 WS Kampen
The Netherlands 05205-15463

National Association for the Deaf
814 Thayer Avenue
Silver Spring, MD 20910

Self Help for Hard-of-Hearing People, Inc.
7910 Woodmont Avenue, Suite 1200
Bethesda, MD 20814

16

Speech, Language, and Literacy Development

Topics

- Speech Characteristics
- Language
- Literacy
- Children Who Use Cochlear Implants
- Speech and Language Evaluation: General Principles

- Assessing Speech Skills: Intelligibility, Segmentals, and Suprasegmentals
- Assessing Language Skills
- Speech and Language Therapy
- Final Remarks
- Key Chapter Points

In many ways, hearing loss has more far-reaching consequences for children than for adults. Not only may children not hear or understand the speech of others, but their own speech and language acquisition likely will be delayed as a result of their hearing loss. In this chapter, we will consider their speech, language, and literacy development.

Recent data about children who have used cochlear implants for a prolonged period of time also will be presented so that we may contrast their speech, language and reading skills with children who have similar hearing losses but use hearing aids. In this chapter, you will learn that the advent of cochlear implants has had a dramatic effect on the outlook of speech, language, and literacy development in children who have significant hearing loss.

SPEECH CHARACTERISTICS

Segmental errors: errors in speech sounds.

Suprasegmental errors: errors in speech rhythm and prosody, the pitch, rate, intensity, and duration imposed on phonemes and words.

Overall intelligibility, *segmental errors* (errors in the sounds of speech), and *suprasegmental errors* (errors in speech rhythm and prosody) are often considered when compiling a description of children's speech (Figure 16–1). As a general rule, children with more residual hearing speak better and produce fewer segmental and suprasegmental errors than children with less residual hearing. However, how well a child speaks also depends on numerous other factors, including the speech therapy received, motivation to speak, the consistency of appropriate amplification use, the age of first receiving hearing aids, and the child's speech environment. For example, does the child hear speech often? Do those around the youngster provide good speech models? Is reinforcement provided when the child tries to speak?

Children who have mild to moderate hearing losses tend to have only mild speech and language difficulties (Elfenbein, Hardin-Jones, & Davis, 1994), particularly if they use appropriate amplification. For this reason, in this chapter we will focus on children who have more significant hearing losses. Additional information about children with less severe hearing loss can be found in Blair, Peterson, and Viehweg (1985), Davis (1990), McClure (1977), and Reich, Hambleton, and Houldin (1977).

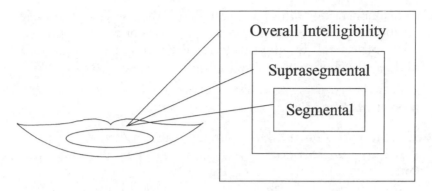

Figure 16–1. Speech proficiency is determined with a consideration of overall intelligibility, segmental errors, and suprasegmental errors.

Overall Intelligibility

Most children with profound hearing impairments are difficult to understand. On average, you will rarely identify more than 20% of the words they say (John & Howarth, 1965; Markides, 1970; Monsen, 1978).

Research suggests that children with significant hearing loss demonstrate different developmental patterns than normally hearing children and shows that they reach a plateau in their speech skills relatively early in their development. For example, the phonetic repertoires of deaf infants have been found to be restricted when compared to their normally hearing peers (Lach, Ling, Ling, & Ship, 1970; Stoel-Gammon, 1988). Children who have been studied longitudinally between the ages of 11 and 14 years demonstrate little change in the average number and types of vowel and diphthong errors they make over time (McGarr, 1987). Although children may be idiosyncratic in many aspects of the speech production, many demonstrate similar error patterns when speaking.

Segmental Errors

Children with hearing impairments produce many segmental errors, both when speaking vowels and diphthongs and when speaking consonants. Markides (1970) attempted to quantify the articulatory errors. In a group of hearing-aid users who had a mean hearing level of 95-dB HL, 56% of all vowels and diphthongs and 72% of all consonants were rated by a group of listeners as deviant. Not surprisingly, there exists an inverse relationship between the number of vowel and consonant errors and overall intelligibility: As the number of errors in a child's speech increases, intelligibility decreases (Smith, 1975).

Vowel Production

Children who have significant hearing losses and who use hearing aids most commonly neutralize vowels, so a child might intend to say "Me too!" but instead produce, "Mah tah!" Some physiological studies have focused on how the tongue moves during vowel production. These studies suggest that talkers with profound hearing loss may not move their tongue bodies in the anterior-posterior (front-back) dimension as much as normally hearing talkers and may rely primarily on jaw displacement for distinguishing vowel height (e.g., the low vowel /a/ versus the high vowel /ɪ/) (Dagenais & Critz-Crosby, 1992; Tye-Murray, 1987, 1991). This restricted tongue movement is no doubt a primary component underlying the perceptual phenomenon of neutralized vowels.

A list of vowel error types includes the following (Smith, 1975):

■ Neutralizations
■ Substitutions
■ Dipthongizations
■ Prolongations
■ Nasalizations

Consonant Production

Children who have severe and profound hearing losses and who use hearing aids tend to produce characteristic consonantal errors. These errors include voiced/voiceless confusions, substitutions, omissions, distortions, and errors in consonant clusters (Hudgins & Numbers, 1942; Smith, 1975). For example, a child might intend to speak the word *boat*, but actually say "poe." In this production, the youngster substituted the voiceless /p/ for the voiced /b/ and omitted the final /t/ sound. Many children produce consonants that are visible on the face more accurately than consonants that are not visible. For instance, a child is more likely to produce the word *pat* correctly than the word *cat*. The /p/ entails visible lip closure, whereas the tongue dorsum closing gesture for /k/ cannot be seen. Apparently, a child with a significant hearing impairment relies heavily on visual information for acquiring speech.

Manner of production errors are common. Affricatives, fricatives, glides, and laterals are especially difficult for many children to produce (Nober, 1967; Osberger, Robbins, Lybolt, Kent,
& Peters, 1986).

The Roles of Auditory Information in Speech Acquisition

To understand the difficulties children with minimal hearing
capability have in developing intelligible speech, it is helpful to
think about the ways in which auditory information helps us
learn to talk. Auditory information plays at least five important
roles during a child's acquisition of speech:

1. *Auditory information potentiates the development of specific principles of articulatory organization.* By listening to the speech of
   others in their community, children learn how to regulate
   their speech breathing, they learn how to flex and extend
   their tongue bodies, and they learn how to alternate rhyth-
   mically between vowels and consonants. Children who cannot hear often do not learn to (a) manage their breath
   streams for speech, (b) rotate their tongue forward and backward in the mouth to establish vowel postures, and (c) move
   the articulators smoothly and continuously from one articulatory posture to the next.
2. *By listening to others, children learn how to produce specific
   speech events.* For instance, they learn to distinguish /p/ with
   a relatively rapid velocity opening gesture and /w/ with a
   slow velocity gesture.
3. *Children develop a system of phonological performance* (i.e., they
   learn the phonemes of their language community) through
   listening. Often children who cannot hear do not acquire
   some sounds in their language, especially those associated
   with high-frequency auditory information, such as /s/ and
   /ʃ/.
4. *Auditory feedback informs children about the consequences of their
   articulatory gestures, and how these consequences compare to
   sounds produced by other talkers.* For example, if a talker ex-
   plodes air through his lips, he learns that this will produce a
   plosive sound. If he does it with too much vigor, he will hear
   a sound that may be inappropriately loud, when compared
   to other talkers of his language. It is not uncommon for a
   deaf talker to produce a slight popping sound when producing plosives.

continued

5. *Auditory feedback may provide information for monitoring ongoing speech production and for detecting errors* . For instance, you might hear yourself say "See went," and then quickly correct yourself and say "She went." Deaf talkers are unable to monitor themselves in this way.

When a child does not have a sensory mechanism that fulfills these five roles, acquiring speech and maintaining appropriate articulatory patterns is a formidable task (Tye-Murray, Spencer, & Woodworth, 1995).

Suprasegmental Errors

Children with significant hearing loss tend to have a distinctive speech quality. Their speech often sounds breathy, labored, staccato, and arrhythmic. Errors in suprasegmental patterns contribute to this aberrant speech quality. These include errors in stress, speaking rate, coarticulation, breath control, pitch, and intensity.

Stress

Many children place equal stress on all syllables or stress words inappropriately. For instance, the word *baby* may be produced with the stress on the second syllable instead of the first, as in "bah-BEE." Research suggests that talkers with significant hearing loss may be able to produce the articulatory maneuvers necessary for producing appropriate stress, for example, greater jaw and lip displacement for stressed syllables and less displacement for unstressed syllables. As such, the absence of auditory feedback may not limit children's potential to produce stress appropriately, but other factors such as unfamiliarity with stress patterns may come into play (Robb & Pang-Chang, 1992; Tye-Murray & Folkins, 1990).

Speaking Rate

Typically, children with severe and profound losses speak very slowly, pausing often, both within words and between words (Hudgins, 1934; Nickerson, 1975). They may insert extraneous sounds and prolong words (John & Howarth, 1964). Voelker (1938) found that children with profound hearing loss spoke 70 words per minute, as compared to 164 words per minute spoken by children with normal hearing.

Coarticulation

Many children do not coarticulate sounds in the same way as normally hearing talkers (Angelocci, Kopp, & Hollbrook, 1964). For instance, a child might say the word *basket* as "ba-a-sa-ka-a-ta." In this production, the child has articulated each sound as if it were an isolated unit.

Normally hearing talkers tend to begin preparing for an upcoming vowel position during a preceding consonant position, such that the jaw is in a higher position during the /p/ that precedes the /i/ in the word *peep*, and is in a lower position during the /p/ that precedes the /a/ in the word *pop*. Talkers with profound hearing loss tend not to demonstrate this coarticulatory effect (Tye-Murray, Zimmermann, & Folkins, 1987). Acoustic studies also support the lack of coarticulation (Monsen, 1976; Rothman, 1976). For example, the acoustic characteristics associated with consonant-vowel segments of monosyllables tend to be similar, regardless of phonetic context.

Breath control

Most hard-of-hearing and deaf children produce relatively few syllables per breath, as they often manage their airflow inefficiently. In fact, often the first objectives in a speech therapy curriculum is to establish better breath control in the young deaf talker (Ling, 1976).

Adult talkers who have profound and prelingual hearing loss demonstrate normal respiratory and aerodynamic behaviors for nonspeech tasks and aberrant behaviors for speech (Forner & Hixon, 1977; Itoh, Horii, Daniloff, & Binnie, 1982). Poor breathing behavior correlates highly with poor speech intelligibility (Hudgins & Numbers, 1942).

Deaf talkers often inefficiently manage the speech airstream, as characterized by higher air volume expenditure during connected speech (Forner & Hixon, 1977; Metz, Whitehead, & Whitehead, 1984). For example, they demonstrate higher air consumption and shorter durations for sustained vowels, and higher airflow rates than normally hearing talkers. This means that they let out more breath when speaking a syllable than do normally hearing talkers. Unstable airflow also occurs (Hutchinson & Smith, 1976; Whitehead & Barefoot, 1983). McGarr and Lofqvist (1982) suggested that air wastage may occur because deaf talkers fail to establish biomechanical resistance either with the larynx and/or other supralaryngeal articulators.

Voice Quality

Children's voice quality may be unpleasant. Their pitch may sound excessively high or variable (Angelocci, Kopp, & Holbrook, 1964; Boone, 1977). Some children speak with a monotone. Pitch breaks, with pitch abruptly changing from high to low, are common.

Intensity

Children may speak too softly or too loudly and often their intensity may fluctuate inappropriately. It is not surprising that children often cannot adjust their speaking intensity as a function of context. That is, they may not raise intensity when talking in a noisy gymnasium nor lower it when speaking in a quiet library.

LANGUAGE

In light of the many segmental and suprasegmental errors, it is not surprising that many children with severe hearing impairments have poor intelligibility. When these speech problems coexist with language problems, communication becomes difficult indeed. In this section, we will focus specifically on the kinds of language problems many children with significant loss manifest.

Regardless of which communication mode they use most frequently, be it simultaneous communication, aural/oral , ASL, or Cued Speech, most children who are profoundly deaf do not learn the English language very well. One way to appreciate how hearing impairment affects language development is to compare normally hearing and hard-of-hearing groups. 8-year-old normally hearing children have a better knowledge of grammar than do adults with profound hearing loss. Moreover, most adults with significant hearing loss never acquire a vocabulary better than that of a normally hearing fourth grader (Bamford & Saunders, 1991).

We often categorize language difficulties as either problems of form (syntax and morphology), content (semantics and vocabulary), or pragmatics (use).

Form

The list comprising problems of *form* is extensive (see Seyfried & Kricos, 1996). Children with hearing loss may overuse nouns and verbs and rarely use adverbs, prepositions, or pronouns. They may omit function words. Most of their sentences have a simple subject-verb-object structure, and their sentences have few words compared to those produced by normally hearing children. Compound or complex sentences are rare, as are morphemes that mark plurality or past tense. In telling a story about her cat, one child said, "Socks jump. Cup fall over. Mess big. Mom mad about Socks." In this narrative, the child omitted functions words such as *was* and tense markers such as *ed.* Her syntactic structures were simple. Although you might follow her story, you probably will think that her sentences sound telegraphic.

Sometimes children order their words incorrectly. A child may say, "Saw cat big," meaning that she saw a big cat.

Not only do they rarely speak compound or complex sentences, children with significant hearing loss usually cannot interpret them when they speechread or read. For example, you might say to a child, "The cat was chased by the dog." The child may interpret this sentence as though it were in the active tense. Thus the meaning becomes: *The cat chased the dog.*

You might speak a nominal sentence to a child, such as, "The ending of the school year saddened the teacher." The child might interpret it in an objective sense, and derive this meaning: *The school year saddened the teacher.*

Children with significant hearing loss sometimes show similar developmental trends as normally hearing children, albeit delayed. Deaf children between the ages of 5 and 7 years, often acquire syntactic structures in the same order as normally hearing children, but at a much slower rate. However, children who show a great degree of language delay are at higher risk of following deviant patterns of development (Levitt, McGarr, & Geffner, 1987). That is, they are likely to follow developmental patterns that are different than those of normally hearing children.

Content

Perhaps one of the most pervasive language problems among children with hearing loss is a restricted vocabulary. Children

Form: Proper use of the elements of lauguage, such as nouns and verbs, prepositions, and so on.

Content: extent of vocabulary and use of words.

often learn only common everyday words. They may have gaps in their vocabularies, wherein they do not know words relating to an entire concept, such as outer space. Hence, words such as *planet, Martian, star, spacemen,* and *rocket* may be unfamiliar. They often use words in limited ways. For instance, a child may use a word such as *happy* as a predicate (e.g., *The boy is happy*) but not as a modifier (e.g., *The happy boy is here*). Many children cannot identify synonyms and antonyms or understand idioms such as *She was mad as a hornet.*

Longitudinal studies of the vocabulary of young deaf children reveal delays when compared to those of normally hearing children. For instance, White and White (1987) studied 46 prelingually deaf infants over a 3-year period. The infants ranged in age between 8 and 30 months at the time of entry into the study. By the third year, children had attained a receptive and expressive vocabulary that matched those of normally hearing children who are only 1 year of age.

Pragmatics

Pragmatics: The study of how language is used.

Children with a hearing impairment sometimes use questions inappropriately. For instance, one child's first question to a new acquaintance was, "How much money does your father make?" A child may not know how to initiate or maintain a conversation or know how to repair breakdowns in communication. In some circumstances, the child may nod and bluff, pretending to understand.

A child also may not know many of the social graces of conversation. For example, he or she may not know how to take turns while conversing, how to acknowledge that the message has been heard, and how to change the topic of conversation. Overall, the child probably will not use language functionally as well as his normally hearing peers. In the following conversation, a child with hearing loss introduced a topic abruptly, and did not respond to the adult's request for clarification:

Adult:	"Do you want to come with me?"
Child:	"Car fell off table, boom!"
Adult:	"What did you say?"
Child:	"Mine."

These inappropriate responses may relate both to the child's hearing loss (he may not have recognized the adult's utterances) and his unfamiliarity with conversational rules.

In general, there at least three reasons why some children do not learn conversational pragmatics very well. These are the following:

■ **First, they do not receive extensive practice in using language.** Their unfamiliarity with many language structures and reduced vocabulary limit their ability to converse. Moreover, if they do not use an aural/oral communication mode, they have fewer conversational partners to interact with because few normally hearing persons know manually coded English or ASL.
■ **Second, they cannot overhear their parents or other people talking.** Thus, they do not receive the everyday, incidental models of how to use language.
■ **Third, they do not receive the same formal instruction as normally hearing children.** For instance, a parent may carefully explain the rules of politeness to a child with normal hearing (do not interrupt, say "thank you"; let someone else say something). The parent may not explain the rules to her child with a hearing loss, either because of the child's limited language or because of the parent's limited skill in using *manually coded English* or ASL.

LITERACY

Literacy is an issue closely related to language development. Literacy is indexed by performance on reading and writing measures. Given many children's difficulties with using English language, it is not surprising that many also have difficulty in learning to read and comprehend and to compose written text.

Reading

Deaf and hard-of-hearing children who use hearing aids often show delays and/or differences when compared to normally hearing children. The average reading and writing level of deaf high school students is at a third or fourth grade level (Allen, 1986) and rarely does a deaf or hard-of-hearing student

A child using **manually coded Engliish** or ASL may not receive the same language experiences as a normally hearing child since few people in the child's environment will be familiar with these means of communication.

exceed a 7.5 grade reading level (Trybus & Krachmer, 1977). Reading difficulties are a resilient problem: There has been little improvement in the average reading performance of hard-of-hearing children relative to their normally hearing peers over the past 80 years (LaSasso & Mobley, in press; Paul, 1998).

Reading problems no doubt stem largely from an inadequate language system. Deficits in vocabulary and unfamiliarity with groups of related words (as in the planets, and space-related terms) and unfamiliarity with complex syntactic structures interfere with deaf children's ability to understand printed text.

Other factors that compound the reading task include deficits in experience and world knowledge (Quigley & Paul, 1986) and perhaps, deficits in children's abilities to take on another's (i.e., the author's) point of view. For example, if a child has never overheard a news report on television, he or she may have difficulty in reading articles related to current events. If a child has difficulty in viewing the world from another's perspective, he or she may not be able to digest fictional stories and narratives.

In addition, there appears to be a reciprocal relationship between a child's ability to use oral English language (i.e., "orality" or aural/oral communication skills) and reading performance (Geers & Moog, 1989). Paul (1998) suggests that this relationship may relate to a child's working knowledge of the alphabet principle, which is the basis of English print, as well as the development of skills related to the conversational-based form of language (Paul, in press). For example, skills related to the conversational-based form of language may include a child's ability to carry on a meaningful dialogue with an adult or another child.

Finally, additional factors that may affect reading performance include the type of instruction a child has received. For instance, children who have been educated with a whole-word (or look-say) type of instruction may have different reading skills than children who have been educated with a phonetic-based system (letter analysis). The design of the curriculum, the expertise of the teacher(s), and the involvement of the family may also interact with reading performance.

Writing

Deaf children often lag behind their normally hearing peers in writing skills. Their writing samples often contain syntactic errors, such as omission of articles, inappropriate use of pronouns, and omission of bound morphemes (e.g., *'s* and *-ed*). Deaf writers tend to use a preponderance of subject-verb-object sentences, and rarely construct complex syntactic structures. Rarely do deaf writers use synonyms, antonyms, metaphors, or cohesive forms of substitution or ellipsis. They may introduce a variety of topics, without elaborating on them (Yoshinaga-Itano, Snyder, & Mayberry, 1996).

Some children have difficulty in writing narratives, in which there is a clear beginning, middle, and end to their story. Sometimes they have difficulty in focusing on the important parameters of a story. For example, a third-grade boy, when asked to write a story about a girl holding a scorched dress and an iron, wrote the following sample:

> *Girl have red sweater. Hair yellow. Girl work hard!*

In this example, the child appears to have focused on surface details of the picture rather than the underlying story line. The child also used inappropriate verb tense (e.g., *have* instead of *has*) and omitted function words. Most children progress beyond this level of expression and often demonstrate gains in their narrative skills (including semantic linkages by use of surface structure and topic and event, connectors, logical sequence, temporal sequencing, physical causality, and psychological causality) between the ages of 7 and 18 years of age, although they rarely achieve the competency of normally hearing age-matched peers (Yoshinaga-Itano & Downey, 1996).

CHILDREN WHO USE COCHLEAR IMPLANTS

In the foregoing discussion, we have been concerned with children who use hearing aids. Children who have a significant hearing loss but who use cochlear implants represent a relatively new group of children, a group that performs more similarly to children who have better hearing than to children who have a profound hearing loss. In this section, we will consider the speech, language, and literacy of young cochlear-implant users.

Implantation of children with multichannel cochlear implants was approved by the FDA in 1990. We are now in a time period when longitudinal information about their performance is becoming available, and we now can make statements about their long-term performance.

Speech

Children who use cochlear implants typically tend to speak better than children who use hearing aids, and you may recognize considerably more than 20% of their words (Osberger, Robbins, Todd, Riley, & Miyamoto, 1994; Tobey, Geers, & Brenner, 1994).

Vowel Production

There is evidence that children with prolonged cochlear-implant experience achieve better vowel production than children who use hearing aids and who have similar hearing losses. Figure 16–2 shows the vowel production of 36 children who have prelingual deafness and use cochlear implants (Tye-Murray, Tomblin, & Spencer, 1997). These data were collected between 1990 and 1997 as part of the University of Iowa Hospitals' Cochlear Implant Program. The children were 5 years, 6 months of age on average at the time of implantation, with a range of 2 years to 11 years. The children use simultaneous communication and attended public school in their local communities. To have been included in the study, they had to have worn their cochlear implants for at least 5 years. They were tested one time before implantation, and then every year there-

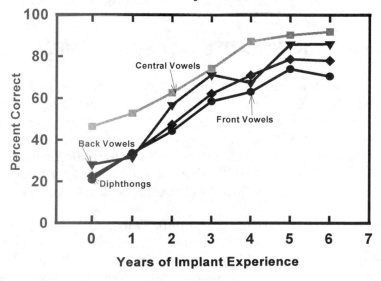

Figure 16–2. Vowel production over time for 36 young cochlear-implant users.

after. Data were obtained during a story-retell task, a task that will be described in more detail later in the chapter.

Percent correct results are plotted as a function of place of articulation, and averaged across children. Figure 16–2 suggests that, after 5 or 6 years of implant use, children produce vowels with about 80% accuracy, on average. This is considerably better than the 44% accuracy levels reported by Markides (1970) for young hearing-aid users.

Consonant production

Receipt of a cochlear implant also enhances a child's ability to produce consonants. Figures 16–3 and 16–4 portray a description of the 36 children's consonant production, as a function of both place and manner of production.

Figure 16–3 indicates that after 6 years of device experience, children who use cochlear implants produced consonants with about 70% accuracy, which is better than the 28% accuracy level reported by Markides (1970) for hearing-aid users. Interestingly, just like children who have similar hearing losses but

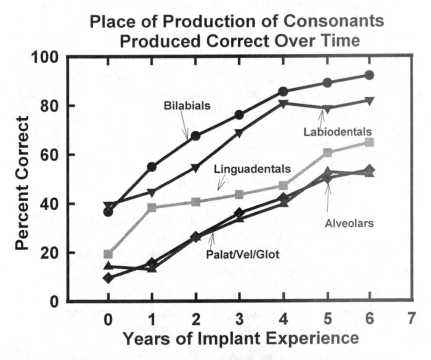

Figure 16-3. Consonant production over time as a function of place of articulation from 36 young cochlear-implant users (Palat = palatals, Vel = velars, Glot = glottals).

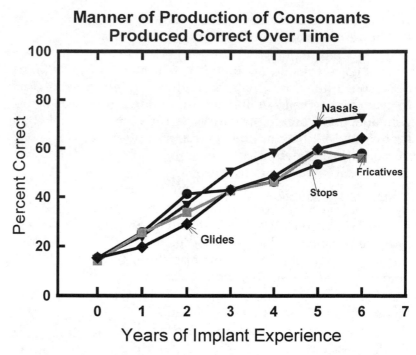

Figure 16–4. Consonant production over time as a function of manner of articulation from 36 young cochlear-implant users.

who use hearing aids, the young cochlear-implant users tended to produce the more visible bilabial consonants correctly more often than the less visible palatals, velars, and glottals. The relatively good overall performance and the exceptionally good production of more visible sounds suggests that young cochlear-implant users rely both on the auditory and visual signals for acquiring consonant sounds.

Figure 16–4 presents manner of consonant production over time. The young cochlear-implant users showed about the same amount of improvement for all manner classes. Perhaps the most interesting finding shown in this figure relates to the production of fricatives. By the sixth year of cochlear-implant use, children produced such sounds as /s/ and /z/ with almost 60% accuracy. Many children with similar losses who use hearing-aids never acquire these sounds (Smith, 1975).

Relationship Between Hearing Abilities and Segmental Speech Production in Cochlear-Implant Users

In addition to completing a speech test, the children in the cochlear-implant study described here also completed the *Word In-*

telligibility Picture Index (WIPI) (Ross & Lerman, 1971), which is a 6-choice monosyllabic word recognition task. This test was scored by percent phonemes correct.

Figure 16–5 illustrates the relationship between speech production (in a sentence-imitation task rather than a story-retell task) and performance on the WIPI. The data were collected after each child had accumulated 5 years of experience with their cochlear implants. There is a strong relationship between children's abilities to produce phonemes and their abilities to recognize them. A Pearson correlation, which tests how well one set of data predicts another, was $r = .88$, which is a remarkably strong correlation. No doubt many factors affect children's speech acquisition with a cochlear implant, including family commitment to the cochlear implant process and a child's intervention plan. However, the findings in Figure 16–5 suggest a direct correspondence exists between a child's ability to speak and a child's ability to recognize speech sounds.

Suprasegmental speech production

Children who use cochlear implants tend to produce fewer suprasegmental errors than children who have similar hearing

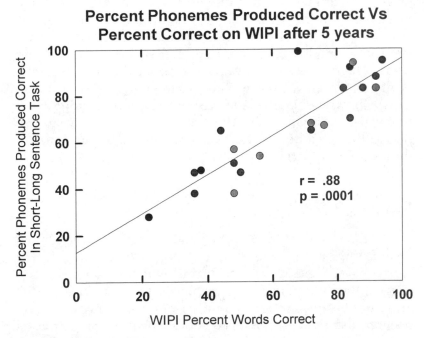

Figure 16–5. The relationship between children's speech production and speech recognition skills after 5 years of cochlear-implant experience.

losses but who use hearing aids (Tye-Murray, Spencer, & Woodworth, 1995). In fact, clinicians sometimes notice changes in the voice quality of children within the first year after they receive a cochlear implant, and these changes often precede changes in segmental speech production.

Language: Content and Form

Children who receive cochlear implants may have accelerated and enhanced language acquisition, although researchers are only now beginning to explore this issue in depth. Tomblin, Spencer, Tyler, and Gantz (submitted for publication) looked at the syntax of a group of 29 young cochlear-implant users and a comparable group of 29 young hearing-aid users with a measure called the *Index of Productive Syntax* (IPSyn) (Scarborough, 1990). They determined that the cochlear-implant users demonstrated greater rates of growth in English grammar over time than did the hearing-aid users.

Not many investigators have looked at vocabulary acquisition in young cochlear-implant users. Geers and Moog (1994) studied 12 young cochlear-implant users and 12 hearing-aid users over a period of three years. They found that the children who used cochlear implants had higher levels of expressive vocabulary than children who used hearing aids. However, it is important to note that the cochlear-implant users still were significantly delayed when compared to their normally-hearing peers. Their vocabulary levels were about those of normally hearing children who were three years younger. Waltzman et al. (1997), who obtained language data from 38 children who received their cochlear implants before the age of 5 years, reported that they demonstrated 4 years of vocabulary growth during a 3-year period.

Reading

Given that children who use cochlear implants often show greater improvements in their language skills than children who use hearing aids, it is not surprising that preliminary data suggest they go on to develop superior reading skills (this is an issue that has not been studied in depth) (Figure 16–6). Spencer and Tomblin (1997) studied 34 cochlear-implant users who have prelingual deafness. At the time they were tested, they had 62 months of implant experience, with a range of 24 to 108 months. They ranged in grade level from kindergarten

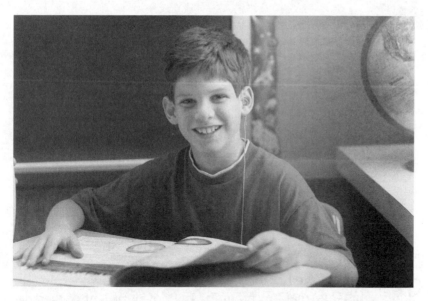

Figure 16–6. Use of a cochlear implant appears to lead to better reading skills than use of conventional amplification. This is probably because enhanced hearing capacity allows children to acquire English language more readily, which in turn has a saluatory effect on literacy. (Photograph by Patti Gabriel, courtesy of Central Institute for the Deaf)

to senior high school. On average, they were at the fourth grade level. The investigators also tested a comparable group of hearing-aid users. Children completed the *Woodcock Reading Mastery Test*, which assess children's ability to comprehend short two- to three-sentence paragraphs. The investigators found that 50% of the children who used cochlear implants were reading at grade level. They achieved higher reading levels than the hearing-aid users and exhibited faster performance growth rates over time.

SPEECH AND LANGUAGE EVALUATION: GENERAL PRINCIPLES

Speech-language evaluation: assessment of speech and language performance.

Now that we have described speech, language, and literacy development, let us now turn our attention to the assessment of speech and language performance. First we will consider general principles, then more specific issues.

There are several general principles to remember when testing the speech and language of children who have hearing loss. The principles pertain to the following topics:

■ Task type
■ Mode of communication
■ Rapport
■ Test procedures
■ Test norms

The first principle is that children often use speech and language differently in one setting than in another, and they perform differently on varying tasks. For example, children are more likely to produce a sound correctly when they imitate their speech-language pathologist than when they tell a story to their classmates. For this reason, it is wise to construct a profile of the child's speech and language proficiency from numerous formal and informal measures. By using a variety of speech tasks, a clinician can determine how robust certain skills are and whether they have generalized to real-world settings. This information can guide the development of therapy objectives and can be used to evaluate progress.

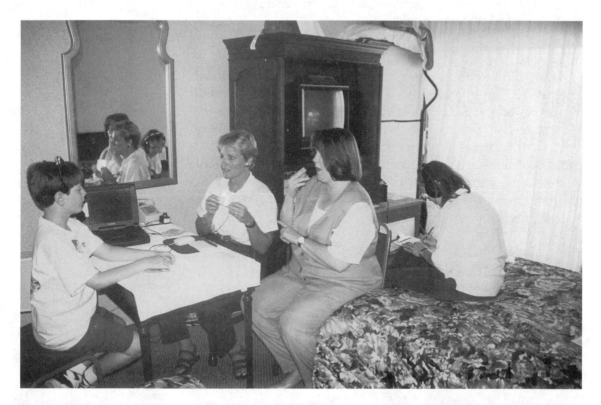

Figure 16–7. A speech and language evaluation usually is performed with a child's preferred mode of communication (in this picture, simultaneous communication). Here, an interpreter cues the messages of a speech-language pathologist, who does not know Cued speech. (Photograph by Kim Readmond, Central Institute for the Deaf)

The second principle to remember when evaluating speech and language is that the evaluation should be performed with a child's preferred mode of communication (Figure 16–7). For example, the youth may use *simultaneous communication*. If the speech-language pathologist does not know the child's sign system, then a sign language interpreter should be secured. The child must understand the tasks and the test items to provide a true reflection of speech and language skills.

The third principle is that, before formally evaluating a child, a rapport must be established between tester and child. You may find that many children with hearing losses are shy about using their voices, especially among strangers. If children do not feel comfortable in the tester's presence, they will not provide speech or language samples that represent their true skills. In fact, they may not provide samples at all!

Fourth, it is important to select specific test procedures that are appropriate for the child's age and language. For example, if an articulation test has picture cards, the child must have the vocabulary necessary to name the pictures.

Finally, the speech-language pathologist should try to use at least some tests that have been developed for children with hearing loss (although this may not always be possible, because few tests are available). For children who use simultaneous communication, you will find that many tests have not been designed to be administered with sign. Moreover, norms of many tests reflect the performance of normally hearing children and not children with hearing loss.

Simultaneous communication: an educational approach used with children with severe and profound hearing loss that integrates aural/oral communication and manual communication.

ASSESSING SPEECH SKILLS: INTELLIGIBILITY, SEGMENTALS, AND SUPRASEGMENTALS

Now that we have considered general principles for a speech-language evaluation, let us review procedures for assessing speech. The evaluation may include an overall assessment of intelligibility. It also may include assessment of segmentals and suprasegmentals.

Speech Intelligibility

To assess speech intelligibility, a speech sample first must be collected and then evaluated. To obtain a speech sample, the speech-language pathologist might ask a child to perform any or all of the following tasks:

■ **Imitate a series of isolated words or sentences.** For example, a speech-language pathologist might say, "The boy saw the cat," and the child then repeats the sentence. This procedure typically elicits a child's best performance (Figure 16-8).

■ **Create a citation speech sample.** A speech-language pathologist might instruct a child, "Tell me the name of the picture," or, "Tell me what is happening here." The child then speaks the name or describes what is occurring in the picture. This task is highly structured like an imitated-sentence task, but the child does not receive a speech and/or vocabulary model to imitate.

■ **Retell a story.** A speech-language pathologist may show the pictures in Figure 16–9 to a child one at a

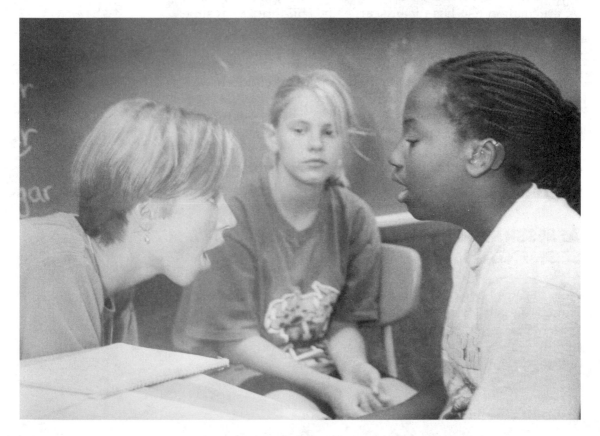

Figure 16–8. One way to collect a speech sample from a child is to use an imitation task. Theclinician speaks an utterance and the child imitates it. (Photograph by Marcus Kosa, courtesy of Central Institute for the Deaf)

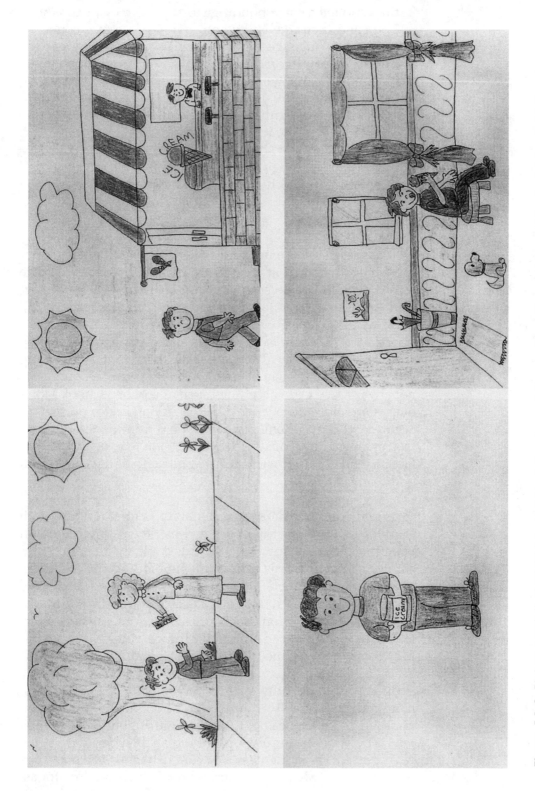

Figure 16–9. Picture cards that might be used to elicit a story-retell speech and language sample. A clinician first tells a story, using a prepared text that corresponds to each picture in the picture series (here, organized clockwise, beginning with the top left-hand corner). Then the child tells the story back.

time and tell a corresponding story, picture by picture. The child then retells the story. This procedure constrains the language that children use in the sample, but still allows for the evaluation of spontaneous speech and language production.

■ **Speak spontaneously, using continuous speech.** A speech-language pathologist might observe informally a child in therapy, in the classroom, or on the playground while he or she speaks to other children. In the therapy session, they may engage in casual conversation, and the speech-language pathologist pays close attention to the child's articulation proficiency and language structures.

Once a speech sample has been collected, overall intelligibility can be evaluated in at least three different ways. First, the recordings can be played to a group of listeners, who can assign each sample a value from a rating scale (Johnson, 1975). For example, *1* on a 5-point scale might correspond to *I understood none of the child's message,* and 5 correspond to *I understood all of the child's message.* There are some disadvantages to using rating scales. A group of listeners must be assembled, which is not always easy to do in settings such as a public school. Moreover, some have questioned whether rating scales present an accurate portrait of children who vary from one another in their intelligibility (Samar & Metz, 1988). It may be that judges have a tendency to cluster scores at one end of the continuum or the other.

A second way to evaluate intelligibility is to play the speech samples to a group of listeners and ask them to write down what they hear. The number of words correctly identified constitutes a percent words correct intelligibility score. The listeners also might estimate how much of the child's speech they understood, such as 10% of the words, 20%, and so forth. Although the transcription procedure also requires a panel of listeners to be assembled, it has high face validity because it shows how many of their words can be identified by listeners.

A third way to quantify speech intelligibility is for a speech-language pathologist to transcribe phonetically the spoken message and reference the spoken transcription to the printed text. The speech-language pathologist then can determine what percentage of the words or sounds were spoken correctly. This is probably the most commonly used procedure for assessing intelligibility in clinical and educational settings.

Measures of speech intelligibility vary as a function of several different variables (Figure 16–10). For instance:

■ A child will be more intelligible when reading a paragraph than speaking a list of unrelated sentences.
■ Listeners will understand more of a child's speech if they have heard the speech of other children with hearing loss before, than if they are naive listeners.
■ Listeners will recognize more speech if they can hear and see children rather than only hear them.

When recording intelligibility scores it is wise to comment on these variables, especially if the child's progress is to be monitored over time. If this is not done, the child's intelligibility score might improve because of a change in an extraneous variable. This may be misinterpreted as an improvement in the child's speaking proficiency.

Segmentals

Segmental speech testing determines which sounds children can articulate and which sounds they cannot. Variables to consider when selecting test procedures include context, methodology, and whether to use conventional tests of articulation.

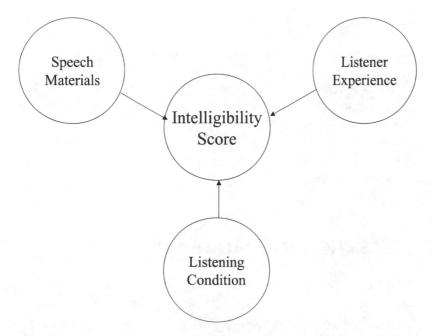

Figure 16–10. Factors that may affect a speech intelligibility score.

Segmental speech production can be evaluated in with a variety of contexts, including nonsense syllables, isolated words, sentences, and spontaneous speech. It is common to evaluate how well children produce various features of articulation, such as place and manner.

Methodologically, a child may imitate the speech-language pathologist or might produce the sounds by naming picture cards or reading printed words aloud. The child also may speak spontaneously, and then the speech-language pathologist can determine what sounds were produced in a set number of words (say, the first 200 words spoken by the child).

Often, conventional articulation tests are used to assess segmental speech skills, such as the *Goldman-Fristoe Test of Articulation* (Goldman & Fristoe, 1969) and the *Test of Minimal Articulation Competence* (T-MAC) (Secord, 1981). Some speech-language pathologists modify the tests by eliminating test words that are not in the child's vocabulary. If modifications are made, they should be recorded alongside the child's scores. Tests designed specifically for children with hearing loss include the *Phonologic Level Speech Evaluation* (Ling, 1976), the *CID Phonetic Inventory* (Moog, 1988), and the *Speech Intelligibility Evaluation* (SPINE) (Monsen, 1981).

Suprasegmentals

Suprasegmental speech skills can be evaluated by rating children's spontaneous speech as described by Subtelny, Orlando, and Whitehead (1981) or by asking them to perform specific speech tasks. For instance, a speech-language pathologist might determine whether a child can sustain the vowel /a/ for 5 seconds (to assess breath management) or whether the child can speak two-syllable phrases with correct stress and pitch variation (to assess his or her ability to imitate stress patterns) (Levitt, 1987).

ASSESSING LANGUAGE SKILLS

Table 16–1 presents examples of language tests sometimes used with children who are hearing impaired. They are organized according to whether they primarily assess form, content, or pragmatics.

Table 16-1. Language tests that are sometimes used to test children who have hearing loss. Assessment instruments that were designed specifically for hard-of-hearing children and teenagers are denoted with an asterisk (*).

Form
Rhode Island Test of Language Structure (RITLS) (Engen & Engen, 1983)
Grammatical Analysis of Elicited Language (GAEL) (Moog & Geers, 1979)
Grammatical Analysis of Elicited Language, pre-sentence level (GAEL-p) (Moog, Kozak, & Geers, 1983)
Test of Syntactic Ability (TSA) (Quigley, Monranelli, & Wilbur, 1976)
Written Language Syntax Test (WLST) (Berry, 1981)
Berko Morphology Test (Berko, 1984)
Test for Auditory Comprehension of Language (TACL) (Carrow, 1973)
Developmental Sentence Analysis (DSA) (Lee, 1974)
Index of Productive Syntax (IPSyn) (Scarborough, 1990)

Content
Semantic content analysis (Kretschmer and Kretschmer, 1978)
Peabody Picture Vocabulary Test—Revised (PPVT-R) (Dunn & Dunn, 1981)
Reynell Developmental Language Scales (Reynell, 1977)

Function
Pragmatic content analysis (Kretschmer & Kretschmer, 1978)
Performative content analysis (Hasenstab & Tobey, 1991)

Assessment procedures generally can be classified as checklists (e.g., Moog & Geers, 1975), tests (e.g., Quigley, Monranelli, & Wilbur, 1976) or language sample analyses (e.g., Kretschmer & Kretschmer, 1978). In compiling a checklist, a speech-language pathologist checks whether a particular behavior is present. For example, the speech-language pathologist might check *yes* or *no* for the statement, *The child recognizes the meaning of subject-verb-object sentences.*

Many tests contain items that assess formally a child's ability to use language structures. For example, if negation is assessed, the child might be asked to change the sentence, *He will go* to *He will not go.*

Language sample analyses usually are performed on samples of both the child's receptive and expressive language. A clinician might describe the semantic classes children use and recognize, their complex sentence productions, and their communication proficiency.

SPEECH AND LANGUAGE THERAPY

Still Holds True Today

G. Sibley Haycock (1933) wrote a book about teaching speech to children who have significant hearing loss in the early part of the 20th century. This book had enormous influence both in the time it was written, and subsequently influenced the development of more modern curriculums (e.g., Ling, 1976). The goal of the program outlined in the book was to promote natural speech in deaf children. To this end, it was suggested that children be

taught by such methods as will give to [their speech] the following characteristics:

■ In general, the movements of the mechanisms involved must be correctly controlled and become, through practice and habit, more or less automatic. In particular, the breathing and the vocalization must be correct in method and controlled in action; and the consonants and the vowels must be easily and smoothly produced and correct as to sound, according to the locally accepted standard of pronunciation.
■ The constituent phonetic elements composing words must be rendered with due regard to their relationship to one another.
■ Words must be properly accented.
■ Words in sentences must be given the measure of emphasis required by the meaning they are intended to convey.
■ The speech must be duly phrased, and uttered with ease and fluency.
■ The voice should express emotional quality.
■ The rate of the speech must approximate to the normal.
■ The sentences must be marked by a rise and fall of the voice, giving to the speech a certain amount of tunefulness. (p. 18)

These goals still are relevant to today's speech curricula.

Most children with significant hearing loss need abundant amounts of speech and language therapy. Speech and language skills often do not emerge spontaneously. Concerted attention over many years must be placed on developing skills if a child is to learn to speak and use English.

Speech Therapy

Goals for a comprehensive speech-development program may include the following (Carney & Moeller, 1998, p. S62):

■ Increase vocalizations that have appropriate timing characteristics and that require numerous vocal tract movements.
■ Expand phonetic and phonemic repertoires.
■ Establish link between audition and speech production.
■ Improve suprasegmental aspects of speech.
■ Increase speech intelligibility.

Results from the speech evaluation are used to select therapy goals. The phonetic transcriptions of elicited and spontaneous speech may be used for phoneme and phonological error pattern analysis. Phonetic error analysis yields an inventory of sounds a child can produce, as well as a catalogue of the child's deletions, substitutions, and distortions. Phonological error analysis reveals phonological process errors. These may include final consonant deletions, cluster reductions, and frontings. Therapy goals may focus on increasing a child's phonetic repertoire and on reducing phonological process errors. Auditory modeling is used extensively, sometimes in conjunction with a visual and tactile supplement (Tye-Murray, Spencer, Witt, & Bedia, 1997).

Therapy curricula often differ according to the way speech is presented to the child and how feedback is provided. For instance, in an auditory approach, children may receive instructions and correction about their speech via the auditory modality primarily, although often, no attempt is made to limit children's use of nonauditory cues, such as natural facial cues. In a more visual approach, visual stimuli are presented purposefully to supplement the auditory signal. A visual program may entail the use of mirrors, cued speech, or graphic symbols that are paired with specific speech sounds or prosodic features.

Probably the most widely implemented speech therapy program based on an auditory approach was developed by Daniel Ling (1976). This program rests on the premise that there is a hierarchy of speech skills. The most effective and efficient way to learn how to talk is to learn skills in an appropriate sequence and to build on an existing skill to develop a new one. For instance, before a child can learn specific speech sounds, he or she must first learn to regulate voice level and pitch. A child should be able to speak homophenous syllable strings, such as *bee-bee-bee*, before being asked to speak heterogeneous strings, such as *bee-boo-bee-boo*.

Visual methods include the Northampton Charts, developed at Clark School for the Deaf in 1885 and updated in 1925. Sounds are associated with a letter, and the sounds are represented on charts, which are on display during the therapy session, and even in the classroom throughout the day. Visual methods also include the use of computer-based visual feedback systems, such as the IBM Speech Viewer (IBM, 1988). Computer-based visual aids may present a visual response to a child's production, indicating the "goodness" of production or overall accuracy. For instance, a child may sustain phonation into a microphone connected to the computer, and a balloon shown on the computer monitor is shown growing in size throughout the duration of phonation.

Language Therapy

Therapy goals in language development may include the following (Carney & Moeller, 1998):

■ Increase communication between parent and child.
■ Promote an understanding of complex concepts and discourse units.
■ Enhance vocabulary growth.
■ Increase world knowledge.
■ Enhance self-expression.
■ Enhance growth in use of language syntax and pragmatics.
■ Develop narrative skills.

A number of curricula have been developed for promoting language growth. Language curricula vary from highly structured to naturalistic. Most modern curricula advocate more naturalistic methods. Therapy goals often are based on information about the language development of normally hearing children, and goals are reinforced throughout the day, whether at school or at home.

Content, form, and pragmatics are addressed in the development of a language intervention plan. Special emphasis may be placed on vocabulary development if the child is younger, and children might be encouraged to use conjunctions, pronouns, and modals.

If a child is of school age, concerted attention may be placed on the development of syntax and semantics. The speech-language pathologist may spend time observing the child in the classroom. The speech-language pathologist then makes specific recommendations about how the classroom teacher might reinforce speech and language therapy goals in a naturalistic setting and incorporate goals into the academic curriculum. The classroom observation also may reveal specific language error patterns that the child is producing outside of the therapy setting.

FINAL REMARKS

In this chapter, we have considered speech and language development and, to a lesser extent, reading. Often, a primary concern of a speech and hearing professional who works with children is to foster growth in these areas. Speech and hearing professionals are often concerned with nurturing a child's social skills too. These social skills may include knowledge about how to behave politely, how to cooperate with peers, and how to follow rules. Many children who have hearing loss experience common social problems. These may include (Schum & Gfeller, 1994):

■ A preference for playing with children younger than self
■ Social isolation
■ Naiveté about peer interests and customs
■ Limited understanding about internal states such as feelings
■ Difficulty in empathizing
■ Feelings of frustration or intimidation during social interactions

Several useful discussions about the development of social skills are available in the literature, as are ways to alleviate such social difficulties as those listed above (Gfeller & Schum, 1994; Paul & Jackson, 1993; Quigley & Smith, 1982; Schloss & Smith, 1990; Schum, 1991; Schum & Gfeller, 1991).

KEY CHAPTER POINTS

✔ Children with hearing loss may make characteristic speech errors, such as neutralizing vowels and omitting final consonants. These errors are primary factors in their overall low intelligibility levels.

✔ They often have problems in content, form, and pragmatics of language. For instance, they have reduced vocabulary and have mastered fewer syntactic structures than normally hearing children.

✔ Children who are hard-of-hearing often have difficulty in reading. Many deaf adults never attain better than a fourth grade reading level.

✔ Evidence suggests that receipt of a cochlear implant may enhance and accelerate speech, language, and literacy growth.

✔ A speech and language evaluation is performed in order to develop a hierarchy of speech-language therapy objectives.

Parent-Centered Conversation and Language Instruction[1]

Topics

- Parent-Centered Language Intervention

- Fostering Language Use Through Conversation

- Parental Use of Repair Strategies

- Final Remarks

- Key Chapter Points

- Key Resources

[1]Parts of Chapter 17 were adapted from *Let's Converse: A How-to Guide to Develop and Expand Conversational Skills of Children and Teenagers Who are Hearing Impaired* by N. Tye-Murray, 1994, Washington, DC: Alexander Graham Bell Association for the Deaf.

This chapter concerns the ways parents or children's primary caretakers may facilitate conversational interactions with their child. The guiding premise is that satisfying conversational interactions between children and their parents will nurture children's language and speech development and advance their social, emotional, and intellectual growth. The speech and hearing professional may play a significant role in helping parents learn how to support conversation and language development. In this chapter, we first will consider language and then conversation, although there is really no clear distinction between the ways in which a parent fosters one versus the other.

When providing instruction to parents, it is important to remember that they know their child better than anyone, including all speech and hearing professionals. Your role is to provide information and empower parents to use their own talents, knowledge, and experiences to foster language growth and conversational skills. Communication patterns emerge in the context of the family system, and the most effective strategies for encouraging communication growth are those that are symbiotic with the family milieu.

PARENT-CENTERED LANGUAGE INTERVENTION

For younger children in particular, a clinician may spend time with a child's family, discussing ways to stimulate language practice in the home. Adults in a child's everyday life have a prime opportunity to stimulate a child's language production. The techniques listed in Figure 17–1 represent ways that parents can stimulate their child's language development (adapted from Spencer, 1994, pp. 51–84; also Tye-Murray, Spencer, Witt, & Bedia, 1996, p. 67). These techniques are simple for parents to implement, and yet are highly effective in expanding language competency. Speech and hearing professionals and other people who interact often with children who have hearing loss also may find these techniques helpful in stimulating their young child's speech and language growth in both everyday and clinical settings. The language stimulation techniques include:

1. **Signaling expectation:** The first technique is to signal expectations. Wait for the child's response. During an interaction, often, after you say something, indicate that a response is expected, by tilting the head and raising eyebrows. This is

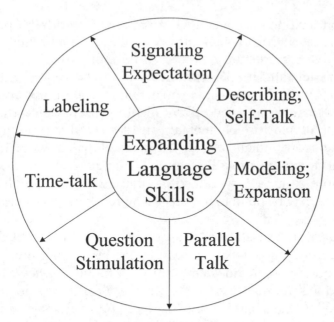

Figure 17–1. Language-stimulation techniques that parents and primary care-takers can use to expand children's language skills.

an effective means of generating a verbal response from the child. It also establishes a turn-taking pattern. For instance, a parent might say, "Hmmm, you have a block. I wonder what you are going to do with it." Then instead of continuing, she or he may look expectantly at the child, and wait for a reply.

2. **Describing; self-talk:** The second technique is called *describing* and self-talk. In implementing this technique, adults use an event or an idea the child is interested in and describe various aspects of it. Also, adults may use *self-talk*, and speak aloud about what they are doing or what they are thinking. In this way, they illustrate that language can be used to organize, analyze, and direct actions by thinking aloud through the process. For example, using the child's preferred communication mode, an adult may say, "I am unpacking my groceries. I'll take out the beef. Hmmm, let's have hamburgers tonight."

3. **Modeling and expansion:** When using a *modeling* or *expansion* language-stimulation technique, an adult copies the meaning of a child's utterances but modifies or expands the grammar of the message. For example a child might say, "Scissors." Her mother may then expand the utterance by saying, "You want the scissors. You can cut with the scissors." Some of the benefits of using modeling and expan-

Describing: an adult uses an event a child is interested in to talk about various aspects of the event.

In **self-talk**, adults talk aloud about what they are doing or thinking.

Modeling: an instructor demonstrates a desired behavior and a student attempts to imitate it.

Expansion: a language stimulation technique in which an adult copies the meaning of a child's utterance but expands the grammar of the message.

sion include (a) the child's message is reinforced, (b) new language structures are introduced, and (c) an imitation of the correct structure is prompted from the child.

Parallel talk: A language-stimulation technique in which an adult matches language to an activity a child is performing.

4. **Parallel talk:** In using the technique of *parallel talk*, an adult matches language to an activity a child is performing. For example, as a child plays silently with a stuffed animal, an adult may use parallel talk and say, "You are holding the bear. Now you are feeding the bear. Oh, you hug the bear." This technique provides a model of language structures and also a commentary. It invites dialogue. For example, the child may respond to the preceding remarks with, "Yes, this is my bear!"

5. **Question stimulation:** If used optimally, the use of questions is a potent means of stimulating language growth. Use of questions provides children with models of how to ask and answer questions. For example, a child may point to a bowl on the table and say, "Cereal?" A parent may respond, "Do you want some cereal?" and thereby provide a model of how to make a request. Although questions can be useful tools in promoting questions, a string of questions can squelch a child's active participation. The Key Resources section suggests how parents might best use questions to provide children with language models and to stimulate language and conversational growth.

Time-talk: A language-stimulation technique in which an adult purposely incorporates time-related language into the conversation.

6. **Time-talk:** The sixth language-stimulation technique is called *time-talk*. When using this strategy, link time words to events or routines that are significant to a child for the purpose of helping children develop the concepts and language of time. For example, adults can use time-talk and sequence events in their conversations, and use such time-related words as *before, during,* and *after.* A grandmother might say, "First, we will add sugar. Second, we will add an egg. Third, we will stir," demonstrating the use of time words, *first, second,* and *third.*

Labeling: A language-stimulation technique in which an adult provides names to objects, actions, and events.

7. **Labeling:** The final technique is to use labels. In using *labeling,* an adult provides names to objects, actions, and events. For instance, a child may pick up a toy cup. A parent might use labeling and comment, "That's a cup."

It will not be very useful to simply hand a list like that presented above to parents and say, "Try these at home." If possible, concomitant instruction should accompany these ideas. Parents may need explicit guidance in how to use language-stimulation techniques. Instruction can be provided in a variety of ways, ranging from less structured to more structured (Figure

17–2). You may find that even mainstream classroom teachers benefit from either less-structured or more-structured instruction in how to use language-stimulation techniques, particularly if they have a child who is hard-of-hearing in their classroom for the first time.

Less-Structured Instruction

You might want to shape parents' language-stimulation behaviors in an informal manner, using a fairly unstructured format. For example, you might observe parent and child as they engage in a conversation during a play session in the home or clinical setting. Afterward, you might say to the mother, "You seemed very attentive to Tim's focus of attention as you played with the Lego pieces. I like the way you named the colors of each piece he picked up." With this remark, you have given the mother positive reinforcement and provided instruction about how to increase vocabulary through the use of labeling. No doubt, such a remark would also serve to bolster her self-confidence and sense of satisfaction about the play session.

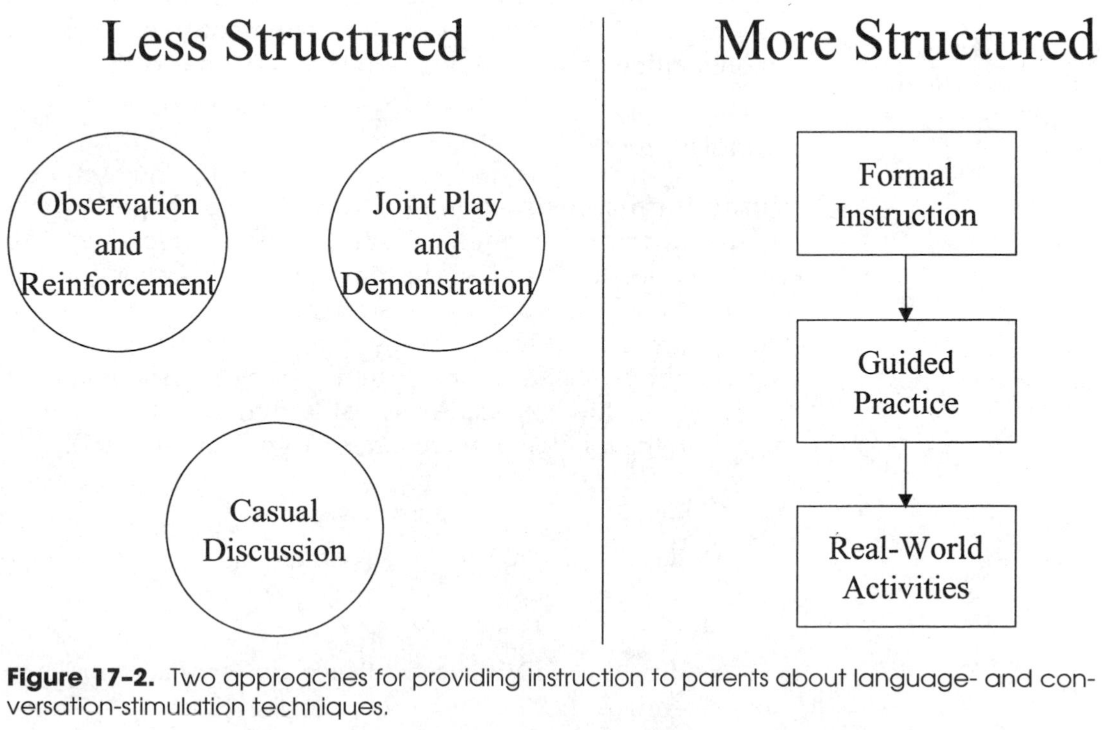

Less-structured instruction: informal shaping of language-stimulation behaviors, often during play.

Less Structured | **More Structured**

Observation and Reinforcement

Joint Play and Demonstration

Casual Discussion

Formal Instruction

↓

Guided Practice

↓

Real-World Activities

Figure 17–2. Two approaches for providing instruction to parents about language- and conversation-stimulation techniques.

During an informal play session, a clinician also might join in with the parent (however, one must be careful not to take over the play session). The clinician might demonstrate language-expansion techniques and suggest additional activities. Parents can observe the effectiveness of a technique, and realize that it probably is not beyond their abilities to implement it ("Hey, I can do that!").

Other less-structured activities may be casual discussions. For instance, a parent might ask you questions about language development, and you might discuss techniques informally.

In these less-structured kinds of interactions, it is extremely important that the clinician exercise tact and respect for the parent. Whenever possible, one should avoid being judgmental of the parent, critical, or negative. The goal is to empower and enable parents to facilitate language growth; criticism or an undue display of professional expertise will only sabotage a clinician's well-intentioned efforts.

More structured instruction: formal or more systematic instruction for parents and caregivers in language stimulation behaviors.

More-Structured Instruction

Instruction for parents or primary caregivers can be more structured and systematic. In this case, a speech and hearing professional might provide formal instruction, guided learning, and real-world practice, just as in a communication strategies training program (Chapter 4). Instruction can occur in either a one-on-one setting or in a parent group forum (Figure 17–2).

Formal Instruction

During formal instruction, a clinician might begin by discussing each of the language-stimulation strategies and reviewing related examples. The clinician might provide audio- or videotaped examples of the strategies in use. For example, the first topic in Table 17–1 is signaling expectations. Two film clips might be shown to the parent group, the first where an adult signals low expectations that her child will communicate, as in the following interchange (from Spencer, 1994):

Child:	(Points toward crayons)
Mother:	"What are you pointing at?"
Child:	(Grabs a color)
Mother:	"You wanted the color. Here's some paper, too."

Mother:	"What are you drawing? It looks like a cat."
Child:	(Continues drawing)
Mother:	"Here is the black. You can color the tail black." (p. 52)

In this first film clip, the mother asks questions, but does not expect her child to answer them. She does not pause and allow the child to initiate a remark. By providing the paper and crayon to her child, she has eliminated the need for him to ask for them. A second film clip demonstrates how an adult can signal higher expectations for communication, and thereby elicit more language from her child (Spencer, 1994):

Child:	(Points toward crayons)
Mother:	"What?" (looks around expectantly)
Child:	"Ka."
Mother:	"Color?"

Table 17–1. Workbook exercises an aural rehabilitation specialist might give to parents so they may practice modeling and expansion.

Modeling and Expansion

On the lines below are some typical utterances a child might say. Beside each utterance, write your own expansion model.

Child's utterance   **Your expansion model**

1. "More." _____

2. "Give." _____

3. "Cup." _____

4. "My turn." _____

Possible expansions could include:

1. You want more juice.
2. Give the baby some juice.
3. Let's pour the juice in the cup.
4. It's your turn to pour.

Child:	"Cala."
Mother:	"Color. Green or black?" (waits)
Child:	"Bak."
Mother:	(Gives the child the black crayon. . . waits)
Child:	"Papa."
Mother:	"Paper—here's a big piece." (Holds paper up)
Child:	"Mine."
Mother:	"Draw me a picture." (pp. 52–53)

After parents view this second clip, parents and clinicians can talk about how the mother frequently pauses and allows time for her child to talk. She uses facial expressions that signal expectation for more information and establishes a turn-taking pattern.

Parental Influences

Parents' interaction styles may impinge on a child's development. A number of investigations have demonstrated that caregivers who interact with children who have a hearing loss behave differently than caregivers who interact with normally hearing children (Cole, 1993). They talk less, repeat themselves more often, provide fewer expansions, present shorter utterances, and present simpler grammatical structures. Interestingly, interaction styles correlate with language achievement. Language development has an inverse relationship with caregivers' use of imperatives and topic changes and with caregivers' frequency of negative remarks (Bromwich, 1981).

Audio- and videotaped examples are highly effective means of providing formal instruction about language nurturing. In the event that no film clips are available, printed transcripts like the one presented here can be discussed. Example transcripts for the other language-stimulation techniques appear in the Key Resources section at the end of the chapter.

Guided Practice

Means for providing guided practice include group discussions, role-playing, and self-critique. For example, in a group discussion, parents might share ideas about how they interest their children in using language in the home environment. They might reflect about how they interact with their child and discuss the techniques they use with one another.

Home-training programs can also provide guided-learning experiences. Parents may receive printed materials to read at home and workbook activities that provide guided-learning for the printed materials. An example of a workbook exercise that might be used in a home-training program appears in Table 17–1.

Real-World Activities

For real-world practice, the third component of a more structured program, parents might tape-record themselves while playing with their child at home and then review the tapes, checking to see whether they have implemented language-expansion techniques (Andrews & Andrews, 1990). This will help them be more mindful of their language-stimulation efforts and also will provide an opportunity to appreciate the success of their efforts.

When assigning a real-world practice activity, a clinician may want to adhere to the following guidelines (see Andrews & Andrews, 1990, p. 67):

- **The activity should be something already practiced and discussed.** It should address something that is relevant to a family and something that has been discussed between clinician and family.
- **An assignment should be given in rewarding contexts.** The clinician might say, "Susan seems to be learning the names of colors now that you are labeling them at home. You seem to be very consistent with this. Now, this week, try to have her spontaneously name colors, perhaps by pausing and waiting for her to talk."
- **Ask the parent whether the assignment is possible, and whether it is appropriate.** We once asked a busy mother to follow a complex calendar of activities. After

3 days, she called us and began the conversation with, "I hate this—I just can't do it." Clearly, we should have talked to her more extensively beforehand, and anticipated her concerns and minimized problems.

■ **Demonstrate the assignment, and then ask the parent to try it, preferably with the child.** This will ensure that there is no confusion about the assignment and also will provide you with a first-hand look at how well the strategy works between parent and child, and will let you know whether the assignment is appropriate.

■ **Provide the assignment in writing.** This will ensure there is no confusion as to what to do and will provide a back-up in case the parent forgets what you discussed.

Real-world practice might be monitored by asking parents to keep a journal about their communication interactions with their child on a daily basis for a set number of weeks. They also can complete daily checklists, indicating whether they consciously performed any of the techniques during that day.

FOSTERING LANGUAGE USE THROUGH CONVERSATION

Now that we have considered language-stimulation techniques and training activities for parents, we will consider ways that parents can nurture conversational skills in their children and how they may learn to use repair strategies effectively. Procedures for providing instruction to parents are like those we just considered for encouraging language strategies. Both less-structured and more-structured procedures are appropriate, and some parents may benefit from formal instruction, guided learning, and real-world practice in developing their conversational skills and learning to use repair strategies in an optimal way.

The underlying premise for conversation-centered instruction is the belief that the best way for parents to stimulate language growth in the home is in the context of conversation. Conversations require children to use language for the purposes of expressing meaning and receiving messages, and do so in situations that are relevant and motivating.

Table 17–2 lists some guidelines that a speech and hearing professional might review with parents. These guidelines concern ways to facilitate conversation with a hard-of-hearing child. These are not rigid *do's* and *don'ts* of conversation but, if followed, often will stimulate a child to converse. The guidelines are as follows:

1. **Allow a child to choose what to talk about and respond to his or her communicative attempts.** The phrase to remember when using this strategy is *stay attuned to the child*. An adult can observe the child's focus of attention, and try to talk about what a child is doing and topics that interest the youngster. Remarks should be contingent upon the child's utterances. For instance, if a child says, "This my car," a father can comment, "I bet the car can go fast." He probably should not respond, "Hand me that jeep over there." If a child is primarily nonverbal, and there are no spoken (or signed) remarks that invite a response, a conversational partner can acknowledge the child's facial expressions, gestures, and unintelligible vocalizations as if they were conversational turns. For example, a child's pointing finger may elicit the remark, "Oh, you want a block," from the child's parent.

2. **Encourage a child to tell narratives and stories, and to give directions.** The second suggested guideline pertains to the use of connected discourse in conversation. During conversations, we take extended turns, telling narratives and stories. Encourage your child to tell narratives with such phrases as, *Tell me more, Then what happened?* and *Who did this?* Visual props can be used, such as a quickly drawn sketch, to encourage a child to tell the *who, what, where, when,* and *why* in reference to the picture.

Table 17–2. Some conversational strategies for adults who interact with children who have hearing loss.

---

1. Allow your child to choose what to talk about, and respond to the communicative attempts.

2. Encourage your child to tell narratives and stories, and to give directions.

3. Organize your messages.

4. Speak with clear speech.

5. Speak positively and avoid critical language.

6. Do not overcontrol your conversations.

Organized messages:
communications that are
not wordy and do not use
complex verbiage;
terminology is precise

Telegraphic speech is
characterized by the
omission of function words.

Clear speech: using a
somewhat slowed
speaking rate and good
but not exaggerated
enunciation of words when
conversing with someone
with a hearing loss.

3. **Organize your messages.** The third guideline requires adults to use meta-communication skills, and to think about *how* they will say *what* they are going to say. This guideline encourages adult conversational partners to organize their messages. What is an organized message? An *organized message* is not verbose and does not have complex verbiage (e.g., the sentence, *The sweater which we bought last Christmas is still in the box under the bed*, is an example of complex verbiage). Important key words and phrases are repeated, and terminology is precise (e.g., *The book is on the table*, rather than, *It's over there*). Telegraphic speech is avoided. *Telegraphic speech* is flagged by the omission of function words such as *of , to*, or *the*. An example of a telegraphic utterance is the sentence, *Boy fall on table, got ouch, and cry*. Not only does such an utterance not promote conversation, it also presents a poor language model.

4. **Speak with clear speech.** *Clear speech* is an important technique to remember when conversing with a child who has hearing loss. Clear speech is characterized by a somewhat slowed speaking rate and good (although not exaggerated) enunciation. Keywords are emphasized, and pauses are inserted at clause boundaries.

5. **Speak positively and avoid critical language.** Critical language is characterized by casting the child in a negative light, or being unduly critical of the child's actions and behaviors. A child who is continually told, "You can't do this" or "You shouldn't do that" (remarks which exemplify negative language) or scolded in ways such as, "You left your backpack again? Can't you be more responsible?" (a remark which exemplifies critical language) soon will lose interest in engaging in conversation. By using positive language and using such words as *can* rather than *cannot* and *do* rather than *don't*, children might be motivated to participate in conversational interchanges.

6. **Do not overcontrol your conversations.** The final guideline is not to overcontrol a conversation with a child who has hearing loss. Table 17–3 presents examples of dialogue that demonstrate overcontrolling conversational moves and turns. Adults who overcontrol their conversations may ask too many questions, they may not respond to their child's utterances, may label excessively (e.g., *Ball. That's a ball. Bat. That's a wooden bat*), they may often correct their child's speech production or language, they may recurrently ask their child to imitate their speech and language models, and they may often change the topic of conversation. Children may respond to these behaviors by becoming passive, helpless, or withdrawing from the conversation.

Table 17–3. Examples of dialogue in which an adult employed over-controlling behaviors during a conversation with a hard-of-hearing child.

Example 1

Child:	"I read my book."
Adult:	"Susan was looking for you."

Comment: Adults who overcontrol conversational often change the topic of conversation. For instance, an adult may not respond to a child's previous remark or attend to the child's focus of attention. When this happens frequently in the course of a conversation, the adult often becomes the "chief" and the child becomes a "junior partner" in the conversational interchange (Fey, Warr-Leeper, Webber, & Disher, 1988). In this interchange, the adult might have responded to the child's remark with, "We'll have to go to the library for another one." Such an acknowledgment might have opened the door for a discussion about what books to check out next.

Example 2

Child:	"Red cup full."
Mother (originally responded):	"Tom, say, 'My cup is full.'"

Comment: Adults may overcontrol conversations when they too frequently correct a child's speech production and language. With her remark, the mother above is no longer conversing with her child, she is giving a language lesson. If corrections occur too frequently, children may become frustrated and may begin to ignore the conversational partner and withdraw from the conversation.

Example 3

Father:	"What's in the bag?"
Daughter:	"My papers."
Father:	"Where did you get the bag?"
Daughter:	"School."
Father:	"What's that on it?"
Daughter:	"My name."

Comment: In this conversation, the father was in complete control. He asked a rapid succession of questions while his daughter passively responded with one word answers. The answer to one question did not influence what the father said next. For instance, he would probably have asked, "What's that on it?" regardless of how his daughter had answered his previous question, "Where did you get the bag?" If he would have commented instead, "Your papers! You must have worked hard today," the daughter might have taken charge and told her father about her school work. In short, she may have become an active conversational partner, and spoken longer utterances.

The six guidelines for promoting conversational interactions are simple to follow. In summary, adults might allow their children to select what to talk about, either by listening to their children or by attending to the children's focus of attention. They may model how to tell narratives and ask their children to tell them stories, encouraging them to follow a clear progression from beginning, to middle, to end. Finally, effective conversational partners can learn to speak with organized messages and not overcontrol their conversations. As with the language techniques we just considered, you might present these strategies first with formal instruction, then guided practice, and finally, real-world instruction.

PARENTAL USE OF REPAIR STRATEGIES

To have a successful conversation with their children, parents should be able to repair breakdowns in communication. Part of an aural rehabilitation plan for a child also may include providing training to parents about the use of repair strategies, both expressive and receptive. Repairing breakdowns in communication requires effort and patience on the part of conversational partners. However, the effective use of repair strategies can promote successful conversational interactions and lead to rewarding interchanges.

In Chapter 2, it was suggested that repair strategies provide explicit instruction to the communication partner (in the context of this chapter, a child) about what to do immediately following a communication breakdown. An expressive repair strategy can be used by an adult when the child has not understood the adult's message. A receptive repair strategy can be used when a parent does not understand something a child has said (and/or signed). In this section, we will consider expressive and receptive repair strategies.

Expressive Repair Strategies

Communication breakdowns during conversation should never be considered as the "fault" of either an adult or the child. However, adults can minimize the likelihood of communication breakdowns by considering their child's needs and abilities as they formulate their messages. A parent might ask him- or herself, "What are my child's cognitive abilities?" or "Does my child have the appropriate background knowledge and language level to understand this message?" The parent might attend to the child's emotional state (e.g., Is my child relaxed, mad, or tired?), and consider whether a message is supported by either linguistic or physical context. For example, does their message introduce a new topic? Is it supported by something concrete in the room? Lastly, parents can ensure that their child is aware of the *who* and the *what* of the message and make sure that their messages are appropriate both for the child's linguistic sophistication and his or her communication mode (Fey, Warr-Leeper, Webber, & Disher, 1988).

During the initial phase of a communication strategies training program, you might want to discuss how parents know when their child does not recognize a message. A clinician will often emphasize that children with hearing impairment often respond just like children with normal hearing when they do not understand a message (Table 17–4). Children may appear inattentive, they may smile or respond inappropriately, or they may bluff and pretend to understand. In most cases (but not necessarily all), parents will want to respond to these signals of

Table 17–4. Means by which children may signal a communication breakdown.

Children may demonstrate:

- Confused facial expressions
- Inattentiveness
- Disinterest
- Frustration
- Inappropriate responses
- Bluffing
- Use of verbal prompts ("What?"; "Huh?")
- Body gestures (shoulder shrug; raised hands)
- Hesitation
- Smiling

communication breakdown by using any one of the expressive repair strategies presented in Table 17–5.

When using the *repeat* repair strategy, parents simply repeat their original message, as in this interchange:

Parent: "What did you do with your backpack?"

Table 17–5. Expressive repair strategies parents may use when their child does not recognize their message and examples of each.

Expressive Repair Strategies for Parents:

■ **Repeat**
Original sentence: *How are you?*
Repair strategy: *How are you?*

■ **Rephrase**
A. Substitute less visible words with more visible words.
B. Substitute words that are better specified by context.
C. Change sentence structure.
   Original sentence: *My soda can is on the table.*
   Repair strategy: *My pop is over there.*

■ **Simplify**
A. Use fewer words.
B. Use more commonplace words.
C. Use two sentences.
   Original sentence: *The yellow carton is in the closet.*
   Repair strategy: *The box is in the closet.*

■ **Elaborate**
A. Provide more information.
B. Repeat important keywords.
   Original sentence: *Marla called to ask about school.*
   Repair strategy: *Marla telephoned. Marla asked about school.*

■ **Say a key word**
Original sentence: *The kids are playing soccer.*
Repair strategy: Kids. *The kids are playing soccer.*

■ **Choice-question (present a closed response set)**
Original sentence: *Who was at the party?*
Repair strategy: *Was the whole class at the party?*

■ **Build-from-the-known**
Original sentence: Take the lamp into the dining room.
Repair strategy: *Here's the lamp. There's the dining room. Take the lamp into the dining room.*

■ **Provide feedback**
Original sentence: *Bring me the glove.*
Repair strategy: *Not the mug, the glove.*

Child: "Huh?"

Parent: "What did you do with your backpack?"

Repeating a message might help a child recognize it; if he or she did not grasp it the first time around, hearing it a second time might be helpful. However, research suggests that other repair strategies may be even more helpful, especially when several interchanges must occur before the child recognizes the parent's message.

Other expressive repair strategies that parents may be encouraged to use during a communication strategies training program entail restructuring their original messages, either by rephrasing them, simplifying them, or elaborating them. A message may be rephrased in at least three ways. Parents may use words that are more visible on the face, they may use words that are better specified by context, or they may use a different sentence structure. Message simplification may be accomplished by using more commonplace words (e.g., using the word *sweater* instead of *cardigan*), by using fewer words, or by using more simple syntactic structures. As the name implies, the elaborate repair strategy entails providing more information and/or repeating important key words.

Besides repeating or restructuring unrecognized messages, parents may be encouraged to use any one of four other repair strategies. These include repeating a key word, building-from-the-known (wherein the parent starts with something the child knows or understands, and then builds on that knowledge base), or providing feedback. Examples of each of these types of repair strategies appear in Table 17–5.

Questions Parents Often Ask About Using Expressive Repair Strategies (Tye-Murray, 1992b)

1. **What should I do if my child listens to only half of what I say before he starts to respond or he stops paying attention before I am through delivering my message?**

Response: Indicate the length of your message, and use hand gestures to indicate where you are in the message as you deliver it. For instance, you might say, "There are three things we

(continued)

can do. (Holding up one finger) First, we can. . .(Holding up two fingers) Second, we can . . . This prepares the child for the length of the message and lets the youngster know where you are in your delivery.

Do not lecture or admonish your child . . . This certainly is not going to encourage a child to attend, nor will insisting that the child pay attention when he or she would rather be doing something else.

2. Which repair strategies should I use?

Response: No one repair strategy is appropriate for every situation. Usually a mixture of repair strategies is most effective. Your choice of repair strategies will depend in part on the age of your child and in part on your personal conversational style. For instance, elaborating a message may not be appropriate when the child is under 4 years of age. You may experience problems rephrasing a message, so for *you*, repeating important key words might be a better repair strategy to use than the rephrase repair strategy.

Receptive Repair Strategies for Parents

Parents may tell you that they feel comfortable in repairing communication breakdowns when their child does not understand something they say. The true difficulties arise when they do not understand their child's messages. In fact, the most valuable component of a communication strategies training program designed for parents may well be the component that deals with the use of receptive repair strategies.

Did You Say . . .

When you restate a message, you demonstrate that you are at least trying to understand it. You also provide a child with important information. By knowing what you recognized, the child can better supply the missing information. You might ask, "Did you say Jean is at the door?" The child can then indicate whether you have understood the message correctly. If you do not have a clue about what your child is talking about, you can focus on the child's nonverbal cues. For instance, if he or she talks quickly and with great animation, you might say, "You seem excited. Am I right?" In this instance, you have observed that something exciting has happened. Pinning a name to an emotional state not only helps to rectify breakdowns in communication, it also demonstrates that you recognize the child's feelings, and that you have comprehended the nonverbal message. This can be a source of encouragement for the child to try to repair the communication breakdown.

When discussing receptive repair strategies with parents, it is again important to stress that communication breakdown is not the "fault" of either the parent or the child (e.g., "I wish I was better able to guess what my child means" or "I wish my child had better language"). However, parents can minimize difficulties by focusing attention on their children as they present a message, by paying attention to children's body movements and environmental and contextual clues and by relying on stored information about the conversational topic and their children.

Receptive repair strategies that might be reviewed during a communication strategies training program are outlined in Table 17–6. The first strategy is the *repeat* repair strategy. The adult asks the child to present the message again. Parents should be encouraged to use this strategy sparingly. If a parent continually asks, "What?" or says, "Tell me again," the child may become frustrated and simply say, "Never mind."

When using the tell-me-more strategy, the next strategy listed in Table 17–6, parents encourage their children to provide additional information, as in this example:

Child: "Dana took dog boom."

Parent: "When did she do that?"

Child: "In there. It's mine!"

Parent: "She has it now?"

Child: "Yeah."

By using the tell-me-more receptive repair strategy, the parent gradually sorted out the problem by probing for more information. Similarly, the parents can learn to use the *did-you-say strategy* and the *tell me in a different way strategy*. For instance, a parent may say, "Show me" or "Draw a picture for me." When using these strategies, parents may either restate the message to confirm it or ask the children to alter how they present the message.

Did-you-say strategy: a conversational repair strategy that involves restating the message.

Tell-me-in-a-different-way strategy: a conversational repair strategy that asks speakers to alter their presentation of the message.

Table 17–6. Receptive repair strategies parents may use when they do not recognize their child's message.

Receptive Repair Strategies for Parents:

■ **Ask the child to repeat the message.**
Examples: *Tell me again.*

What did you say?

Repeat that please.

■ **Encourage the child to provide more information.**
Examples: *When did this happen?*

What happened next?

How do you feel about this?

■ **Restate what they might have said.**
Examples: *Did you say?*

I think you said....

You seem excited. Am I right?

■ **Ask the child to change the delivery of the message**
Examples: *Show me.*

Please look at me so I can see your face.

Can you slow down a little?

Questions Parents Often Ask About Using Receptive Repair Strategies (Tye-Murray, 1992b)

1. How can I encourage family members and strangers to use receptive repair strategies with my child?

Response: Relatives and strangers often do not know what to do when they cannot recognize the speech of a child who has a hearing impairment. Sometimes they pretend to understand. Alternatively, they may begin to address all of their remarks to you, and expect you to act as a go-between. Sometimes you can instruct relatives about how to use receptive repair strategies, although this is not always possible or successful. The most straightforward way to handle this problem is to teach children to repair breakdowns in communication themselves. Children must learn to take social responsibility for signaling the occurrence of breakdowns and develop effective skills to rectify them.

2. Should I try to understand everything my child says?

Response: Quite simply, the answer to this question is *no*. Excessive use of receptive repair strategies may lead to your over-controlling the conversation . . . When interacting with a child who has a significant hearing impairment, you must be willing to conjecture and accept ambiguity, and occasionally endure puzzlement about what your child is attempting to express. If you halt the conversation too many times to confirm a message, your child may become increasingly passive and withdrawn from the conversational interchange . . . rely on intelligent guessing sometimes, and allow the child to have some unhindered turns in a conversation before [you] intervene to confirm the child's message.

FINAL REMARKS

In this chapter, we have just scratched the surface of ways parents can promote language and conversational skills in their children. We have considered how adults can communicate so children will attend to what they say, and how they may listen and respond so children will want to communicate and be able to communicate. The discussion has been confined to language and the mechanics of conversation. However, to converse effectively and to learn language, children must also have world knowledge. Some children experience difficulty when engaging in conversations because they lack a base of information about the world and about how people function in the world. This reduced knowledge base limits what they can understand and what they can talk about. Gfeller (1994) presented a program that describes how parents and other adults in a child's life can facilitate the acquisition of general world information, as well as information about the community, family culture, and the mass media.

Family Dynamics

A parent-centered program may touch on the subject of discipline and the hard-of-hearing child. Families often need understanding and support from a clinician, and this requires that the clinician understands the dynamics of the family. Sometimes, the following family dynamics may be in place:

(continued)

Regardless of the cause of the child's hearing loss, parents find themselves needing to give the deaf child much of their time and attention. Siblings become aware of this inequity and often feel resentful and jealous of their hearing-impaired sibling. There is a great variability in how parents interact with their deaf child. Some parents state that they have the same expectations in terms of behavior and achievement for both their deaf and hearing children. They set limits and enforce consequences for inappropriate behavior; many parents have difficulty in achieving this. Two factors get in the way. Foremost is communication. It is often easier for the parent to do the task than to spend the time getting the child's attention and making sure the task is understood and then completed. Less obvious are the emotions the parents have towards the child. The parent may feel as though the child has suffered enough, and therefore places less demands on the child. The child gets out of doing what siblings are expected to do. This often impacts on the personality of the child, who may grow up always expecting special treatment. (Kravitz & Selekman, 1992, p. 593)

KEY CHAPTER POINTS

✔ Parents and caregivers can use a variety of techniques to promote language growth. These include modeling and expansion.

✔ Questions should be asked judiciously. An ineffective use of questions can lead to adults over-controlling their conversations with children.

✔ Enjoyable conversational interactions are some of the most effective means to promote language growth in children. Parents and caregivers can learn techniques that will facilitate conversation. These techniques include responding to communicative intents and avoiding the use of critical or negative language.

✔ Parents can learn to use expressive and receptive repair strategies to rectify communication breakdowns.

KEY RESOURCES

Asking Questions[1]

Although questions can be useful tools in promoting questions, a string of questions can squelch a child's active participation in a conversation. A child will more likely participate in a conversation if an adult makes comments and acknowledgments, in addition to asking questions. When making a *comment*, the adult introduces new information or new ideas. In making an *acknowledgment*, the adult acknowledges that he or she is paying attention and understands what the child is saying (Adam et al., 1990). Ways to ask questions effectively include the five guidelines listed below. An aural-rehabilitation specialist might review these guidelines with parents, and provide examples during a discussion about how to foster a child's language growth through conversation.

1. **Do not ask questions with a right answer in mind.** Be willing to accept a variety of responses. If you are willing only to accept a particular response, your child will perceive you have a blueprint for the conversation in mind, and the child's task is to identify and follow it.
2. **If you are asking a series of questions, allow your next question to be influenced by the child's response to a previous question.** Children must know that you are listening to what they have to say, and that they are helping direct the conversation. In short, your next question should be contingent on your child's response to your previous question.
3. **Do not be in a hurry to answer your own questions.** A child needs time to recognize your words and to formulate a reply. Be patient in waiting for a response. Avoid asking questions in this way: "Who gave you the Valentine's card? I bet Susan gave it to you."
4. **Do not limit your questions to those that can be answered with a yes-no response.** *Yes-no* questions require minimal involvement on a child's part. *Wh-questions* (who, what, where, when, why) are more likely to result in a child's active participation in the conversation. If you use a *yes-no* question, try pairing it with a *wh-question*. For example, "What did you do today? (pause, and if no response) Did you have gym class?" (Bodner-Johnson, 1991).

5. **Avoid asking rote questions that require a pat response.** A child should have an opportunity to provide a response that develops the conversation. Do not ask questions in this way: "You went to the movie? Did you see the big screen? Was the room dark?" The answer is "Of course!" to all three questions.

Research supports this discussion. A group of investigators analyzed conversational interactions between 16 elementary school teachers and their deaf students (Wood, Wood, Griffiths, Howarth, & Howarth, 1982). They transcribed every word a teacher and student said during a conversation (they used oral/aural communication) and then coded their utterances. When the teachers asked questions, students usually answered them and then stopped. Only for 14% of the questions did children elaborate their responses, and they rarely initiated additional conversation. The fewer the questions asked by a teacher during a conversation, the more likely a child was to elaborate an answer and to speak in longer utterances throughout the conversation. In short, children talked more when their teachers questioned less. A general rule that may be useful is this:

Questions should not be avoided entirely. They should be integrated into the conversation with other comments and acknowledgments, and used occasionally for modeling purposes.

Transcripts for Instructing Adults About Language-Stimulation Techniques

Technique: Describing

Child: (picking up toy car) "My."

Adult: "You are picking up your car."

Child: "Car."

Adult: "That's a race car."

Child: (pushes car along the floor)

Adult: "See how fast the car goes. Look, it hit the chair!"

Technique: Self-talk (providing an ongoing commentary)

Adult: "I am looking for my keys. Hmmm, I thought I put them in my purse. No, they are not here. Maybe they are in the drawer. I will open it. Yes, here they are. Phew, I am relieved to find them."

Technique: Modeling and Expansion

Child: "Bowl."

Adult: "You want a cereal bowl. Here it is."

Child: "Dah."

Adult: "Pudding. Let's put the pudding in the bowl."

Technique: Parallel talk

Child: (Playing with bean-bag stuffed animals)

Adult: "The tiger is hiding under the box. I wonder who he is hiding from."

Child: (Moves toy cat toward box)

Adult: "The cat is looking for the tiger. Maybe they are playing hide-and-seek."

Child: (Throws box off of toy tiger)

Adult: "He found him! The cat found the tiger."

Technique: Question stimulation (question-stimulation phrases are in italics)

Child: "Dah?"

Adult: "*Do you want the cookie?* "

Child:	" My cookie."
Adult:	"No, that's not your cookie. *Whose cookie is this? Whose cookie?*"
Child:	"Who cookie?"
Adult:	"That's Daddy's cookie."

Technique: Time-talk (time-related words are in italics)

Adult:	(looking at scrap book) "Here are the new pictures. Here is a picture of our jack-o-lantern."
Child:	"Halloween."
Adult:	"Yes, Halloween was *last week*. We made a jack-o-lantern."
Child:	"I want Halloween now."
Adult:	"*Today?* No, we have to *wait a whole year*. Halloween won't come again until *next year*."

Techniques: Labeling

Child:	"Dah."
Adult:	"Crayon."
Child:	"Blue."
Adult:	"Here's the blue crayon."

18

Management of Cochlear Implants in Children[1]

Topics

Overview

Initial Contact

Preliminary Counseling

Formal Evaluation

Surgery

The Cochlear Implant Fitting

■ Follow-up Visits

■ Aural Rehabilitation

■ Case Study

■ Final Remarks

■ Key Chapter Points

[1]Parts of this chapter are from "Aural Rehabilitation and Patient Management" by N. Tye-Murray, 1993. In R. S. Tyler (Ed.), *Cochlear Implants: Audiological Foundations* (pp. 87–144). San Diego, CA: Singular Publishing Group.

Children and their families require support and assistance from a variety of professionals before and after the child receives a cochlear implant. In this chapter we will consider the support and aural rehabilitation that speech and hearing professionals provide during and following the implantation process.

> ## Who Makes the Decision About Getting a Cochlear Implant?
>
> When the child is very young, the parents are responsible for making the decision as to whether a child will be a candidate for cochlear implantation and receives an implant once the implant team has determined that the child is an appropriate candidate. They also are responsible for ensuring that the child uses the cochlear implant following the implantation surgery and ensuring that the child receives appropriate aural rehabilitation services. Your role as a speech and hearing professional is to assist in determining whether the child is an appropriate candidate or not. If candidacy is affirmed, then you may provide additional information and counseling to parents that will assist them in making a decision.
>
> When the child is older, he or she also participates in the decision as to whether to receive a cochlear implant. Especially if the child is a young teenager, careful consideration must be given to the youth's expectations and desires. If the adolescent is not committed to making the cochlear implant a successful endeavor, he or she will not likely receive benefit. Negative peer pressure and a desire to identify with the Deaf Culture are some reasons why older children may not want a cochlear implant. Moreover, a disinterest in acquiring speech and listening skills, and a firm commitment to sign, might dissuade older children and adolescents.

OVERVIEW

A cochlear implant service delivery model usually includes seven components. These components are summarized in Table 18–1. They include: initial contact, preimplant counseling, formal evaluation, surgery, fitting, follow-up evaluation, and aural rehabilitation. The key members of a *cochlear implant team* who interact with the child and family are also indicated for each component. The team minimally is comprised of a clinical coordinator, an audiologist, and a surgeon. It usually includes a speech-language pathologist, a psychologist, an educator and/or an aural rehabilitation specialist.

Key members of a **cochlear implant team** include an otolaryngologist, audiologist, speech-language pathologist, psychologist, educator, and/or aural rehabilitation specialist.

Table 18-1. Seven stages of the cochlear implant process and the professionals who may be involved with each stage.

Stage	Professional(s)	Description
Initial contact	Clinical coordinator	Parent receives general information about cochlear implants and candidacy; may be scheduled for an appointment at the cochlear implant center
Preimplant counseling	Speech and hearing professional (usually an audiologist)	Family and child (and educator) receive specific in formation about candidacy, benefits, commitments, and costs and are asked to consider such issues as culture and communication mode
Formal evaluation	Audiologist, surgeon, speech-language pathologist, psychologist, educator	Perform medical, hearing, speech, language, and psychological evaluation to determine candidacy, and evaluate the educational environment and adequacy for support of auditory skill development
Surgery	Surgeon	The internal hardware of the cochlear implant is implanted
Fitting/tune-up	Audiologist	The device is fitted on the child and a map is created; parents (and child) receive instruction about care and maintenance
Follow-up	Audiologist and other members of the cochlear implant team	Any problems are explored, and new develop ments about cochlear implants are reviewed with the family
Aural rehabilitation	Speech and hearing professionals in both the medical and educational centers and educators	The child receives long-term speech perception training and speech and language therapy

INITIAL CONTACT

The first step toward obtaining a cochlear implant is taken by a child's parents or primary caregivers. They may have read a newspaper article or talked to a speech and hearing professional or teacher and desire more information about cochlear implants and candidacy. The parents may have observed other children in their child's classroom who use cochlear implants and been impressed by their progress. A parent might contact the clinical coordinator at the cochlear implant center and ask questions like those listed in Table 18–2.

The clinical coordinator sends printed materials and schedules an appointment for a preliminary counseling session or formal evaluation. The printed materials may cover the following topics in a cursory fashion: the functions of a cochlear implant, how the cochlear implant differs from a hearing aid, who is a cochlear implant candidate, the reasons why some children may receive more benefit than others, the kinds of benefits that can be expected, and the limitations of a cochlear implant.

PRELIMINARY COUNSELING

Counseling for the family, and child if he or she is old enough to understand the candidacy process, is critical. If the child is in an educational setting, then the child's teacher is often invited to the preliminary counseling session. The educator should

Table 18–2. Questions parents may ask during the initial contact.

- Is my child an appropriate candidate?
- How does a cochlear implant work? How does it differ from a hearing aid?
- Will the cochlear implant help my child to talk/hear better?
- Can a cochlear implant electrocute my child? Is it dangerous to use?
- Can my child still play sports if he/she gets one?
- How old does my child need to be?
- Will the cochlear implant last my child's entire lifetime? What happens if it "wears out?"
- Is the cochlear implant waterproof? Will my child be able to take a bath or shower?
- What happens if my child gets hit in the head?
- How often do the devices break?
- How much do they cost? Will my insurance pay for it?
- What's involved in obtaining a cochlear implant?
- Will my child still need to change communication mode? Is signing allowed with a cochlear implant?
- Will my child have to go to a special school for implanted children?
- Are cochlear implants hard to take care of?

be an integral part in the implant process. The educator can provide information about how the child performs in the school setting and ultimately will play a major role in ensuring that the child receives optimal benefit from the device.

The Role of the Educator

Receipt of a cochlear implant is just a first step in an aural rehabilitation plan. Postimplant aural rehabilitation in an educational setting is an important subsequent step.

The educator plays an essential role in maximizing the child's benefits from using a device. The Network of Educators of Children with Cochlear Implants (NECCI), a professional organization of speech and hearing professionals and educators, has created guidelines that delineate the role of the educator in the cochlear implant process (NECCI News, 1992; Nevins & Chute, 1996). Some of these guidelines suggest the following:

■ An educator who is familiar with aural rehabilitation should be involved in every stage of the cochlear implant process, from preimplant counseling to formal evaluation to follow-up and aural rehabilitation.

■ An educator can provide a bridge of communication between the child's family, the cochlear-implant center, and the educational setting. Networking and clear communication among the significant people in a child's life are the most effective means to optimize his or her effective use of the cochlear implant.

■ All children who receive a cochlear implant require an intensive and long-term program of aural rehabilitation provided in the context of a child's educational program. The educator must play a primary role in coordinating aural rehabilitation services and in providing speech, language, and listening practice in the context of the classroom routine. (If a commitment to an intensive program of auditory skill development is not in place, then the child likely will receive little benefit from the cochlear implant.)

Counseling provides information about obtaining, maintaining, and using a cochlear implant, and for maximizing its benefits. Counseling is ongoing and occurs throughout the cochlear implant process. At one time or another, every member of the cochlear implant team provides counseling. Whether child and family members are at the stage of determining candidacy or of planning aural rehabilitation, they must be aware of what is happening and what will happen, they must be prepared for a variety of outcomes, and they must feel as if they are contributing to the decisions that concern them.

Although counseling is ongoing, a block of time usually is set aside for preliminary counseling, either before or after the formal evaluation. This counseling session is most often conducted by an audiologist. The topics that are included in the preliminary counseling session are summarized in Table 18–3. In the following discussion, we will consider what a speech and hearing professional might tell the family about each of these topics.

Audiological and Medical Candidacy Qualifications

The speech and hearing professional reviews audiological and medical candidacy criteria. All children who receive a cochlear implant must have a profound bilateral sensorineural hearing loss. With the exception of 250 Hz, pure-tone thresholds typically should be no better than 95 dB HL. Candidates should receive minimal benefit from amplification; for instance, the child should recognize few if any words auditorily. The possibility of implanting children with slightly better hearing is being investigated in some implant centers.

All children should have a trial period with appropriate amplification before being considered as a cochlear implant candidate. This trial period should last anywhere from 10 weeks or longer (Cowan & Clark, 1997). This is to ensure that the cochlear implant is the only viable means of providing usable residual hearing to the child. If the child appears to be acquiring speech and language skills with the use of a hearing aid, then candidacy should be questioned.

Table 18–3. Topics that often are reviewed during the preliminary counseling session.

- Audiological and medical candidacy qualifications
- Cochlear implant hardware
- Costs
- Realistic expectations
- Commitments
- Cultural considerations
- Communication mode

The exception to this trial-period policy pertains to the child who has incurred a hearing loss following meningitis. Ossification of the cochlea often occurs after such an infection. If computerized axial tomography (a CAT scan) indicates ossification, then the trial period might be shortened or even bypassed.

The Food and Drug Administration recently approved the Cochlear Corporation cochlear implant for implantation in children as young as 18 months of age. Prior to this, the earliest age was 2 years. Although there are exceptions, infants and younger babies are usually not implanted because hearing status is difficult to determine and ability to benefit from amplification cannot be ruled out. In addition, Loeb (1989) noted that very young children may be unable to participate in the fitting procedure, thereby making electrical thresholds and comfort levels of stimulation difficult to determine. However, some centers are providing cochlear implants to children younger than 18 months, on a limited basis, and it is likely that this practice will become more commonplace in the near future.

Scientific data show a correlation between duration of deafness and benefit, with children who receive cochlear implants after a short period of deafness performing better on measures of speech perception than those who receive one after a longer period (Tyler, 1993). Such findings have led to more children below the age of 2 years receiving cochlear implants.

Good general health, no chronic ear disease, and an unobstructed cochlea are often prerequisites for most cochlear implants. The presence of other disabilities, such as blindness or mental retardation, may require special consideration but does not necessarily preclude implantation.

The Cochlear-Implant Hardware

A brief overview of the cochlear implant hardware is important so that the family will appreciate what the device will look like, how it will be worn, and what will be involved in maintaining it in good working order. This can be established with the aid of photographs like that shown in Figure 18–1 and by letting the family and child meet other young cochlear implant users.

When cochlear implants were first approved for children by the Food and Drug Administration (FDA) in 1990, the devices had included speech processors that were about the size of an oversized deck of cards. This speech processor could be worn

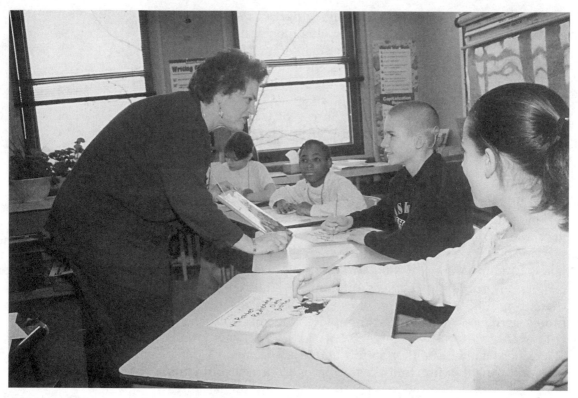

Figure 18–1. A child wearing a cochlear implant. Parents and child should have an appreciation of how the child will wear the cochlear implant and what it will look like before the cochlear implant surgery. (Photograph by Kim Readmond, Central Institute for the Deaf)

in a variety of ways, including in a chest harness or a fanny pack. New developments have led to a miniaturization of the speech processor, so that you may soon see children who wear their speech processors behind their ear, in a fashion similar to a behind-the-ear hearing aid.

Costs and Reimbursements

Costs and reimbursement issues are discussed in great detail prior to implantation. The cochlear implant and surgery are very expensive. Costs include coverage for the formal evaluation, hospitalization, surgery, the device itself, fitting, follow-up visits, and aural rehabilitation. The family should expect some expenses related to cochlear implant maintenance annually because problems with the device hardware are not uncommon. For instance, a microphone may have to be replaced frequently, especially with very young users who are physically active.

In some instances, the family's medical insurance policy will pay for some of the costs related to obtaining a cochlear implant. Because many policies are negotiated individually, and benefits change periodically, it is difficult to generalize with accuracy how much of the total costs might be covered by any particular policy. Preauthorization of insurance benefits should be obtained from the provider before significant costs are incurred. The clinical coordinator and the family usually share responsibility in obtaining preauthorization.

Insurance policies can be classified as private, state, and/or federal plans. Private insurance companies (with the exception of many Health Maintenance Organizations [HMOs]) have been the most cooperative in approving coverage of cochlear implants, although there is considerable variability in the extent of authorized benefits. Medicaid, which is jointly funded by the state and federal governments, provides some coverage (for those who cannot afford health insurance) in some states. Finally, federal programs such as Champus (designed for retired and disabled military personnel and their dependents) may pay for some fraction of the costs incurred for cochlear implantation.

Realistic Expectations

The family and child must develop realistic expectations about what the cochlear implant will provide. Otherwise, they may suffer disappointment and frustration and even a sense of betrayal after the child receives the device. Unmet expectations will dampen enthusiasm to participate in follow-up visits and aural rehabilitation, and may even lead to nonuse of the cochlear implant.

All members of the cochlear implant team help the candidate and family members develop realistic expectations, beginning with the clinical coordinator during the initial contact. During the preliminary counseling session, the family's expectations are further probed, and corrected when necessary. The speech and hearing professional who conducts the preliminary counseling session makes it clear that the child will always have a hearing deficit. The cochlear implant is a communication aid and not a bionic ear that will provide normal hearing. The audiologist also explains in laymen's terms how other young users perform.

A questionnaire might be administered to sample family member's expectations about possible benefits of using a device. If responses indicate the presence of unrealistic expectations (e.g., a parent may indicate, *A cochlear implant will solve the difficulties I have in communicating with my child, or My child is going to begin talking shortly after he gets one of these devices*), you will want to work with the family before continuing on to cochlear implant surgery.

Ways to establish realistic expectations include the provision of opportunities for parents to talk with a variety of other parents of young cochlear implant users, some of whom receive more and some of whom receive less benefit from their devices. Scientific data about children's performance with a cochlear implant over time also might be shared with parents; data that indicate the best and poorest performance of groups of children, and average performance. Data about listening, speech, and language might be discussed (see Chapter 15 for examples of databases). When presenting research findings, it is important to do so in a way that is comprehensible and accessible to the parents.

The speech and hearing professional might summarize the following information for parents: First, parents should understand that a number of factors influence a child's performance with a cochlear implant. A child with a postlingual hearing loss will exhibit better listening abilities than one with a prelingual hearing loss, at least for several years following implantation (Dowell & Cowan, 1997; Staller, Dowell, Beiter, & Brimacombe, 1991). Children who are under 5 years of age at the time of implantation are more likely to benefit than older children, especially children who older than 10 years (Osberger et al., 1993; Tye-Murray, Spencer, & Woodworth, 1995). A child who has a hearing loss of short duration likely will show greater benefit than one who has a loss of long duration (Staller et al., 1991). The support system provided by the family, the status of the auditory nerve and cochlea, the child's personality and interest in communication with speech, communication mode and the quality and quantity of aural rehabilitation are other factors that affect amount of benefit.

With these foregoing qualifications, the speech and hearing professional might summarize what we know about the performance of children, on average, heretofore. Most children who have prelingual hearing losses and who receive a cochlear implant achieve some sound awareness and some speech-reading enhancement when using their cochlear implants. Moreover, most children achieve some improvement in their speech and language performance (Geers & Tobey, 1994; Tye-Murray, Spencer, & Woodworth, 1995). Those who receive a great deal of benefit (often referred to as *star performers* in the literature) may achieve open-set word recognition (Fryauf-Berstchy, Tyler, et al., 1997) and may speak clearly enough that most people understand much of what they say (Chapter 16) . Performance on measures of speech and language tend to improve over time, and many children do not demonstrate a plateau in their skill development, even after 5 or more years of cochlear implant use (Tye-Murray, Tomblin, & Spencer, 1997).

One potential pitfall in establishing realistic expectations is that parents may come to expect too little and never challenge their child to listen. Some parents are delighted that, on receiving a cochlear implant, their child begins to respond to environmental sounds and to recognize his or her own name. They do not expect the child to utilize the electrical signal as a means of enhancing speechreading performance, nor for speech listening, even when audiological testing indicates good benefit from the device. To some extent, parents—and teachers—can limit a child's performance by their own limited expectations.

Commitments

Receiving a cochlear implant requires tremendous commitment from the family and child in terms of time, effort, and money. It is important that the magnitude of these commitments is fully comprehended before the family proceeds with implantation.

The child (and parents) must return to the cochlear implant center periodically for device adjustments and audiological evaluation. During the first year of cochlear implant use, return trips may number six or more. They usually occur at least annually thereafter. A visit to the cochlear implant center may require that the parent take leave from work and that the family allocate funds for travel and perhaps lodging, if the cochlear implant center is far from the home.

Parents usually must maintain the device. They must learn how to determine when the device is malfunctioning and how to perform minor repairs, such as replacing a cord. They must have the financial wherewithal to replace nonfunctioning hardware. The parents typically are responsible for handling the device (e.g., placing it on the body, turning it on, and adjusting the level) and storing the device when it is not in use. Unless the child is older, the parents must assume responsibility for ensuring that the child wears the device during all waking hours at the appropriate settings. They may need to instruct the child's teacher about how to handle it.

Receipt of a cochlear implant marks the beginning of an aural rehabilitation process that may last for some years. The family must ensure that the child has a stimulating auditory environment in both the home and school. Ideally, family members should be willing to direct the child's attention toward sounds in the home environment and label them and consistently integrate speech into their communication mode.

Most aural rehabilitation programs for young cochlear implant users involve parents. Although an involved family does not necessarily guarantee a successful cochlear implant user, a child probably will not be a successful user without one. Involved parents demonstrate all or many of the following behaviors. They:

■ Ensure that the child wears the cochlear implant regularly.
■ Ensure that the cochlear implant is in good working order.
■ Provide consistent auditory speech stimulation and a good language model in everyday settings.
■ Stimulate the child's speech and language production.
■ Engage their child frequently in conversation.
■ Maintain regular contact with school personnel.
■ Participate in the development and implementation of the child's educational program.

During the preimplant counseling session, a clinician will stress the importance of parental involvement.

Social Considerations

Parents of cochlear implant candidates need to be aware of the controversy surrounding implantation in children. Many members of the Deaf Community discourage cochlear implant for young prelingually deaf children. Lane (1990) suggested that a cochlear implant may prevent or delay a child from becoming acculturated as a member of the Deaf Community. After receiving a cochlear implant, the child may not learn ASL or socialize with members of the Deaf Community because of the necessity of intense auditory stimulation and an emphasis on oral/aural communication skills during childhood. On the other hand, the child may not develop the oral/aural skills that would allow him or her to integrate easily into the hearing world. Implanted children may someday be "culturally homeless, belonging to neither the Deaf nor the hearing communities" (Evans, 1989, p. 312). A cochlear implant also may delay the parents' acceptance of the child's hearing loss.

The debate about whether children should be implanted seems as vigorous today in the public arena as it was on June 27, 1990 when the FDA approved the marketing of multichannel cochlear implants for implantation in children as young as 2 years of age. At that time, in response to the FDA decision, the National Association for the Deaf (NAD) issued a position statement, that included the denouncement:

> *The NAD deplores the decision of the Food and Drug Administration which was unsound scientifically, procedurally, and ethically.*

The statement went on to call for the FDA to withdraw marketing approval. Similar anger about implant use in children was expressed in a 1994 *New York Times Magazine* article. The reporter (Solomon, 1994), after interviewing numerous members of the Deaf Culture, offered this opinion:

> Cochlear implants remind me, more than anything else, of sex-change surgery. Are transsexuals really members of their chosen sex? Well, they look like that other sex, take on the roles of that other sex, and so on, but they do not have all those internal workings of the other sex, and cannot create children in the organic fashion of members of the chosen sex. Cochlear implants do not allow you to hear, but rather to do something that looks like hearing. (p. 1)

In June, 1997, the *Washington Post* published an indepth article dealing with Deaf Culture and the anger of its members directed toward cochlear implants and toward those who view deafness as a pathology rather than a culture. The reporter summarized current views of children who use cochlear implants, as well as the view that children should be raised by members of their *culture* rather than members of their *family*:

> Deaf Culture activists maintain that those children [who use cochlear implants] are sure to be failures—deprived of the dignity of their deafness and yet never accepted as full members of the hearing world. They say that choosing to implant children is irresponsible, done for the convenience of hearing parents. At the very least, they argue, deaf children should be allowed to wait to make the choice themselves. They recommend that deaf children be raised by the deaf community, using American Sign Language, in one of 85 residential schools scattered across the children. Trying to "fix" a deaf child, they say, is like trying to "fix" someone because he or she speaks Japanese. (Arana-Ward, 1997, p. 8)

Many parents are aware of the controversy surrounding cochlear implantation, even before contacting a cochlear implant center. One role of the speech and hearing professional may be to provide parents with additional information about the controversy, and to provide support whether they opt for or against implantation. Moreover, they can provide parents with concrete data about how children develop and learn with a cochlear implant, data that may serve to counteract unduely negative publicity.

Professionals at many cochlear implant centers encourage parents to meet deaf adults who use ASL. These interactions may help parents appreciate the rich culture afforded by the Deaf Community (and may even lead them to reconsider their decision for cochlear implantation). If their child proves not to benefit very much after receiving a cochlear implant, parents' awareness of the Deaf Community may mollify unrealized hopes.

Communication Mode

A cochlear implant need not affect communication mode, especially during the first year. For instance, if parents and child communicate using simultaneous communication prior to the child's receiving a cochlear implant, they usually continue using simultaneous communication afterward (Spencer, Tye-Murray, & Tomblin, in press).

Even though communication mode often does not change, this is not to say that communication is inconsequential to progress with a cochlear implant. Data suggest that children who are in an educational setting that utilizes aural/oral communication excel in their speech and listening skills, as compared to children who are in a simultaneous communication classroom placement (Dowell, 1997; Osberger, 1994). In addition, children who use primarily ASL tend to receive little benefit from use of an implant.

FORMAL EVALUATION

The formal evaluation includes extensive audiological testing and medical examination. It may last from 1 to 5 days. It always includes audiological teaching and a medical examination and often includes a psychological and educational evaluation.

Audiological Testing

The audiological testing usually occurs first. The test battery usually includes unaided threshold testing, aided threshold testing, speech recognition testing, and impedance testing. If the child is under the age of 5 years, testing may also include auditory brain stem response audiometry.

Tests of speech recognition must indicate that the child receives no benefit, or limited benefit, from a conventional hearing aid. The tests used to determine benefit from hearing-aid use vary as a function of the child's age and language skills. Tests that may be used to determine speech recognition skills include the *CID Early Speech Perception (ESP) Tests* (Moog & Geers, 1990), the *Northwestern University Children's Perception of Speech* (NU-CHIPS) test (Elliott & Katz, 1980), and the *Word Intelligibility by Picture Identification* (WIPI) test (Ross & Lerman, 1971). These tests were designed to assess word recognition in a closed-set format.

Medical Examination

The medical examination includes a medical history and physical examination to assess general health and to determine whether the child can undergo general anesthesia. A CT scan of the temporal bone of the skull determines the status of the inner ear. Ideally, the cochlea should be structurally normal, although there have been reports which children with cochlear deformities have been implanted successfully (Firszt, Novak, Reeder, & Proctor, 1991). It is desirable that the cochlea be free of bone growth. However, there have been instances in which existing bone growth has been removed during the surgery and the patient subsequently received benefit from the cochlear implant (Balkany, Gantz, & Nadol, 1988). If the otologist determines that medical reasons exist that preclude implantation of an electrode (such as a cochlea structural anomaly), the remainder of the formal evaluation is canceled. If the child is found to have otitis media, then surgery will not be considered until the condition is resolved.

A speech-language pathologist evaluates the child's language and speech skills. Typically, these measures are not used for determining candidacy, although the language measures may indicate whether the child can participate in the cochlear implant fitting process. Grossly delayed language is cause for concern. This may indicate that the child is not receiving sufficient language stimulation in the home or school environment, which does not bode well for successful cochlear implant use. The language measures may help the audiologist select language-appropriate tests for measuring the child's hearing abilities. Both the language and speech measures can be used to design an aural rehabilitation program following surgery and may indicate secondary benefits of implantation.

Psychological and Educational Evaluation

Two other professionals often are involved in the formal evaluation. An educator often participates, and may be a member of the cochlear implant team or may be from the child's educational setting. The educator evaluates the child's educational placement and considers whether or not there is adequate support for auditory skill development. The educator also may evaluate a child's academic achievement, although performance on these measures may not greatly influence candidacy decisions.

The psychologist may determine whether additional conditions that are disabling are present, such as mental retardation or attention deficit disorder. The psychologist also may help to evaluate whether the family has realistic expectations about the benefits of implantation.

Decision

Once the child has passed through each stage of the formal evaluation, the members of the cochlear-implant team meet and discuss their test results. The parents often are invited to this meeting. If the child meets the audiological and medical criteria, realistic expectations are present, and the child has a home and school environment that supports auditory and speech skills, then implantation is usually recommended. It then falls on the parents to decide whether their child will proceed to the next stage of the process—surgery.

A number of factors can cloud a decision about candidacy. These include the presence of any of the following:

- Emotional disturbance in the child or family members
- Severe behavioral problems
- An unwillingness to commit time or effort on the family's (or child's) part toward making the cochlear implant a successful communication aid
- Unrealistic expectations
- A child's inability to participate in the fitting procedure (say because of limited language or reduced cognitive functioning).
- The presence of other disabilities, such as impaired vision, that cannot be corrected.

There are no cookbook procedures to follow when confounding factors are present. Usually, a decision is reached after much discussion among the team members, the family, the child, and, often, an educator.

SURGERY

Once a child's candidacy is established, surgery is scheduled. Cochlear implant surgery requires general anesthesia and lasts about 2–3 hours. Afterward, the child spends 1 to 5 nights in the hospital.

Regardless of the counseling that has occurred beforehand, children and their families often feel anxious before the surgery. Some worry about the anesthesia, potential surgical complications, the aftermath of surgery, and whether their child will receive benefit from the device. Some parents may experience guilt for inflicting a surgical procedure on their child. As a speech and hearing professional you will want to recognize and acknowledge these feelings, and provide additional counseling when necessary.

Children may feel uncomfortable the day following surgery. Some experience tinnitus or soreness around the ear. On rare occasions, a child will experience nausea and slight vertigo. Most of these after-effects disappear quickly.

Cochlear implant fitting: the process of programming the implant's speech processor.

THE COCHLEAR IMPLANT FITTING

Preparing for the Big Day

The first cochlear implant fitting session is usually the source of both excitement and anxiety for parents and their child. Fryauf-Bertschy (1992, p. 3) notes that some children may be frightened and not know what to expect. They may be aware of their parents' hopes and anxieties, and might find this state of affairs stressful. Fryauf-Bertschy provides the following suggestions to follow in preparation for the first tune-up session:

■ Avoid a big build-up to the first tune-up session. Otherwise, the anticipation may be nerve-wracking for both parents and the child.
■ Leave siblings, grandparents and friends at home. It is usually better if just the parents are present.
■ Be prepared for the child to wear the speech processor by bringing a vest, harness, or pocket T-shirt that will accommodate the device comfortably.
■ Bring the child's earmold that was used with his hearing aid for the implanted ear. The mold will help anchor the microphone and may make the child feel more secure about wearing the microphone/transmitter.
■ Bring along a few of the child's noise-making toys. Once the speech processor is programmed, the child will be able to hear moderately soft sounds. A noise-making toy is a good way to introduce the child to sound.
■ Counsel and prepare friends and family, especially grandparents, that the tune-up is only the first stage of the child's implant experience. The child must learn that sound is meaningful before he will respond to it; this will take months of time and practice. (p. 5)

The child returns to the cochlear implant center about 4 to 6 weeks following surgery for the device fitting. The external components are placed on the child and adjusted so that the child can wear them comfortably. The audiologist then adjusts the stimulus parameters of the speech processor, which determine the signals delivered to the electrodes in the electrode array. The program that is established for the speech processor is called a *map*. The process for establishing a map may be called *mapping* or a *tune-up*. Many cochlear implants interface with a personal computer for the tune-up process (Figure 18–2).

The time necessary to fit and map a cochlear implant varies, depending on the maturity and cooperation of the child. A young child must learn to detect when sound is present and to indicate when it is soft and comfortably loud. Initial thresholds may be high and maximum current levels may be low; these may change as the child becomes accustomed to hearing. In addition, due to a limited attention span, only a few electrodes may be programmed during the initial fitting session. Al-

Tune-up: the process for establishing a map.

Map: the program established for the speech processor.

Mapping: another term used to describe the process for establishing a map.

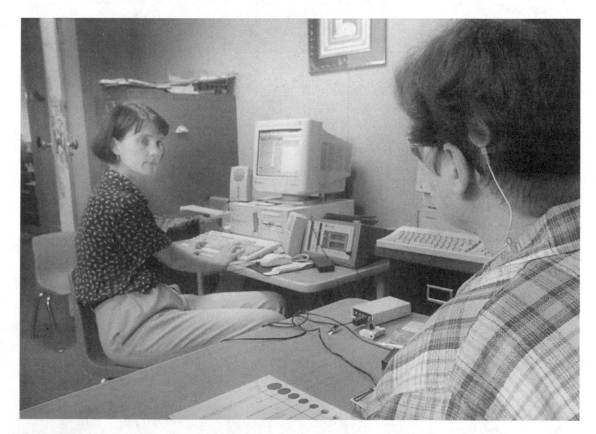

Figure 18–2. An audiologist may use a personal computer when establishing a map for a cochlear implant. (Photograph by Marcus Kosa, courtesy of Central Institute for the Deaf)

though most children can use their cochlear implant after one or two fittings, an optimum fitting may require several months.

When the device is activated, the prelingually deaf child may show no response to sound. Other responses include fright, surprise, rejection, distress, or wonderment. Some children report a sensation in the neck or head.

Dynamic range: the difference between the threshold of stimulation and maximum acceptable loudness.

Threshold: the amount of current that must be passed through an electrode so that the wearer is just aware of a sound sensation.

T-level: another term used for threshold.

Maximum comfort level: the maximum current level that can be introduced before the implant wearer experiences discomfort.

Loudness balancing: programming the speech processor so that stimulation follows the loudness contour of the incoming speech signal.

Pitch ranking determines the ability to discriminate pitch from stimulation of the basal to apical electrodes.

How Do You Establish a Map?

Most cochlear implant maps are established by programming the following parameters:

■ **Dynamic range:** In adjusting the speech processor, each electrode in the electrode array (Chapter 6) is programmed according to the threshold of stimulation and maximum acceptable loudness level. The difference between these two current levels defines a *dynamic range*. An electrical *threshold (T-level)* is the amount of current that must be passed through an electrode so that the child is just aware of a sound sensation. *Maximum comfort level (C-level)* is the maximum current level that can be introduced before the individual experiences discomfort. The thresholds and maximum comfort levels will vary among electrodes and between children, as a function of neuronal survival in the auditory nerve.

■ **Loudness balancing:** Through *loudness balancing*, the speech processor is programmed so that stimulation across electrodes preserves the loudness contour of the speech signal. This is often difficult to perform with children. They must judge the relative loudness of signals presented to different electrodes in the cochlear implant electrode array (see Chapter 6). If the electrodes are not balanced, the child might experience occasional popping sounds and may not hear some speech information.

■ **Pitch and pitch ranking:** Electrodes situated near the basal end of the cochlea are programmed to represent the high-frequency range and those near the apical end represent the low-frequency range. This representation matches the tonotopic organization of the cochlea. *Pitch ranking* determines the ability to discriminate pitch from the

basal to the apical electrodes. During pitch ranking, two electrodes are stimulated, one right after
the other. The child's task is to indicate which
stimulus pulse has a higher or lower pitch. As
with loudness balancing, this too can be a difficult
task for small children to perform.

Parent Instruction

Before leaving the cochlear implant center, parents receive instruction about how to handle the device. Mecklenburg et al.
(1990) presented a list of topics that are reviewed. These are:

- **How is the speech processor turned on and off?**
- **How are the batteries changed?**
- **How long should the batteries last?**
- **Can rechargeable batteries be used?**
- **How is the speech processor tested to see if it's work-
  ing properly?**
- **What does the sensitivity control do?**
- **Can the speech processor be repaired?**
- **How can the speech processor be connected to a ra-
  dio-frequency or infrared transmission system?**
- **How can the telephone signal be fed into the speech
  processor? (p. 214)**

Additional topics of instruction include the warranty, how to
put the device on and take it off, how to troubleshoot the device, and how to perform minor repairs. Simple ways that parents may use to troubleshoot the device and ensure proper
functioning include the following:

- Perform a listening check, with Ling's (1976) Five/Six-
  Sounds Test (described below), to ensure that child is
  receiving sound appropriately.
- If device is not working, check to see if cords are
  plugged in backwards, if a cord is cracked or broken, if
  a battery is inserted improperly, if the battery is dead,
  or if battery contacts are dirty.
- Ensure that the device is kept away from moisture and
  humidity.
- Encourage the child to tell an adult when the device is
  not functioning properly. For example, is the sound
  off? Does it sound muffled? Is there a popping sound?

A schedule for when the child will wear the cochlear implant is established. The child begins by wearing the device in a quiet environment. After a period from 1 week to 2 months, the cochlear implant usually is worn during all waking hours. Parents usually are responsible for enforcing the schedule. Exceptions to regular use include the following:

■ The hardware is in danger of falling off or being damaged, as when the child is playing outside or participating in gym class.
■ The hardware is in danger of getting wet. The child may not wear it outside in the rain or when using the drinking fountain. Cochlear implants are not waterproof.

FOLLOW-UP VISITS

After the first year of cochlear implant use, the child returns to the cochlear implant center annually (or more often). Audiological evaluation indicates whether the cochlear implant is functioning properly and whether performance has changed. Decreased performance is cause for concern because it may signal problems with the device or physiological changes in the auditory system. The audiologist may adjust the speech processor to enhance performance. During the annual visit, the family is advised whether the manufacturer has made new software or other options available for the cochlear implant and the child may be provided with an opportunity to try them.

Children should return to the cochlear implant center whenever problems arise that cannot be fixed by a minor repair. These problems include:

■ An intermittent signal
■ Facial stimulation
■ A change in sound quality
■ Cessation of sound
■ An abnormal popping or squeaking

Sometimes, children will not be aware of changes in their device functioning or will not know how to verbalize that a change has occurred. Parents should be alerted to red flags that may signal a problem. For instance, if a child no longer responds to the sounds he or she once heard, the device may be malfunctioning. Ling's Five Sounds Test (Ling, 1988) may be administered daily for the purpose of assessing whether a child's hearing capacity has changed. For this test, the parent or educator vocalizes the sounds *oo, ee, ah, sh,* and *ss,* with mouth hidden from the child's view. The child's task is to indicate when the sounds are presented, say by clapping. Thus, a parent might say, "Shhh," and the child claps. If the child suddenly is unable to detect a sound that was heretofore audible, than there is reason to suspect a device problem.

Another indicator of a malfunction includes a change in the child's frequency of vocalization, voice quality or articulation accuracy, suggesting that he or she is less able to self-monitor his or her speaking. For example, if a parent of a young child remarks, "He seems so quiet lately. He doesn't hum the way he used to," or "He suddenly sounds monotone," then there is reason to suspect a device problem.

AURAL REHABILITATION

Listening and speech skills do not emerge spontaneously as a result of children receiving cochlear implants and then being exposed to conversation in their everyday environments. A concerted, deliberate rehabilitation effort is required before they learn to utilize the electrical signal from the cochlear implant for the purpose of speech recognition and speech and language acquisition. The aural rehabilitation plan must include participation by the parents, speech and hearing professionals, and educators.

Parents

The aural rehabilitation specialist usually describes informal speech recognition training activities for the parents and child to perform at home. For example, a game of musical chairs can encourage the development of sound detection skills in the young child. Table 18–4 presents sample activities parents might perform during the daily routine. These kinds of activities can provide the child with successful listening experiences, and promote skill growth.

Table 18–4. Routine activities or familiar activities that parents can capitalize on in providing listening practice for their children.

The speech and hearing professional may interact with parents and prepare lists of routine activities they perform regularly with their child in the home environment. They then may discuss how they can incorporate listening practice into these activities. A sample list may include the following:

■ **Getting dressed in the morning.** The child will listen and discriminate between the words *pants* and *sweatshirt*.
■ **Setting the table.** The child will discriminate auditorily between the words *fork* and *napkin*.
■ **Playing favorite games.** The child will discriminate between the words *yellow* and *blue* while playing the game of Candyland.
■ **Playing quietly.** The child will respond to his or her name when a parent calls.

Speech and Hearing Professionals and Educators

Most aural rehabilitation programs extend beyond the boundaries of the family. Speech and hearing professionals and educators play a primary role in helping children to develop listening, speech, and language skills once they have been fitted with their cochlear implants.

An ideal therapy plan integrates auditory goals with goals for speech production, language acquisition, and classroom curriculum. For instance Nevins and Chute (1996) suggested specific procedures for incorporating listening practice into daily classroom routines as well as lessons of science, social studies, reading, language, and other school subjects. The daily roll call may provide opportunity for practice in auditory name recognition. In a science unit, closed sets of vocabulary about the weather can be presented in an audition-only mode; for example, a teacher might say with his or her mouth hidden *clouds* or *lightning* or *thunderstorm*, three words that differ in prosodic pattern (p. 149). The child would be expected to discriminate among the three words.

Administrative support from the child's special education program is essential in case management. This is because there is a critical need for networking among family, classroom teachers, audiologists, speech-language pathologists, and additional cochlear-implant and educational team members. School personnel should be encouraged to call members of the cochlear implant center staff with any questions or comments. Collaborative meetings between education staff and cochlear implant staff are sometimes held via telephone or face-to-face in order to establish information-exchange networks.

Although each child's pattern of progress is individual, the level of therapy should remain high for a prolonged interval, even as long as 5 years or more. The speech and hearing professional has the unique challenge of maintaining the child's interest and motivation to achieve goals over years of therapy time.

Other roles of the speech and hearing professional in an educational setting include the following:

■ To provide information about the cochlear implant and how it works.
■ To evaluate the child's speech and listening performance in the school environment.
■ To provide a school inservice to other professionals in the child's school.
■ To provide instruction to the classroom teacher about how to troubleshoot the device.

CASE STUDY

Now let us consider a case study. This case study provides an example of some of the issues that must be considered when determining cochlear implant candidacy.

Janet Dooley was diagnosed with a bilateral profound hearing loss at 17 months of age. The etiology was unknown, but the loss was believed to have been present at birth. She has worn hearing aids for 4 months, and has been participating in a parent-infant program that utilizes simultaneous communication. Janet has not developed any spoken language, but has developed a sign vocabulary of five words. Her parents are hopeful that a cochlear implant will accelerate her language development and stimulate her speech production. The following issues should be addressed:

■ **Confirmation of hearing status.** An audiologist should perform an extensive audiological assessment, including objective audiological procedures. Aided thresholds can then be determined. Audiological test results should be compared with earlier results to determine whether performance over time is consistent. It is important that accurate information about the magnitude of the hearing loss is available, and it must be determined whether Janet is receiving optimal benefit from the hearing aid.

■ **Evaluation of changes in speech and language.** A comprehensive spoken language assessment should be performed to determine how well Janet is progressing with her hearing aid. A determination can be made as to whether her aided hearing is allowing her to acquire oral communication skills. If she is showing little progress, she may be an appropriate candidate.

■ **Review of educational placement.** Her current parent-infant program should be examined, to determine whether it affords adequate auditory speech stimulation. If it does not, the parents may wish to reconsider placement. The fact that she has shown little progress in her speech skills and language in her current placement suggests that it may not be an optimum placement.

■ **Medical examination.** Impedance testing and an otoscopic examination should be performed to evaluate the health of the middle ear. A CT scan can determine whether the cochlea is normal on either side of the head. A comprehensive medical examination should be performed to rule out any other contraindications to cochlear implant surgery.

■ **Development of realistic expectations.** Janet's parents should be briefed about benefit with a cochlear implant. They can be advised that hearing, speech, and language may not be any better with a cochlear implant than with a hearing aid.

Final Remarks

Speech perception training and speech-language therapy curricula for children who use cochlear implants are, for the most part, not much different in content and organization that those that are appropriate for use with children who use hearing aids. For instance, the techniques and hierarchy of objectives described in Chapters 7 and 9 for auditory training and speechreading training, respectively, are appropriate for children who use either type of listening device. Perhaps the greatest difference you will note when working with children who use the two types of listening devices is that, on average, children who use cochlear implants progress faster in their skill acquisition than children with similar hearing losses who use hearing aids. They also progress farther. Thus a child who uses a cochlear implant may someday perform open-set word recognition exercises in an auditory training program curriculum, whereas a child who uses a hearing aid may advance only to closed-set word recognition exercises. Moreover, children may require less structured language teaching techniques, and instead, may progress with more naturalistic, real-world language instruction than their counterparts who use hearing aids.

KEY CHAPTER POINTS

✔ The cochlear implant service delivery model often has seven key components: initial contact, preimplant counseling, formal evaluation, surgery, fitting, follow-up evaluation, and aural rehabilitation.

✔ Once candidacy is determined, parents are responsible for making the decision about whether the child will receive a cochlear implant.

✔ The preliminary counseling session may occur before or after the formal evaluation. Counseling is critical for the parents and child. They receive information about obtaining, maintaining, and using a cochlear implant, and for maximizing its benefits. Often, the child's educator plays an important role during this stage of the process.

✔ Typically, children must be at least 18 months to 2 years of age before receiving a cochlear implant and have a profound bilateral hearing loss, although there are exceptions. They should be healthy and ideally have no other disabilities other than deafness.

✔ Receiving a cochlear implant requires a tremendous commitment from the family and child, in terms of money, time, and effort. The family needs to be aware of these commitments and be willing to become intimately involved in the aural-rehabilitation plan.

✔ It is important for parents to develop realistic expectations before the cochlear implant surgery. Some parents view the cochlear implant as a "bionic ear," and have inordinately high hopes about what the device can do for their child. These parents may be disappointed by a child's initial results with a cochlear implant and may even become disinterested in postimplant aural rehabilitation.

✔ Cochlear implantation for children has been a controversial issue for many years. Parents need to be aware of the fact that many members of the Deaf Community disapprove of cochlear implants for children, and parents should have some appreciation of the reasons underlying this disapproval. They should also be familiar with data indicating the benefits of cochlear implant use.

✔ Although many children do not change their mode of communication after receiving a cochlear implant, they will receive little benefit if there is not a firm commitment to auditory and speech development in the home and school settings. Children who use primarily ASL likely will receive minimal benefit from receiving a cochlear implant.

✔ During the fitting or tune-up, a map is established for the cochlear implant speech processor. The length of time necessary to fit a child varies, and is contingent upon the child's maturity and cooperation.

✔ A concerted aural rehabilitation effort must follow receipt of a cochlear implant. Children need intensive speech perception training and speech and language therapy after they begin to use a cochlear implant, and for many years thereafter. The curricula appropriate for young cochlear implant users are often similar to those that are appropriate for hearing-aid users who are of similar age, although language instruction may be less formal and more naturalistic.

Glossary

A-weighted scale: A filtering network used in a sound pressure level meter weighted to provide an equal loudness contour at 40 phones; sound level measurements made with this scale are designated with dB(A).

AAA: American Academy of Audiology.

AARP: American Association of Retired Persons.

ABR: Auditory brainstem response.

Acoustic cue: Acoustic information in a segment of speech that conveys phonetic information.

Acoustic feedback: Sound produced when the amplified sound from a device receiver is picked up again by the microphone and reamplified; a high-pitched squeal.

Acquired hearing loss: Hearing loss that is acquired after birth.

Action level: Noise exposure level at which a worker must be enrolled in an occupational hearing conservation program; OSHA defines this level as 85 dBA for an average of 8 hours per day.

Acute otitis media: Inflammation of the middle ear that lasts for 3 weeks or less.

ADA: Americans with Disabilities Act; Academy of Dispensing Audiologists.

Adventitious hearing loss: Hearing loss occurring after birth.

Aggressive conversational style: Conversational style characteristic of some persons who have hearing loss, characterized by hostility, belligerence, and bad attitude.

Aided thresholds: Hearing thresholds obtained from a patient using hearing aids, indicated by an "A" on the audiogram.

Air conduction: Sound travels through the air, enters the external auditory canal, and progresses through the middle ear, inner ear, and then to the brain; air conduction thresholds are represented by a "O" (right ear) and "X" (left ear) on the audiogram.

ALD: Assistive listening device; may be hardwired or wireless; designed to enhance detection and recognition of environmental sounds and speech.

Altered speech: Human speech that is recorded and then altered in some manner.

Alzheimer's disease: Dementia, characterized by progressive neuronal degeneration and mental deterioration.

Ambient noise: Noise in a listening environment.

American Academy of Audiology: AAA; professional society for audiologists, founded in 1988.

American Association of Retired Persons: AARP; Consumer group for persons over the age of 50 years.

American National Standards Institute: ANSI; group that determines standards for measuring instruments, including audiometers.

American Sign Language: ASL; A manual system of communication used by members of the Deaf Culture in the United States; sometimes referred to with the term Ameslan.

American Speech-Language-Hearing Association: ASHA; professional organization of speech and hearing professionals, including speech-language pathologists, audiologists, and speech and hearing scientists.

American Tinnitus Association: ATA; consumer organization for persons who have tinnitus.

Americans with Disabilities Act: ADA; United States law enacted in 1990 to provide equal access to persons with disabilities.

Amplification: Provision of increased intensity of sound.

Analytic speechreading training: An instructional method that focuses the student's attention on speechreading individual speech units.

Anomaly: A structure that is irregular or deviates from the norm, such as a cochlear anomaly.

Anoxia: Deficiency or absence of oxygen in the bodily tissues.

Aperiodic: Not occurring at regular intervals; not periodic.

Apgar score: A numeric value between 1 and 10, assigned to a newborn to describe physical status at birth; determined by the baby's color, heart rate, respiration, muscle tone, and responsiveness.

Articulation: Movement and positioning of the oral cavity structures, including tongue tip, tongue body, jaw, and lips, during speech production.

ASHA: American Speech-Language-Hearing Association.

Assertive conversational style: Conversational style used by some persons with hearing loss, characterized by a respect for the rights of others and assuming responsibility for the success of the conversational interaction.

Assistive listening device: ALD; instrument designed to provide awareness and/or identification of environmental signals and speech and to improve signal-to-noise ratios; usually includes a microphone and a receiver.

ATA: American Tinnitus Association.

Attention deficit disorder: ADD; cognitive deficit that limits an individual's ability to pay attention and stay focused on a task; may involve restlessness, distractibility, and hyperactivity.

Audible: Loud enough to be heard.

Audiogram: A graphic representation of hearing thresholds as a function of stimulus frequency.

Audiologic rehabilitation: Term often used synonymously with aural rehabilitation or aural habilitation; sometimes may entail greater emphasis on the provision and follow-up of listening devices and less emphasis on communication strategies training and speech perception training.

Audiologist: Allied health care professional who has academic accreditation in the practice of audiology; professional who provides an array of services related to hearing evaluation and rehabilitation.

Audiometer: Electronic instrument used for the measurement of hearing sensitivity.

Audiometric zero: Lowest sound pressure level that can just be detected by an average adult ear at any particular frequency; designated as 0 dB Hearing Level (HL) on an audiogram.

Audiovisual: Speech that is presented to both the auditory and visual modalities.

Audition: Hearing.

Auditorily: With audition.

Auditory: Pertaining to hearing.

Auditory brainstem implant: ABI; implant that has an electrode that implants to the juncture of the eighth cranial nerve and the cochlear nucleus in the brainstem; provides crude sound awareness.

Auditory brainstem response: ABR; auditory evoked potential that originates from the eighth cranial nerve and is generated by electrical stimulation of the cochlea via an electrode.

Auditory canal: External auditory meatus.

Auditory feedback: One's own speech signal that is heard while speaking.

Auditory memory: Acquisition, storage, and retrieval of auditory sound patterns in both short-term and long-term form.

Auditory-only: Speech that is presented to only the auditory modality.

Auditory training: Instruction designed to maximize an individual's use of residual hearing by means of both formal and informal listening practice.

Auditory-verbal therapy: An educational approach in which technology, techniques, and strategies are used to enable children to listen and understand spoken language, with a primary emphasis on the auditory modality for learning.

Aural habilitation: Sometimes used synonymously with aural rehabilitation; intervention for persons who have not developed listening, speech, and language skills; may include diagnosis of communication- and hearing-related difficulties, speech perception training, speech and language therapy, manual communication, and educational management.

Aural/oral method: An instructional method used to teach children with significant hearing loss using hearing, speechreading, and spoken language, but not manual communication.

Aural rehabilitation: Intervention aimed at minimizing and alleviating the communication difficulties associated with hearing loss; may include diagnosis of hearing loss and communication handicap, amplification, counseling, communication strategies training, speech perception training, family instruction, speech-language therapy, and educational management.

Auricle: Pinna; external or outer ear.

Automatic gain control: AGC; nonlinear hearing aid compression circuitry that changes gain as signal level changes and/or limits the output of the hearing aid when the level reaches a specified value.

Autosomal recessive inheritance: Transmission of genetic characteristics in which both parents must pass on the genetic characteristic.

Autosome: Any of the 22 pairs of 23 chromosome pairs not related to determination of gender.

Background noise: Extraneous noise that masks the acoustic signal of interest.

Battery: A cell that provides electrical power; set of diagnostic tests.

Behavioral audiometry: Pure-tone and speech audiometry that requires a behavioral response from the patient.

Behind-the-ear hearing aid: BTE; a hearing aid that is worn over the pinna and is coupled to the ear canal by means of an earmold.

Bilateral: On both sides; involving both ears.

Binaural: For both ears.

Binaural advantage: The advantage of using both ears instead of one, such as better hearing thresholds and enhanced listening in the presence of background noise.

Binaural amplification: Use of a hearing aid in each ear.

Body hearing aid: A hearing aid worn on the body; includes a box worn on the torso and a cord connecting to an ear-level receiver.

Bone conduction: Transmission of sound through the bones in the body, particularly the skull.

Bone-conductor: Vibrator or oscillator that is used to transmit sound to the bones of the skull by means of vibration.

BTE: Behind-the-ear hearing aid.

Carrier phrase: In speech audiometry, a phrase that precedes the target word, such as, "Say the word _____."

CAD: Central auditory disorder.

CAT scan: Computerized axial tomography scan.

Central auditory disorder: CAD; functional auditory disorder that is centered in the brainstem or cortex, and not the peripheral hearing system (outer, middle, or inner ear).

Cerumen: Ear wax.

Chronic: Of long-standing duration.

Chronological age: Age of an individual referenced to birth.

CIC: Completely-in-the-canal hearing aid.

Circuit: A combination of electronic components that conveys electronic current.

Circuitry: The parts of an electric circuit.

Classroom acoustics: The background noise and reverberation properties characteristic of a classroom, determined by the size and surfaces of the room, the sound sources inside and outside, furnishings, people, and other factors.

Clear speech: Speech that is at a moderately loud conversational level, characterized by precise but not exaggerated articulation, pausing at appropriate linguistic boundaries, and somewhat slow speaking rate; often used to increase the message recognition of hard-of-hearing listeners.

Closed captioning: Printed text or printed dialog that corresponds to the auditory speech signal from a television program or movie.

Closed-set: A stimulus or response set that contains a fixed number of items, that are known to the patient.

CNT: Could not test.

Coarticulation: The influence of one phoneme on either a preceeding or succeeding phoneme.

Cochlear implant: Device implanted in the skull that permits persons with deafness to receive stimulation of the auditory mechanism; typically comprised of a microphone, a speech processor, and an electrode array that is inserted into the cochlea; directly stimulates the auditory nerve by means of electrical current.

Cochlear-implant team: Group of professionals who are part of the cochlear implant process; usually includes an otolaryngologist, audiologist, and clinical coordinator and may include an educator, aural rehabilitation specialist, speech-language pathologist, psychologist, and/or social worker.

Comfortable loudness level: Intensity level that is comfortable to listen to sound.

Communication: The act of exchanging messages; may entail the use of speech, sign, writing, or hand gestures.

Communication breakdown: Instance in the course of a conversation when one participant does not recognize the message presented by another.

Communication handicap: Psychosocial disadvantages that result from hearing loss, including the limitations that occur in performing the activities of everyday life.

Communication strategies training: Instruction provided to a person with hearing loss or the person's frequent communication partner that pertains to communication strategies and the management of communication difficulties.

Communication strategy: A course of action taken to enhance communication.

Communication disorder: An impairment in one's ability to communicate.

Communication partner: Person with whom one engages in conversation.

Comprehension: A sophisticated level of auditory skill development, characterized by an ability to understand connected speech easily.

Compressed speech: Speech that has had segments removed and then has been compressed in such a way that the frequency composition remains intact.

Compression (in hearing aid circuitry): Nonlinear amplifier gain used to determine and limit output gain as a function of input gain.

Compression ratio: The ratio in decibels between the acoustic input to a hearing-aid amplifier and its auditory output.

Computerized axial tomography: CAT; a computer-generated picture of a section of the brain compiled from sectional radiographs obtained from the same plane.

Concha: The bowl-like depression of the outer ear that forms the mouth of the external ear canal.

Conductive hearing loss: Hearing loss that stems from an impairment in the outer or middle ear and that does not involve the inner ear.

Congenital: Present at birth.

Congenital hearing loss: Hearing loss that exists at or dates from birth; reduced hearing sensitivity related to pre- or perinatal causes.

Consonant-vowel-consonant: CVC; a monosyllabic word structure; CVCs often are used as stimuli in isolated-word speech-recognition tests.

Construct validity: Statistical term meaning the extent to which a test measures what it is supposed to measure, usually a trait or skill (e.g., speech perception).

Constructive strategy: Tactic designed to optimize the listening environment for communication; a kind of facilitative strategy.

Content validity: Statistical term meaning the extent to which a test adequately samples what it is supposed to measure.

Contextual information: Linguistic support available for identifying a target word, phrase, or sentence.

Continuous discourse tracking: CDT; aural rehabilitation technique in which the receiver (listener) attempts to repeat verbatim text that is presented by a sender (speaker); performance is summarized as the number of words repeated per minute.

Conversational fluency: Relates to how smoothly conversation unfolds, and is reflected by the time spent in repairing communication breakdowns, the exchange of information and ideas, and the sharing of speaking time.

Conversational rules: Implicit rules that guide the conduct of participants engaged in conversation.

Conversational turn: During the course of a conversation, the period during which a participant delivers a contribution to the conversation.

Corner audiogram: An audiogram that displays a profound hearing loss, with thresholds measurable only in the low frequencies.

Critical period: The early years of a child's or animal's life in which the language and vocal patterns of the individual's species are acquired most easily.

Cued speech: A system for enhancing speechreading; hand configurations are placed at different mouth and throat positions to distinguish between similar visual speech patterns.

CVC: Consonant-Vowel-Consonant syllable.

Cycling: In speech perception training, coming back to a training objective that has been achieved with some success in order to provide reinforcement and additional learning.

DAC: Digital-to-analog conversion.

DAI: Direct audio input.

Daily log: A procedure for assessing conversational fluency and communication handicap, in which respondents perform a self-monitoring procedure about behaviors of interest and provide self-reports; usually completed more than once, over a set period of time.

dB: Decibel.

Deaf: Having minimal or no hearing.

Deaf Culture: A subculture in society that shares a common language (American Sign Language), beliefs, customs, arts, history, and folklore; primarily comprised of individuals who have prelingual deafness.

Decibel: Logarithmic unit of sound pressure; 1/10th of a Bel; unit for expressing sound intensity.

Dementia: Progressive loss of cognitive function.

Detection: The ability to recognize when a sound is present and when it is absent.

Developmental delay: Lagging behind in development relative to age-matched peers.

Digital hearing aid: Hearing aid that utilizes digital technology to process the signal.

Direct audio input: DAI; hard-wired connection that leads directly from the sound source to the hearing aid or other listening device.

Directional microphone: Microphone that is more sensitive to sound originating from in front of the hearing-aid user than from behind.

Disability: A loss of function.

Discourse: Communication of thoughts by use of language.

Discrimination: In speech-perception training, the ability to distinguish one stimulus from another; in speech-recognition testing, sometimes used to refer to word-recognition ability.

Disorder: An abnormality in functioning.

Dissonance theory: Theory concerning situations in which one's self-perceptions do not coincide with reality.

Distortion: Undesirable change in the audio signal.

DNA: Deoxyribonucleic acid; molecules that carry genetic instructions.

DNT: Did not test.

Dominant hereditary hearing loss: Hearing loss that stems from a genetic characteristic on at least one gene of a pair.

Dominating conversational behaviors: Characteristic of an aggressive conversational style; includes taking extended speaking turns, frequent interruptions, and abrupt topic changes.

Dri-aid kit: A small package used to keep moisture out of the internal components of listening devices.

Drill: Repeated exercises and rote activities.

DSP: Digital signal processing.

DSP hearing aid: Hearing aid that utilizes digital signal processing; signal is converted from an analog to digital signal, the signal is manipulated according to a processing algorithm, and then the signal is converted back into an analog signal.

Dynamic range: The difference in decibels between an individual's threshold of sensitivity for a sound and the level at which the sound becomes uncomfortably loud.

Dysfunction: Abnormal function.

EAR plugs: Etymotic Applied Research plugs; provide ear protection.

Ear protection: Term used to refer to hearing protectors such as ear plugs and ear muffs.

Earache: Pain in the ear.

Earhook: The curved apparatus of a behind-the-ear hearing aid and some other types of listening devices that connects the device case to the earmold, and hooks over the pinna.

Earmold: A device that fits into the concha and directs sound from the earhook of a listening device to the ear canal.

Earmold acoustics: The influence of the earmold's configuration and structure, such as bore length and venting, on the acoustic properties of the sound delivered to the tympanic membrane by a listening device.

Earmold bore: A hole in the earmold through which an amplified audio signal travels.

Earmold impression: Cast made of the concha and ear canal.

Earmold vent: A canal drilled in the earmold for the purpose of aeration or alteration of the audio signal.

Earmuffs: A kind of ear protection, made of earcups that seal around the ear for the purpose of sound attenuation.

Earplug: A kind of ear protection, consisting of a material that is inserted into the ear canal for the purpose of sound attenuation.

Effective gain: Difference in decibels between a patient's aided and unaided thresholds.

Effusion: In the middle ear, exudation of body fluid from the middle ear membranous walls as a result of inflammation.

Eighth cranial nerve: The cranial nerve consisting of an auditory and vestibular branch.

Electroacoustic: Related to the conversion of an acoustic signal to an electrical signal or an electrical signal to an acoustic signal.

Electrode: Metal ball or plate through which electrical stimulation is applied to the body or electrical energy is measured.

Electrode array: Electrodes placed in pairs on a carrier wire and inserted into the cochlea; component of a cochlear implant.

ENT: Ear, nose, and throat.

Equivalent lists: In speech recognition testing, test lists that contain items that are presumed to be equally difficult to recognize.

Evoked potential: Electrical activity generated in the brain in response to a sensory stimulus.

Expanded speech: Recorded speech that is altered by duplicating small segments of the signal so that the speech sounds as if it were produced with a slow speaking rate; no additional spectral information is introduced.

Expansion: Language-stimulation technique in which an adult copies the meaning of a child's utterance but modifies or expands the grammar of the message.

Expressive repair strategy: Tactic taken by an individual when a communication partner has not understood one of his or her messages.

External auditory meatus: External ear canal.

External ear canal: The canal of the outer ear leading from the concha to the tympanic membrane.

Eyeglass hearing aid: Style of hearing aid in which the hearing aid is housed in the temple piece of a pair of eyeglasses.

f_0: Fundamental frequency.

F1: First formant.

F2: Second formant

Facilitative communication strategy: A strategy used to facilitate communication; includes means taken to instruct the talker, structure the listening environment, enhance the structure of the received message, and affect the speech recognition performance of the individual using the strategy.

Familial deafness: Deafness reoccurring in members of the same family.

FDA: Food and Drug Administration.

Fetal alcohol syndrome: Syndrome found in children whose mothers abused alcohol while the child was in utero; children who have the syndrome may have mental retardation, low birth weight, unusual eye spacing, chronic otitis media, and sensorineural hearing loss.

Filter: In listening devices, a component that differentially amplifies and attenuates certain bands of frequencies in the incoming signal.

Filtered speech: Speech that has been passed through filter banks for the purpose of removing or amplifying frequency bands in the signal.

Fingerspelling: A kind of manual communication, in which words are spelled letter-by-letter using standard hand configurations.

5-dB rule: Noise protection rule that specifies that the intensity level of a sound can be increased by 5 dB for every 50% reduction in the length of presentation of the sound.

Flat audiogram: Audiogram configuration in which the thresholds across frequencies are similar.

Fluctuating hearing loss: Hearing loss that varies in magnitude over time.

FM: Frequency modulation.

FM auditory trainer: Classroom assistive listening device in which the teacher wears a microphone and the signal is transmitted to the student(s) by means of frequency modulated radio waves.

FM boot: A small boot-like device worn on the bottom of a user's hearing aid that contains an FM receiver; used as part of an FM assistive listening device.

FM system: An assistive listening device that conveys sound from a sound source to a listener by means of a sinusoidally varying carrier wave; designed to enhance signal-to-noise ratio.

Food and Drug Administration: FDA; U.S. government agency that oversees the regulation of medical devices such as hearing aids and cochlear implants.

Formal instruction: The first stage in a communication-strategies training program, in which individuals receive information about various types of communication strategies and other appropriate listening and speaking behaviors.

Formal training: In reference to speech perception training, highly structured activities that may involve drill, usually scheduled to occur during designated times of the day, either in a one-on-one lesson format or in a small group.

Formant: A resonance in the vocal tract that results in some frequencies in the speech signal having more energy than other frequencies.

Formant 1: The first frequency band above the fundamental frequency that demonstrates high energy in the speech signal.

Formant 2: The second frequency band above the fundamental frequency that demonstrates high energy in the speech signal.

Formant transition: Segment in the speech signal that displays rapid change in the frequency or spectral composition of the formants.

Frequency: The number of regularly repeated events in a given unit of time; usually measured in cycles per second and expressed in Hertz (Hz).

Frequency of usage: A measure indicating how often a particular word occurs during everyday conversation.

Frequency response: Output characteristics of a listening device; denoted as gain as a function of frequency.

Frequent communication partner: A particular person with whom another often converses; often a family member.

Fricative: Speech sound generated by creating turbulent airflow through a constriction in the oral cavity.

Full-on gain: Hearing aid setting that results in the maximum acoustic output.

Functional gain: Difference in decibels between unaided and aided thresholds.

Fundamental frequency: F_0; in speech, the lowest frequency in the speech output; voice pitch.

Gain: In hearing aids, the difference in decibels between the input level of an acoustic signal and the output level.

Gene: DNA structure that is the unit of heredity.

Genetic: Concerning heredity.

Genetic counseling: Providing information to prospective parents about the likelihood of an inherited condition or disorder in their children.

Genotype: The genetic make-up of an individual.

Geriatric: Concerning the aging process.

Guided learning: The second stage in a communication strategies training program, in which individuals use conversational strategies in a structured setting.

Habilitation: Program or intervention aimed at the initial development of skills and abilities.

HAE: Hearing aid evaluation.

HAO: Hearing aid orientation.

Hair cells: Sensory cells in the cochlea that attach to the nerve endings of the eighth cranial nerve.

Handicap: Obstacles to everyday functioning that result from a disability.

Hard-of-hearing: HOH; having a hearing loss; usually not used to refer to a profound hearing loss.

Hard-wired: Tethered by a wire or cord.

Head shadow: Attenuation of sound to one ear because of the presence of the head between the ear and the sound source.

Headphone: Earphone.

Hearing aid: An electronic listening device designed to amplify and deliver sound from the environment to the listener; includes a microphone, amplifier, and receiver.

Hearing aid evaluation: HAE; procedure wherein an appropriate hearing aid is selected for an individual.

Hearing aid orientation: HAO; process of instructing a patient (and a patient's family member) to handle, use, and maintain a new hearing aid.

Hearing conservation: Prevention or reduction of hearing loss through a program of identifying and minimizing risk, monitoring hearing sensitivity, education, and providing protection from noise exposure.

Hearing disability: Functional limitations imposed on an individual as a result of hearing loss.

Hearing disorder: A disturbance of the auditory structures and/or auditory functioning.

Hearing handicap: Difficulties in everyday functioning that arise as a result of hearing loss.

Hearing impairment: Abnormal or reduced hearing sensitivity; hearing loss.

Hearing level: HL; decibel level referenced to audiometric zero.

Hearing loss: Abnormal or reduced hearing sensitivity; hearing impairment.

Hearing loss, mild: Hearing thresholds between 25 and 40 dB HL.

Hearing loss, moderate: Hearing thresholds between 40 and 55 dB HL.

Hearing loss, moderate-to-severe: Hearing thresholds between 55 and 70 dB HL.

Hearing loss, severe: Hearing thresholds between 70 and 90 dB HL.

Hearing loss, profound: Hearing loss greater than 90 dB HL.

Hearing protection: Devices designed to minimize the risk of noise-induced hearing loss.

Hearing threshold: Level of intensity at which a sound is just audible to an individual.

High-pass filtered speech: Speech that has been passed through filter banks, leaving the higher but not the lower frequencies.

HL: Hearing level.

Homophenes: Words that look identical on the mouth.

HMO: Health maintenance organization.

Identification: The ability to label auditory stimuli.

IEP: Individualized educational plan.

IFSP: Individualized family service plan.

Impairment: Reduced or abnormal function.

Impedance audiometry: Battery of measures designed to assess middle ear functioning, including tympanometry and acoustic reflex threshold determination; immittance audiometry.

Impression: Cast made of the concha and/or ear canal for the purpose of creating an earmold or a hearing aid.

Impulse noise: A burst of sound, as produced by a gunshot or an explosion; has an instantaneous rise time and short duration.

Informal training: In reference to speech perception training, activities that occur during the daily routine, often incorporated into other activities, such as conversation or academic learning.

Interactive communication behaviors: Consistent with an assertive conversational style; includes a sharing of responsibility for advancing a topic of conversation, choosing what to talk about, showing interest, and responding to remarks appropriately.

Interdisciplinary team: A group of professionals with different expertise working together for the purpose of providing assessment and intervention in a coordinated and cooperative fashion.

Internal components: Components of a cochlear implant that are implanted within the skull.

In-the-canal hearing aid: ITC hearing aid; hearing aid that fits in the external ear canal, with only a partial filling of the concha.

In-the-ear hearing aid: ITE hearing aid; hearing aid that fits into the concha of the ear.

Incidence: Frequency of occurrence.

Individualized education plan: IEP; federally mandated plan for providing education to children with disabilities, updated once a year.

Individualized family service plan: IFSP; federally mandated plan for the education of preschool children with an emphasis on family involvement, updated annually.

Individuals with Disabilities Education Act: IDEA; U.S. Public Laws 94-142 and 99-457, which mandate free and appropriate education for all children with disabilities over the age of 3 years, and encourages services for children below 3 years of age.

Induction loop: A length of wire surrounding the circumference of a room or table that conducts electrical energy from an amplifier, and thus creates a magnetic field; the current flow from an induction loop can induce the telecoil in a hearing aid for the purpose of providing amplified sound to the user.

Industrial audiometry: Assessment of hearing at regular intervals for the purpose of assessing the effects of noise exposure, as well as the measurement of industrial noise levels.

Infrared system: Assistive listening device that broadcasts from the sound source to a receiver/amplifier by means of infrared light waves.

Inner ear: Part of the hearing mechanism that houses the structures for hearing and balance and includes the cochlea, vestibules, and semicircular canals.

Input signal: Acoustic signal that enters a listening device.

Insertion gain: Hearing aid gain.

Instructional strategy: Instruction provided to a communication partner so that the person converses in a way that maximizes the hard-of-hearing person's recognition of messages and minimizes the possibility of communication breakdown; a kind of facilitative communication strategy.

Intelligibility: The degree to which speech can be recognized.

Interleave: To interweave patterns of signals.

Interleave processing: A cochlear implant processing strategy whereby trains of pulses are delivered across electrodes in the electrode array in a nonsimultaneous fashion.

Interview: An assessment procedure to assess conversational fluency and communication handicap, in which individuals talk about their conversational problems and they consider possible reasons as to why communication breakdowns happen.

Intraural: Between the two ears.

Ipsilateral: Pertaining to the same side.

ITC hearing aid: In-the-canal hearing aid.

ITE hearing aid: In-the-ear hearing aid.

JND: Just noticeable difference.

Just noticeable difference: JND; the smallest increment of stimulus change in which the stimulus can be perceived as different; difference limen.

K-AMP circuit: Hearing-aid circuit designed to provide more gain for moderate-level sound, no gain for high-intensity sound, and compression limiting for the highest level sound; also often more amplification for high frequencies.

Kinesthetic: Relating to the perception of movement, position, and tension of body parts.

Kneepoint: Point on an input-output function of a hearing aid where compression is activated.

Labeling: A language-stimulation technique in which an adult provides names to objects, actions, and events.

Language: Complex system of symbols that are used in a rule-governed fashion for the purpose of communication.

LDL: Loudness discomfort level.

Learning disability: LD; a lack of ability in an area of learning that is inconsistent with an individual's cognitive capacity and is not a result of a deficit in sensory, motor, or emotional disorder.

Learning effect: Performance on a test improves as a function of familiarity with the test procedures and test items and not because of a change in ability.

Level: Intensity of sound.

Lexical: Concerning the lexicon.

Lexical neighbors: Words that are phonemically (or visually) similar.

Lexicon: All of the units of meaning, such as words and morphemes, in a given language.

Life factors: Conditions that help define one's life, such as relationships, family, and vocation.

Limited set: The response items in a stimulus or response set are limited by situational or contextual cues, for example, words related to summer.

Linear amplification: Hearing aid amplification system in which there is a one-to-one correspondence between the input and output until the maximum output level is reached.

Linked adjacency pairs: Two remarks that often are linked in conversation, as when one communication partner asks, "How are you?" and another responds, "Fine, thank you."

Lipreading: The process of recognizing speech using only the visual speech signal and other visual cues, such as facial expression.

Listening check: Informal assessment of whether a listening device is functioning appropriately.

Live-voice testing: Stimuli in a test of speech recognition are presented by a talker in real time.

Loudness: Perception of the intensity of a sound.

Loudness comfort level: Level at which sound is perceived to be comfortably loud.

Loudness discomfort level: LDL; level at which sound is perceived to be uncomfortably loud.

Low-pass filtered speech: Speech that has been passed through filter banks, leaving the lower, but not the higher, frequencies.

Lucite: Material often used for constructing earmolds.

Magnetic loop: Induction loop.

Mainstreaming: Reassignment of children with disabilities from a special education classroom to a classroom in the regular school environment.

Maladaptive strategy: Inappropriate behavioral mechanisms for coping with the difficulties caused in conversation by hearing loss, such as avoidance behavior.

Managed care: A health care reimbursement plan in which an organization intercedes between patient and provider and determines the kind and extent of services that will be provided.

Manner of articulation: Classification of a speech sound as a function of how it is produced in the oral cavity (e.g., glide).

Manual alphabet: Series of hand configurations that correspond to each letter in the alphabet; used to fingerspell words in manual communication.

Manual communication: Communication modes that entail the use of fingerspelling, signs, and gestures.

Map: Specifications of threshold, suprathreshold, and frequency by which the speech processor of a cochlear implant processes the speech signal and delivers it in electrical form to the electrodes in the electrode array.

Masker: For tinnitus, an electronic listening device that delivers low-level noise to the ear for the purpose of masking the presence of tinnitus.

Masking: Noise that interferes with the perception of another sound.

Maximum power output: MPO; maximum level intensity that a hearing aid can produce; SSPL.

MCL: Most comfortable loudness.

Mean length speaking turn: MLT; used in the assessment of conversational interactions, computed by determining the average number of words a person speaks during a set number of conversational turns.

Meningitis: A common cause of childhood deafness caused by bacterial or viral inflammation of the meninges.

Mental age: Intellectual age.

Mental retardation: Intellectual function is below normal range.

Message-tailoring strategy: Phrasing one's remarks in a way that constrains the responses of a communication partner; a kind of facilitative communication strategy.

Metalinguistic: To think about and attend to the use of language.

Microphone: Transducer that converts an audio signal into an electronic signal.

Middle ear: Portion of the hearing mechanism extending from the tympanic membrane to the oval window of the cochlea; includes the ossicles and middle ear cavity.

Mimetic: Imitating or copying the movements.

Mixed hearing loss: A hearing loss that has a conductive and sensorineural component.

Mobile unit: A mobile van that is equipped to screen hearing; used for educational and on-site industrial hearing screening programs.

Modality: Any of the five senses, including audition and vision.

Modeling: An instructor demonstrates a desired behavior and a student attempts to imitate it.

Monaural: Concerning one ear.

Monosyllabic word: A word comprised of one syllable.

Morpheme: Smallest unit of language that conveys meaning.

Most comfortable loudness: MCL; level at which sound is most comfortable for a listener, usually measured in dB HL.

Multichannel: More than one channel of information; often used to describe cochlear implants that present different channels of information to different regions of the cochlea.

Multidisciplinary team: A group of professionals with different expertise contributing to the assessment, intervention, and management program for a particular individual.

Multiple-memory hearing aid: A hearing aid that can be programmed to process the speech signal in more than one way, so that the user can adjust the processing strategy for different listening environments.

Multisensory approach: Educational approach for deaf children that emphasizes the use of vision, residual hearing, and touch to enhance communication.

Myringitis: Inflammation of the tympanic membrane.

NAD: National Association of the Deaf.

National Association of the Deaf: NAD; advocacy group for members of the Deaf Culture.

NECCI: Network of Educators of Children with Cochlear Implants.

Neckloop: A transducer worn around the neck as part of an FM assistive device system, consisting of a cord from a receiver; transmits signals via magnetic induction to the telecoil of the user's hearing aid.

Neonatal: Concerning the first 4 weeks of life.

Network of Educators of Children with Cochlear Implants: NECCI; professional organization of speech and hearing professionals and educators who are involved with children who receive and use cochlear implants.

NIHL: Noise-induced hearing loss.

Noise: Unwanted sound.

Noise exposure: Level of noise and duration of exposure.

Noise-induced hearing loss: NIHL; sensorineural hearing loss that is the result of exposure to excessive levels of sound; auditory trauma caused by loud sound and resulting in permanent hearing loss.

Noise-induced permanent threshold shift: NIPTS; Permanent decrease in an individual's hearing thresholds as a result of exposure to excessive sound levels.

Noise-induced temporary threshold shift: NITTS; transient shift in an individual's hearing thresholds as a result of exposure to excessive sound levels; temporary threshold shift.

Noise reduction: The difference in sound pressure level of a noise, measured at two different locations.

Noninteractive communication behaviors: Characteristic of a passive conversational style; includes failure to contribute to the development of a conversational topic, minimal response to turn-taking signals, and a proclivity to bluff.

Nonlinear amplification: Amplification system that does not provide a one-to-one correspondence between input and output at all input levels.

Nonsense syllable: Single syllable of speech that has no meaning.

Nonspecific repair strategy: A repair strategy used to repair a communication breakdown that does not provide specific instruction to the communication partner about what to do next: *what, huh, pardon*.

Norm: Standards derived from a sample of the population of interest, thought to represent typical values of the characteristic under study or test.

NR: No response.

OAE: Otoacoustic emission.

Objective: Physically measurable.

Occlusion effect: Enhancement of the level of low-frequency sound in bone-conducted signals as a result of occlusion of the ear canal.

Occupational hearing loss: Noise-induced hearing loss incurred on the job.

Occupational Safety and Health Act: U.S. federal legislation passed in 1970 to ensure safe and healthy work environments; resulted in the establishment of OSHA, NIOSH, and OSHRC.

Occupational Safety and Health Administration: OSHA; Federal agency that regulates occupational health and safety hazards and establishes and enforces minimum standards for industrial hearing conservation programs.

OHCP: Occupational hearing conservation program.

Omnidirectional microphone: Microphone that is sensitive to sound coming from all directions.

Open-set: Testing or training task that does not provide a set of choices to the patient.

Oral interpreter: A professional who silently repeats a talker's message as it is spoken, so that a hard-of-hearing person may lipread the message.

Oralism: Method of instruction for deaf children that emphasizes spoken language skills to the exclusion of manual communication.

OSHA: Occupational Safety and Health Administration.

Ossification: A conversion of tissue into bone.

Otitis media: Inflammation of the middle ear.

Oto: Otolaryngology.

Otoacoustic emission: OAE; low-level sound emitted by the cochlear spontaneously on presentation of an auditory stimulus.

Otolaryngologist: Physician who specializes in the diagnosis and treatment of diseases and conditions of the ear, nose, and throat.

Otologist: Physician who specializes in the diagnosis and treatment of diseases and conditions of the ear.

Otoscope: Instrument for visual examination of the external ear and tympanic membrane.

Ototoxic: Having a poisonous effect on the structures of the ear, particularly the hair cells in the cochlea and vestibular organs.

Outer ear: Peripheral part of the auditory mechanism that includes the pinna, the concha, the external auditory canal, and lateral wall of the tympanic membrane.

Output: Energy or information exiting from a listening device.

Output limiting: Limiting the output of a listening device by means of peak-clipping or compression.

Parallel talk: A language-stimulation technique, wherein an adult matches language to an activity a child is performing.

Passive conversational style: Conversational style of some persons who have hearing loss, characterized by withdrawal from conversation, frequent bluffing, and avoidance of social interactions.

Patient orientation: An orientation centered on the patient's background, current status, needs, and wants, on which the design and delivery of rehabilitative services are based.

Perilingual: In reference to hearing loss, loss acquired during the stage of spoken language acquisition.

Phenotype: Visible expression of a genotype of an individual.

Phoneme: A speech sound.

Phonetic alphabet: Symbols that represent the sounds of a spoken language.

Phonetically balanced word lists: PB word lists; sets of words that contain speech sounds with the same frequency of occurrence as in everyday conversation.

Pinna: Auricle; the cartilaginous structures of the outer ear.

PL 101-336: Americans with Disabilities Act (ADA) of 1990.

PL 101-431: Television Decoder Circuitry Act of 1990.

PL 94-142: Individuals with Disabilities Education Act of 1975.

Place of articulation: Classification of a speech sound according to where in the oral cavity it is produced (e.g., bilabial).

Play audiometry: Behavioral method for testing the hearing thresholds of young children, in which correct identification of a stimulus presentation is rewarded by allowing the child to perform a play-oriented activity.

Plosive: Stop-consonant speech sound that is produced by creating an oral cavity closure, building air pressure behind the closure, and then releasing it (e.g., /p, t, k/).

Postlingual: In reference to hearing loss, loss incurred after the acquisition of spoken language.

Postnatal: After birth.

Pragmatics: The study of how language is used.

Prelingual: In reference to hearing loss, loss is incurred before the acquisition of spoken language.

Presbycusis: Age-related hearing loss.

Prescribed gain: Gain and frequency response of a hearing aid that are determined by use of a prescriptive formula.

Prescriptive hearing-aid fitting: Strategy for fitting hearing aids by using a formula to calculate the desired gain and frequency response; formula incorporates pure-tone audiometric thresholds and, usually, information about uncomfortable loudness levels.

Probe microphone: Microphone transducer that is inserted into the external ear canal for the purpose of measuring sound near the tympanic membrane.

Processing strategy: Strategy used by cochlear implants to determine how the input signal is processed, including the degree of amplification of different frequency bands and the manner in which the signal is delivered by different electrodes in the electrode array; process used to transform the speech signal into a pattern of electrical stimulation.

Program: The setting of a speech processor or hearing aid according to the user's measured thresholds, comfort levels, and other subjective responses to stimulation.

Programmable hearing aid: Hearing aid in which several parameters of the instrument, such as gain, are under computer control.

Progressive: Advancing; occurring over time.

Prosody: Suprasegmental aspects of the speech signal, including fluctuations in voice pitch, rhythm, rate, intensity, and stress patterns; intonation.

Psychic costs: Nonmonetary costs that relate to psychosocial well-being.

PTA: Pure-tone average.

Pure-tone average: PTA: Average of hearing thresholds at 500 Hz, 1000 Hz, and 2000 Hz.

Questionnaires: A procedure to assess conversational fluency and communication handicap, in which respondents provide subjective information about their listening and communication difficulties.

Real-ear gain: Gain of a hearing aid at the tympanic membrane, measured with a probe-microphone; the difference between the SPL in the external ear canal and the SPL at the field reference point for a specified sound field.

Real-time captioning: Captioning of a person's speech in real-time using computer technology.

Real-world practice: The third stage in a communication strategies training exercise, practice of a new skill or behavior in an everyday environment.

Receiver: Component that converts electrical energy into acoustic energy, as in a hearing aid; or component of an FM system worn by the listener that receives FM signals from a transmitter; or individual who receives a message from a sender.

Receptive repair strategy: Tactic taken by an individual when he or she has not understood a message presented by a communication partner.

Rehabilitation: Intervention designed for the reteaching of particular skills.

Reinforcement: Something desirable, such as a sticker or privilege, provided to a student after he or she performs a training activity or behaves in a desired manner.

Reliability: Extent to which a test yields similar results with repeated administration.

Relay system: System used by persons with significant hearing loss to use the telephone; individual contacts a relay operator who serves to transmit messages between caller and person called by means of teletype and/or voice.

Remote control: Hand-held device that permits adjustments in the volume or changes in the program of a programmable hearing aid.

Repair strategies: Tactics implemented by a participant in a conversation to rectify breakdowns in communication.

Residual hearing: The hearing remaining in a person who has hearing loss.

Reverberation: Prolongation of an auditory signal by multiple reflections in a closed environment; amount of echo in an enclosed space.

Role-play: Individuals participate in hypothetical real-world situations.

S/N ratio: Signal-to-noise ratio.

Sales orientation: An orientation to providing rehabilitation services in which emphasis is placed on persuading the patient to pursue and procure services, interventions, and listening devices.

Saturation: Level at which an amplifier no longer provides an increase in output compared to input.

Screening: The use of tests that are quick and easy to administer to a large group for the purpose of identifying individuals who require further diagnostic testing.

SDT: Speech detection threshold.

Seeing Essential English: SEE1; a manual communication system that incorporates some signs of American Sign Language and some English syntax.

Segmental: Pertaining to the sounds of speech.

Self Help for Hard of Hearing People: SHHH; organization for adults who have hearing loss.

Self-talk: Language-stimulation technique in which an adult describes what he or she is doing or thinking for the purpose of promoting language development in a child.

Semantic: Related to meaning, and the relationship between units of language and their referents.

Sender: Individual who presents a message, as opposed to a *receiver*.

Senile: Related to old age.

Sensation level: SL; the intensity level of a sound in dB expressed in reference to the individual's threshold for the sound.

Sensorineural hearing loss: SNHL; hearing loss with a cochlear or retrocochlear origin.

Sign language: System of manual communication in which hand configurations, positions, and movements are used to express concepts and linguistic information.

Signal processing: Manipulation of various parameters of the signal.

Signal-to-noise ratio: S/N ratio; the level of a signal relative to a background of noise, usually expressed in dB.

Signed English: Manual communication system that utilizes English word order and syntax.

Signing Exact English: SEE2; a simplified version of Seeing Essential English.

Silica gel: Agent that absorbs moisture, often used in the storage of hearing aids.

Simultaneous communication: Educational approach used with individuals with severe and profound hearing loss that integrates aural/oral communication and manual communication; total communication.

SL: Sensational level.

SLP: Speech-language pathologist.

SNHL: Sensorineural hearing loss.

Sociolinguistics: The branch of linguistics that concerns the effects of social and cultural differences within a language community on its use of language and conversational patterns.

Sound field: A free-field environment where sound is propagated.

Sound field testing: Determination of hearing sensitivity or speech recognition ability with the stimuli presented through loudspeakers, often used in pediatric testing or hearing-aid evaluations.

Sound level: The intensity of a sound expressed in decibels.

Sound level meter: An instrument designed to measure the intensity of sound in dB according to an accepted standard.

Sound pressure level: SPL; magnitude of sound energy relative to a reference pressure, 0.0002 dynes/cm^2.

Sound-proof: Impenetrable by acoustic energy.

Speech: Coordination of respiration, phonation, articulation, and resonation for the purpose of producing spoken language.

Speech audiometry: Measurement of speech listening skills, including speech awareness and speech recognition.

Speech-language pathology: Professional discipline related to the study, diagnosis, and treatment of speech and language disorders.

Speech reception threshold: SRT; threshold level for speech recognition, that is the lowest presentation level for spondee words at which 50% can be identified correctly.

Speech recognition: The ability to perceive and identify speech units.

Speechreading: Speech recognition using auditory and visual cues.

Speechreading enhancement: The difference or ratio between speech recognition performance in an audition-only condition and an audition-plus-vision condition.

Specific repair strategy: Repair strategy used to rectify a communication breakdown that provides explicit instruction to the communication partner about what to do next.

SPL: Sound pressure level.

Spondee: Two-syllable word with equal stress on each syllable.

Spondee threshold: ST; speech reception threshold.

SRT: Speech reception threshold.

SSPL90: Saturation sound pressure level 90; eletroacoustic assessment of a hearing aid's maximum level of output signal, expressed as a frequency response curve to a 90 dB signal, with the hearing aid volume control set to full-on.

ST: Speech threshold.

Stage of life: Phases in the life cycle, including childhood, young adulthood, middle age, and old age.

Stimulus: Something that can evoke or elicit a response.

Stop consonant: Plosive; speech sound produced by building up air pressure behind a closure in the oral cavity and then releasing it (e.g., /p, t, k/).

Structured communication interaction: Simulated conversation that reflects some of the communication difficulties a person with hearing loss may experience during everyday conversation; for example, TOPICON.

Sudden hearing loss: Hearing loss that is incurred suddenly; acute and rapid onset.

Suprasegmentals: Prosodic aspects of speech; variations in pitch, rate, intensity, and duration superimposed on phonemes and words.

Syndrome: Collection of conditions that co-occur as a result from a single cause and constitute a distinct clinical entity.

Syntax: Word order in a given language.

Synthesized speech: Speech generated by computer.

T-switch: Telecoil switch.

Tactile aid: Vibrotactile aid; aid that transduces sound to vibration and delivers it to the skin for the purpose of sound awareness and gross sound identification.

Target gain: In hearing-aid fitting, the prescribed gain for each frequency against which the actual hearing-aid output is compared.

TDD: Telecommunication device for the deaf.

Telecoil: T coil; induction coil often in a hearing aid that receives electromagnetic signals from a telephone or a loop amplification system.

Telecoil switch: T-switch; switch on a hearing aid that activates the telecoil.

Telecommunication device for the deaf: TDD; TT (text telephone); TTY; telephone device for persons with deafness or significant hearing loss in which messages are typed on a keyboard; transmitted over telephone wires, and displayed on a small monitor screen.

Telegraphic speech: Spoken language patterns that are characterized by the omission of function words and, sometimes, incorrect word order.

Telephone amplifier: Assistive listening device designed to increase the intensity of a signal emanating from a telephone receiver.

Television Decoder Circuitry Act: U.S. Public Law 101-336 of 1990; act that requires all televisions with a 13-inch diagonal screen or wider to contain circuitry necessary for closed captioning.

Temporary threshold shift: TTS; transient hearing loss following exposure to excessive noise.

Test-retest reliability: Measure of test consistency from one presentation to the next.

3-dB rule: Time-intensity tradeoff that states for every 50% decrease in noise-exposure, a 3 dB-A increase in noise level is permitted without increasing the risk of noise-induced hearing loss.

Threshold: Level at which a stimulus or change in a stimulus can just be detected.

Threshold shift: Change in hearing sensitivity expressed in dB.

Time-compressed speech: Speech that has been accelerated by means of removing segments from the waveform and compressing the remaining segments together, without changing its frequency composition.

Time-talk: A language-stimulation techniques wherein an adult purposely incorporates time-related language into conversation.

Time-weighted average: TWA; index of daily noise exposure that is the product of durations of exposure relative to the allowable durations of exposure for a particular sound level.

Tinnitus: Sensation of noise in the head without an external cause.

Tinnitus masker: Electronic hearing aid that generates and outputs noise at low levels for the purpose of masking an individual's tinnitus.

Transmitter: A device that emits electromagnetic rays; a component of an FM system that modulates the frequency of a radio signal in an audio frequency signal and transmits the waves through air to an amplifier/receiver.

TT: Text telephone; TDD.

TTS: Temporary threshold shift.

TTY: Teletypewriter; less-frequently used term than TDD or TT.

Tune-up: Mapping; establishing a map for a cochlear implant speech processor.

TWA: Time-weighted average.

Tx: Therapy or treatment.

Tympanogram: Graph of middle ear immittance as a function of air pressure in the external auditory canal.

UCL: Uncomfortable loudness.

UL: Uncomfortable level.

ULL: Uncomfortable loudness level.

Uncomfortable level: UL; level at which sound is judged to be so loud as to be uncomfortable to the listener.

Uncomfortable loudness level: ULL; UCL; intensity level at which a listener judges a sound to be uncomfortably loud; loudness discomfort level.

Unilateral: Pertaining to one side.

Unisensory: Unimodal; used to referred to an educational philosophy in which stimulation is presented primarily through the auditory modality.

Use gain: Amount of gain provided by a hearing aid when the volume control is set where it is commonly used.

Vent: Bore drilled into an earmold that permits the passage of sound and air; used for aeration of the external auditory canal or for acoustic modification of the amplified sound.

Vertigo: Dizziness, including a sensation of spinning or whirling.

Vibrotactile: Pertaining to the detection of vibrations through the sense of touch.

Vibrotactile hearing aid: An assistive listening device that converts acoustic energy into vibratory patterns that are delivered to the skin.

Videotaped scenarios: Videotaped examples of communication interactions, which may include use of communications strategies and language-stimulation techniques.

Viseme: Groups of speech sounds that appear identical on the lips (e.g., /p, m, b/).

Visual alerting systems: Assistive devices that include alarm clocks, doorbells, and smoke detectors in which the alerting mechanism is a flashing light.

Visual reinforcement audiometry: VRA; audiometric technique used with young children in which a correct response to a stimulus presentation is reinforced by a visual reward, such as the activation of a lighted toy.

Volume control: Manual or automatic control used to adjust the output of a listening device.

Voicing: Classification of a speech sound according to whether it is produced with or without voice (e.g., /b/ versus /p/).

VRA: Visual reinforcement audiometry.

Weighting scale: Sound level meter filtering network, in which the measurement of one band of frequencies is emphasized over another (e.g., dBA scale).

White noise: Noise having energy at all frequencies audible to the human ear.

Wide-band noise: White noise.

Wireless system: An assistive listening device in which wires are not necessary to connect the sound source to the listener; includes FM and infrared systems.

Word recognition: Ability to perceive and identify a word.

Word-recognition score: Percent words correct.

References

Adam, A. J., Fortier, P., Schiel, G., Smith, M., Soland, C., & Stone, P. (1990). *Listening to learn: A handbook for parents with hearing-impaired children.* Washington, DC: Alexander Graham Bell Association for the Deaf.

Albers, A. (1970). *The world of sound.* New York, NY: A. S. Barnes and Company.

Alcantara, J. I., Cowan, R. S. C., Blamey, P. J., & Clark, G. M. (1990). A comparison of two training strategies for speech recognition with an electrotactile speech processor. *Journal of Speech and Hearing Research, 33,* 195–204.

Allen, T. E. (1986). Patterns of academic achievement among hearing impaired students: 1974 and 1983. In A. N. Schildroth & M. A. Karchmer (Eds.), *Deaf children in America* (pp. 161–206). San Diego, CA: College-Hill Press.

Allen, W. (1998). WU leads quest to map genetic code. *St. Louis Post Dispatch,* No.19, 1.

Alpiner, J. G., & Garstecki, D. C. (1996). Audiologic rehabilitation for adults: Assessment and management. In R. L. Schow & M. A. Nerbonne (Eds.), *Introduction to audiologic rehabilitation* (3rd ed., pp. 361–412). Needham Heights, MA: Allyn and Bacon.

Anders, G. (1997). Doctors learn to bridge cultural gaps. *The Wall Street Journal* Sep 4, n177.

Andrews, J. R., & Andrews, M. A. (1990). *Family based treatment in communication disorders: A systemic approach.* Sandwich, IL: Janelle Publications, Inc.

Angelocci, A., Kopp, G., & Holbrook, A. (1964). The vowel formants of deaf and normal-hearing eleven to fourteen year old boys. *Journal of Speech and Hearing Disorders, 29,* 156–170.

Arana-Ward, M. (1997). As technology advances, a bitter debate divides the deaf. *Washington Post,* May 11, A1.

Armstrong, T.L. (1991). The relationship between gender and psychological distress in hard-of-hearing people. Paper presented to the American Public Health Association, Washington, D.C.

Axelsson, A., & Clark, W. W. (1995). Hearing conservation programs: Nonserved occupations/populations. In T. Morata & D. Dunn (Eds.), *Occupational hearing loss: State of the art reviews* (Vol. 10, pp. 657–663). Philadelphia, PA: Hanley and Belfus.

Bellis, T. J. (1996). *Assessment and management of central auditory processing disorders in the educational setting: From science to practice.* San Diego, CA: Singular Publishing Group.

Bench, J., & Bamford, J. (1979). *Speech-hearing tests and the spoken language of hearing-impaired children.* London, England: Academic Press.

Benguerel, A. P., & Pichora-Fuller, K. (1982). Coarticulation effects in lipreading. *Journal of Speech and Hearing Research, 25,* 600–607.

Berger, K. W. (1972). *Speechreading: Principles and methods.* Baltimore, MD: National Education Press.

Berko, J. (1984). The child's learning of English morphology. *Word, 14,* 150–177.

Bernstein, L. E., Demorest, M. E., Coulter, D. C., & O'Connell, M. P. (1991). Lipreading sentences with vibrotactile vocoders: Performance of normal-hearing and hearing-impaired subjects. *Journal of the Acoustical Society of America, 90,* 29712984.

Berry, S. (1981). *Written Language Syntax Test.* Washington, DC: Gallaudet College Press.

Binnie, C. A. (1991). New perspectives in audiological rehabilitation. In G. A. Studebaker, F. H. Bess, & L. B. Beck (Eds.), *The Vanderbilt Hearing-aid Report II* (pp. 233–243). Parkton, MD: York Press.

Binnie, C. A. (1994). The future of audiological rehabilitation: Overview and forecast. *Journal of the Academy of Rehabilitative Audiology, 27*(Suppl.), 1324.

Binnie, C. A., Montgomery, A. A., & Jackson, P. L. (1974). Auditory and visual contribution to the perception of consonants. *Journal of Speech and Hearing Research, 17,* 619–630.

Blair, J., Petersen, M., & Viehweg, S. (1985). The effects of mild hearing loss on academic performance of young schoolage children. *Volta Review, 87,* 87–93.

Blamey, P. J., & Alcantara, J. I. (1994). Research in auditory training. *Journal of the Academy of Rehabilitative Audiology, 27*(Suppl.), 161–192.

Blood, G. W., Blood, I. M., & Danhauer, J. L. (1978). Listeners' impression of normal-hearing and hearing-impaired children. *Journal of Communication Disorders, 11,* 513–518.

Boone, D. (1977). *The voice and voice therapy* (2nd ed.). Englewood Cliffs, NJ: Prentice-Hall.

Boothroyd, A. (1984). Auditory perception of speech contrasts by subjects with sensorineural hearing loss. *Journal of Speech and Hearing Research, 27,* 134144.

Boothroyd, A. (1991). Assessment of speech perception capacity in profoundly deaf children. *The American Journal of Otology, 12*(Suppl.), 67–72.

Brackett, D. (1990). Developing an individualized education program for the mainstreamed hearing-impaired student. In M. Ross (Ed.), *Hearing-impaired children in the mainstream* (pp. 81–94). Parkton, MD: York Press.

Brainerd, S. H., & Frankel, B. G. (1985). The relationship between audiometric and selfreport measures of hearing handicap. *Ear and Hearing, 6,* 89–92.

Bransford, J. D., & Franks, J. J. (1979). The abstraction of linguistic ideas. *Cognitive Psychology, 2,* 331–350.

Bromwich, R. (1981). *Working with parents and infants: An interactional approach.* Baltimore, MD: University Park Press.

Broadcaster. (1991). Cochlear Implants in Children: A position paper of the National Association of the Deaf. Silver Springs, MD: National Association of the Deaf.

Brooks, D. N. (1990). Measures for the assessment of hearing aid provision and rehabilitation. *British Journal of Audiology, 24,* 229–233.

Byrne, D., & Dillon, H. (1986). The National Acoustic Laboratories (NAL) new procedure for selecting the gain and frequency response of a hearing aid. *Ear and Hearing, 7,* 257–265.

Caissie, R., & Rockwell, E. (1994). Communication difficulties experienced by nursing home residents with a hearing loss during conversation with staff members. *Journal of Speech-Language Pathology and Audiology, 18,*127–134.

Carhart, R. (1960). Auditory training. In H. Davis & R. Silverman (Eds.), *Hearing and deafness* (2nd ed., pp. 346–359). New York, NY: Holt, Rinehart and Winston.

Carney, A., & Moeller, M. P. (1998). Treatment efficacy: Hearing loss in children. *Journal of Speech, Language, and Hearing Research, 41*(Suppl.), S61–S84.

Carrow, E. (1973). *Test for Auditory Comprehension of Language.* Lamar, TX: Learning Concepts.

Castle, D. (1988). The oral interpreter. *Volta Review, 90,* 307–313.

Cheesman, M. G. (1997). Speech perception by elderly listeners: Basic knowledge and implications for audiology. *Journal of Speech-Language Pathology and Audiology, 21.*

Cherry, R., & Rubinstein, A. (1988). Speechreading instruction for adults: Issues and practices. *Volta Review, 90,* 289–306.

Clark, J. G. (1994). Understanding, building and maintaining relationships with patients. *Effective counseling in audiology: Perspectives and practice* (pp. 18–37). Englewood Cliffs, NJ: PrenticeHall.

Clark, T. (1994). SKI*HI: Applications for home-based intervention. In J. Rousch & N. Matkin (Eds.), *Infants and toddlers with hearing loss: Family-centered assessment and intervention* (pp. 237–251). Baltimore, MD: York Press.

Clark, W. W. (1991). Noise exposure and hearing loss from leisure-time activities: A review. *Journal of the Acoustical Society of America, 90,* 175–181.

Code of Ethics. (1984). In W. H. Northcott (Ed.), *Oral interpreting: Principles and practices* (pp. 266–269). Baltimore, MD: University Park Press.

Cole, E. B. (1993). *Listening and talking: A guide to promoting spoken language in young hearing-impaired children.* Washington, DC: Alexander Graham Bell Association for the Deaf.

Compton, C. L. (1995). Selecting what's best for the individual. In R. S. Tyler & D. J. Schum (Eds.), *Assistive devices for persons with hearing impairment* (pp. 224–250). Needham Heights, Md: Allyn and Bacon.

Cornett, R. O. (1967). Cued speech. *American Annals of the Deaf, 112,* 313.

Cowie, R., & Douglas-Cowie, E. (1992). *Postlingually acquired deafness: Speech deterioration and the wider consequences.* New York, NY: Mouton de Gruyter.

Cox, R. M., & Alexander, G. C. (1991). Hearing aid benefit in everyday environments. *Ear and Hearing, 12,* 127–139.

Cox, R. M., Alexander, G., & Gilmore, C. (1987). Development of the Connected Speech Test (CST). *Ear and Hearing, 8* 1195–1265.

Craig, W. N. (1964). Effects of preschool training on the development of reading and lipreading skills of deaf children. *American Annals of the Deaf, 109,* 280–296.

Cunningham, W. R., & Brookbank, J. W. (1988). *Gerontology: The psychology, biology, and sociology of aging.* New York: Harper and Row.

Dagenais, P., & Critz-Crosby, P. (1992). Comparing tongue positioning by normal hearing and hearing-impaired children during vowel production. *Journal of Speech and Hearing Research, 35,* 5–44.

Daly, N., Bench, J., & Chappell, H. (1996). Gender differences in speechreadability. *Journal of the Academy of Rehabilitative Audiology, 29,* 27–40.

Dancer, J., Krain, M., Thompson, C., Davis, P., & Glenn, J. (1994). A crosssectional investigation of speechreading in adults: Effects of gender, practice, and education. *Volta Review, 96,* 31–40.

Danhauer, J. L., Johnson, C. E., Kasten, R. N., & Brimacombe, J. A. (1985, March). The hearing aid effect: Summary, conclusions and recommendations. *The Hearing Journal,* pp. 12–14.

Davis, H., & Silverman, R. (1978). *Hearing and deafness* (4th ed.). New York, NY: Holt Rinehart, and Winston.

Davis, J. M. (Ed.). (1990). *Our forgotten children: Hard-of-hearing pupils in the schools* (2nd ed.). Washington, DC: SelfHelp for the Hard of Hearing.

DeFillipo, C. L., & Scott, B. L. (1978). A method for hearing and evaluating the reception of ongoing speech. *Journal of the Acoustical Society of America, 63,* 1186–1192.

DeFillipo, C. L., Sims, D. G., & Gottermeier, L. (1995). Linking visual and kinesthetic imagery in lipreading instruction. *Journal of Speech and Hearing Research, 38,* 244–256.

Demorest, M. E., & Erdman, S. A. (1987). Development of the Communication Profile for the Hearing Impaired. *Journal of Speech and Hearing Disorders, 52,* 129–143.

Demorest, M. E., & Walden, B. E. (1984). Psychometric principles in the selection, interpretation, and evaluation of communication self-assessment inventories. I *Journal of Speech and Hearing Disorders, 54,* 180–188.

Deno, E. (1970). The cascade of special education services. *Exceptional Children, 39,* 495.

Dorman, M. (1993). Speech perception by adults. In R. S. Tyler (Ed.), *Cochlear implants: Audiological foundations* (pp. 145–190). San Diego, CA: Singular Publishing Group, Inc.

Dowell, R., Brown, A., & Mecklenburg, D. (1990). Clinical assessment of implanted deaf adults. In G. Clark, Y. Tong, & J. Patrick (Eds.), *Cochlear prostheses* (pp. 193–206). Edinburgh: Churchill Livingstone.

Downs, M. (1974). Deafness Management Quotient (DMQ). *Hearing and Speech News, 42,* 26–28.

Dunn, L., & Dunn, L. (1981). *Peabody Picture Vocabulary Test—Revised.* Circle Pines, MN: American Guidance Service.

Dunst, C. (1985). Rethinking early intervention. *Analysis and Intervention in Developmental Disabilities, 5,* 165–201.

Elfenbein, J. (1994a). Communication breakdowns in conversations: Childinitiated repair strategies. In N. TyeMurray (Ed.), *Let's converse: A how-to guide to develop and expand the conversational skills of children and teenagers who are hearing impaired* (pp. 123–146). Washington DC: Alexander Graham Bell Association for the Deaf.

Elfenbein, J. (1994b). Children who are hard of hearing. In J. B. Tomblin, H. L. Morris, & D. C. Spriestersbach (Eds.), *Diagnosis in speech-language pathology* (pp. 403424). San Diego, CA: Singular Publishing Group.

Elfenbein, J., Hardin-Jones, M., & Davis, J. (1994). Oral communication skills of hard of hearing children. *Journal of Speech and Hearing Research, 37,* 216217.

Elliott, L., & Katz, D. (1980). *Development of a new children's test of speech discrimination.* St. Louis, MO: Audiotec.

Engen, E., & Engen, T. (1983). *Rhode Island Test of Language Structure Manual.* Baltimore, MD: University Park Press.

Erber, N. P. (1974). Visual perception of speech by deaf children: Recent developments and continuing needs. *Journal of Speech and Hearing Disorders, 39,* 178–185.

Erber, N. P. (1978). *Communication therapy for hearing-impaired adults.* Melbourne, Australia: Clavis Publishing.

Erber, N. P. (1982). *Auditory training.* Washington, DC: Alexander Graham Bell Association for the Deaf.

Erber, N. P. (1992). Adaptive screening of sentence perception in older adults. *Ear and Hearing, 13,* 58–60.

Erber, N. P. (1996). *Communication therapy for adults with sensory loss* (2nd ed.). Melbourne, Australia: Clavis Publishing.

Erber, N. P., & Lind, C. (1994). Communication therapy: Theory and practice. *Journal of the Academy of Rehabilitative Audiology, 27*(Suppl.), 267–287.

Erdman, S. A. (1993). Counseling hearing impaired adults. In J. Alpiner & P. McCarthy (Eds.), *Rehabilitative audiology: Children and adults* (2nd ed., pp. 74–416). Baltimore, MD: Williams and Wilkins.

Erdman, S. A. (1994). Self-assessment: From research focus to research tool. *Journal of the Academy of Rehabilitative Audiology, 27*(Suppl.), 67–92.

Eriksson-Mangold, M., & Carlsson, S. G. (1991). Psychological and somatic distress in relation to hearing disability, hearing handicap, and hearing measurements. *Journal of Psychosomatic Research, 35,* 729–740.

Estabrooks, W. (1994). *Auditory-verbal therapy.* Washington, DC: Alexander Graham Bell Association for the Deaf.

Farrimond, T. (1959). Age differences in the ability to use visual codes in auditory communication. *Language and Speech, 2,* 179.

Feinmesser, M., Tell, L., & Levi, H. (1982). Follow-up of 40,000 infants screened for hearing defect. *Audiology, 21,*197–203.

Fey, M. E., Warr-Leeper, G., Webber, S. A., & Disher, L. M. (1988). Repairing children's repairs: Evaluation and facilitation of children's clarification requests and responses. *Topics in Language Disorders, 8,* 63–84.

Fisher, C. G. (1968). Confusions among visually perceived consonants. *Journal of Speech and Hearing Research, 11,* 796800.

Flexor, C. (1994). Facilitating hearing and listening in young children. San Diego, CA: Singular Publishing Group.

Flexor, C. (1997). Sound-field FM systems: Questions most often asked about classroom amplification. *Hearsay, 11,* 514.

Forner, L., & Hixon, T. (1977). Respiratory kinematics in profoundly hearingimpaired speakers. *Journal of Speech and Hearing Research, 66,* 373–408.

Fryauf-Bertschy, H., Tyler, R., Kelsay, D., Gantz, B., & Woodworth, B. (1997). Cochlear implant use by prelingually deafened children: The influences of age at implant and length of device use. *Journal of Speech Hearing Language Research, 40,* 183–199.

Gagne, J. P., Dinon, D., & Parsons, J. (1991). An evaluation of CAST: A computer-aided speechreading training program. *Journal of Speech and Hearing Research, 34,* 213–221.

Gagne, J. P., Stelmacovich, P., & Youetich, W. (1991). Reactions to requests for clarification used by hearing-impaired individuals. *Volta Review, 93,*129–143.

Gagne, J. P., Tugby, K. G., & Michoud, J.. (1991). Development of a speechreading test on the utilization of contextual cues (STUCC): Preliminary findings with normal-hearing subjects. *Journal of the Academy of Rehabilitative Audiology, 24,* 157–170.

Gagne, J. P., & Wyllie, K. M. (1989). Relative effectiveness of three repair strategies on the visual-identification of misperceived words. *Ear and Hearing, 10,* 368–374.

Garahan, M. B., Waller, J. A., Houghton, M., Tisdale, W. A., & Runge, C. F. (1992). Hearing loss prevalence and management in nursing home residents. *Journal of the American Geriatric Society, 40,* 130134.

Geers, A. E., & Moog, J. S. (1987). Predicting spoken language acquisition in profoundly deaf children. *Journal of Speech and Hearing Disorders, 52,* 84–94.

Geers, A. E., & Moog, J. S. (1992). Speech perception and production skills of students with impaired hearing from oral and total communication education settings. *Journal of Speech and Hearing Research, 35,*1384–1393.

Geers, A. E., & Moog, J. S. (1994). Description of the CID study. *Volta Review, 96,*1–14.

Geers, A., Moog, J., & Schick, B. (1984). Acquisition of spoken and signed English by profoundly deaf children. *Journal of Speech and Hearing Disorders, 49,* 378–388.

Gfeller, K., & Schum, R. (1994). Requisites for conversation: Engendering world knowledge. In N. Tye-Murray (Ed.), *Let's converse: A how-to-guide to develop and expand conversational skills of children and teenagers who are hearing impaired* (pp. 177–212). Washington, DC: Alexander Graham Bell Association for the Deaf.

Giolas, T.G. and Kaplan, H. (1997). Special populations. *Seminars in Hearing,* 18, 199–214.

Glennon, S. L. (1990). Homework activities for social skills training. In P. J. Schloss & M. A. Smith (Eds.), *Teaching social skills to hearing–impaired students* (pp. 85–90). Washington, DC: Alexander Graham Bell Association for the Deaf.

Goldman, R., & Fristoe, M. (1969). *Test of Articulation.* Circle Pines, MN: American Guidance Service.

Gordon-Salant, S. (1987). Consonant recognition and confusion patterns among elderly hearing-impaired subjects. *Ear and Hearing, 8,* 270–276.

Gorlin, R., Toriello, H., & Cohen, M. M. (1995). *Hereditary hearing loss and its syndromes.* [Oxford Monographs on Medical Genetics, No. 28]. New York, NY: Oxford University Press.

Greenberg, M. (1983). Family stress and child competence: The effects of early intervention for families with deaf infants. *American Annals of the Deaf, 128,* 407–417.

Greenberg, M. T., Calderon, R., & Kusche, C. (1984). Early intervention using simultaneous communication with deaf infants: The effects on communicative development. *Child Development, 55,* 607–616.

Greenburg, J. H., & Jenkins, J. J. (1964). Studies in the psychological correlates of the sound system of American English. *Word, 20,* 157–177.

Greenstein, J. (1975). *Methods of fostering language development in deaf infants: Final report (BBB00581).* Washington, DC: Bureau of Education for the Handicapped (DHEW/OE).

Grice, H. P. (1975). Logic and conversation. In P. Cole & J. L. Morgan (Eds.), *Syntax and semantics (3): Speech acts* (pp. 6475). New York, NY: Academic Press.

Groher, M. E. (1989). Modifications in assessment and treatment for the communicatively impaired elderly. In R. Hull & K. Griffin (Eds.), *Communication disorders in aging* (pp. 50–72). Newbury Park, CA: Sage.

Gudmundsen, G. I. (1997). Physical options. In H. Tobin (Ed.), *Practical hearing aid selection and fitting* (pp. 1–16). Washington, DC: Department of Veterans Affairs.

Hanin, L. (1988). *The effects of experience and linguistic context on speechreading.* Unpublished doctoral dissertation, The City University Graduate School, New York, NY.

Haskins, H. A. (1949). *A phonetically balanced test of speech discrimination for children.* Unpublished master's thesis, Northwestern University, Evanston, IL.

Hastenstab, M. S., & Tobey, E. A. (1991). Language development in children receiving Nucleus multichannel cochlear implants. *Ear and Hearing, 12,* 55S–65S.

Haycock, G. S. (1933). *The teaching of speech.* Washington DC: Alexander Graham Bell Association for the Deaf.

Hazard, W. R., Andres, R., Bierman, E. L., & Blass, J. P. (1990). *Principles of geriatric medicine and gerontology* (2nd ed.). New York, NY: McGraw Hill, Inc.

Hazell, J.W. (1990). Tinnitus, III: The practical management of sensorineural tinnitus. *Journal of Otolaryngology, 19,* 11–18.

Hearing Journal, The. (1991). A timeline of the hearing industry. *The Hearing Journal, 50,* 54–72.

Heider, F., & Heider, G. (1940). An experimental investigation of lip reading. *Psychological Monographs,* 232,1–153.

Heller, P. J. (1990). Psycho-educational assessment. In M. Ross (Ed.), *Hearing-impaired children in the mainstream* (pp. 45–60). Baltimore, MD: York Press.

Hé tu, R. (1996). The stigma attached to hearing impairment. *Scandinavian Audiology,* 43, 12–24.

Hé tu, R., Reverin, L., Getty, O. L., Lalande, N. M., & St-Cyr, C. (1990). The reluctance toacknowledge hearing difficulties among hearing-impaired workers. *British Journal of Audiology, 24,* 265–276.

Hirsch, H. V. B., & Spinelli, D. N. (1970). Visual experience modifies distribution of horizontally and vertically oriented receptive fields in cats. *Science, 168,* 869–871.

Hirsh, I. J., Davis, H., Silverman, S. R., Reynolds, E. G., Eldert, E., & Benson, R. W. (1952). Development of materials for speech audiometry. *Journal of Speech and Hearing Disorders, 17,* 321–337.

Honnell, S., Dancer, J., & Gentry, B. (1991). Age and speechreading performance in relation to percent correct, eyeblinks, and written responses. *Volta Review, 93,* 207–231.

Houle, C. O. (1997). *Governing boards.* San Franciso, CA: Jossey-Bass Publishers.

Hudgins, C., & Numbers, F. (1942). An investigation of the intelligibility of speech of the deaf. *Genetic Psychological Monographs, 25,* 289–392.

Hull, R. H. (1995). *Hearing in aging.* San Diego, CA: Singular Publishing Group, Inc.

Humes, L. E. (1996). Speech understanding in the elderly. *Journal of the American Academy of Audiology, 7,* 161–167.

Hutchinson, J., & Smith, L. (1976). Aerodynamic functioning in consonant production by hearing-impaired adults. *Audiology Hearing Education, 2,* 16–19.

IBM. (1988). IBM Personal System/2 Independence Series. *Speech Viewer Application Software User's Guide.* Boca Raton, FL: IBM.

Itoh, M., Horii, Y., Daniloff, R., & Binnie, C. (1982). Selected aerodynamic characteristics of deaf individuals' various speech and nonspeech tasks. *Folia Phoniatrica, 34,* 191–209.

Jackson, P.L. (1992). A psychological and economic profile of the hearing impaired and deaf. In R.H. Hull (Ed.) Aural rehabilitation (2nd Ed.), San Diego, CA: Singular Publishing Group, 42–49.

Jastreboff, P.J. (1990). Phantom auditory perception (tinnitus): Mechanisms of generation and perception. *Neuroscience Research, 8,* 221–254.

Jastreboff, P.J., Gray, W.C. & Gold, S.L. (1996). Neurophysiological approach to tinnitus patients. *American Journal of Otology.*

Jeffers, J., & Barley, M. (1971). *Speechreading (lipreading).* Springfield, IL: Charles C. Thomas.

Jensema, C., & Trybus, R. (1978). *Communication patterns and educational achievement of hearing impaired students* (Series T, No. 2). Washington, DC: Gallaudet College, Office of Demographic Studies.

Jerger, J., Chmiel, R., Wilson, N., & Luchi, R. (1996). Hearing impairment in older adults: New concepts. *Journal of the American Geriatrics Society, 43,* 928935.

John, J., & Howarth, J. (1976). The effect of time distortions on the intelligibility of deaf children's speech. *Language and Speech, 8,* 127–134.

Johnson, D. D. (1975). Communication characteristics of NTID students. *Journal of the Academy of Rehabilitative Audiology, 8,* 17–32.

Johnson, S. M., & Wilhite, G. (1971). Selfobservation as an agent of behavioral change. *Behavior Therapy, 2,* 488–497.

Jones, L., Kyle, J. and Wood, P. (1987). Words apart: Losing your hearing as an adult. NY: Tavistock Publications.

Kalikow, D., Stevens, K., & Elliott, L. (1977). Development of a test of speech intelligibility in noise using sentence materials with controlled word predictability. *Journal of the Acoustical Society of America, 61,* 1337–1351.

Kaplan, H. (1996). Assistive devices for the elderly. *Journal of the American Academy of Audiology, 7,* 203–211.

Kaplan, H., Bally, S. J., & Garretson, C. (1985). *Speechreading: A way to improve understanding.* Washington DC: Gallaudet University Press.

Kaufman, L. (1979). *Perception: The world transformed.* New York, NY: Oxford University Press.

Kichkin, S. (1992). MarkeTrak III. Higher hearing aid sales don't signal better market penetration. *The Hearing Journal, 45,* 47–54.

Kinsella-Meier, M.A. (1996). The process of communication therapy. In M.J. Mosely and S.J. Bally (Eds.) *Communication therapy: An integrated approach to aural rehabilitation,* Washington, D.C.: Gallaudet University Press, 3–23.

Kirchner, R., & Peterson, R. (1980). Multiple impairments among noninstitutionalized blind and visually impaired persons. *Journal of Visual Impairment and Blindness, 74,* 42–44.

Kirk, K. I., Pisoni, D. B., & Osberger, M. J. (1995). Lexical effects on spoken word recognition by pediatric cochlear implant users. *Ear and Hearing, 16,* 470–481.

Knutson, J. F., & Lansing, C. R. (1990). The relationship between communication problems and psychological difficulties in persons with profound acquired hearing loss. Journal of Speech and Hearing Disorders, 55, 656–664.

Kochkin, S. (1997). Professional forum. *Hearing Health, 13,* 21–22.

Kotler, P. H., & Andreasen, A. R. (1996). *Strategic marketing for nonprofit organizations* (5th ed.). Upper Saddle River, NJ: Prentice-Hall.

Kozak, V., & Brooks, B. (1995). *Baby talk.* Unpublished manuscript.

Kravitz, L., & Selekman, J. (1992). Understanding hearing loss in children. *Pediatric Nursing, 18,* 591–594.

Kretschmer, R., & Kretschmer, L. (1978). *Language development and intervention with the hearing impaired.* Baltimore, MD: University Park Press.

Kricos, P. B., & Holmes, A. E. (1996). Efficacy of audiologic rehabilitation for older adults. *Journal of the American Academy of Audiology, 7,* 219–229.

Kricos, P. B., Lesner, S. A., Sandridge, S. A., & Yanke, R. B. (1987). Perceived benefits of amplification as a function of central auditory status in the elderly. *Ear and Hearing, 8,* 337–342.

Kryter, K. D. (1996). *Handbook of hearing and the effects of noise.* New York, NY: Academic Press.

Kuhl, P. K., & Meltzoff, A. N. (1982). The bimodal perception of speech in infancy. *Science, 218,* 1138–1141.

Kyle, J.G., Jones, L.G., and Wood, P.L. (1985). Adjustment to acquired hearing loss: A working model. In H. Orlans (Ed.) *Adjustment to adult hearing loss,* San Diego, CA: College Hill Press.

Lach, R., Ling, D., Ling, L., & Ship, N. (1970). Early speech development in deaf infants. *American Annals of the Deaf, 115,* 522–526.

Lalonde, N.M., Lambert, J. and Riverin, L. (1988). Qualification of the psychosocial disadvantages experienced by workers in a noisy industry and their nearest relatives: Perspectives for rehabilitation. *Audiology, 27,* 196–206.

Lane, H. (1990). *When the mind hears: A history of the deaf.* New York, NY: Random House.

Lane, H. (1984). *When the mind hears: A history of the deaf* New York, NY: Random House.

Lansing, C. R., & Davis, J. M. (1988). Early versus delayed speech perception training for adult cochlear implant users: Initial results. *Journal of the Academy of Rehabilitative Audiology, 21,* 29–41.

Lansing, C. R., & Helgeson, C. L. (1995). Priming the visual recognition of spoken words. *Journal of Speech and Hearing Research, 38,* 1377–1386.

Lee, L. (1974). *Developmental Sentence Analysis.* Evanston, IL: Northwestern University Press.

Lesner, K., Sandridge, S., & Kricos, P. (1987). Training influences on visual consonant and sentence recognition. *Ear and Hearing, 8,* 283–287.

Lesner, S. (1996). Group hearing care for older adults. In P. Kricos & S. Lesner (Eds.), *Hearing care for the older adult: Audiologic rehabilitation* (pp. 203–277). Newton, MA: Butterworth-Heinemann.

Levitt, H. (1987). *Fundamental Speech Skills Test.* New York, NY: City University of New York.

Levitt, H., McGarr, N. S., & Geffner, D. (Eds.). (1987). *Development of language and communication skills in hearingimpaired children.* Washington, DC: ASHA.

Lindblade, D. D., & McDonald, M. (1995). Removing communication barriers for the hearing-impaired elderly. *Medsurgery Nursing, 4,* 370–385.

Ling, D. (1976). *Speech and the hearingimpaired child: Theory and practice.* Washington, DC: Alexander Graham Bell Association for the Deaf.

Luterman, D. (1979). *Counseling parents of hearing-impaired children.* Boston, MA: Little, Brown, and Co.

Luterman, D., & Ross, M. (1991). *When your child is deaf.* Parkton, MD: York Press.

Luxford, W. M., & Brackmann, D. E. (1985). The history of cochlear implants. In R. F. Gray (Ed.), *Cochlear implants* (pp. 1–26). San Diego, CA: College-Hill Press, Inc.

Lynch, E. D., Lee, M. K., Morrow, J. E., Welcsh, P. L., Leon, P. E., & King, M. C. (1997). Nonsyndromic deafness DFNA1 associated with mutation of a human homolog of the drosophila gene diaphanous. *Science, 278,* 1315–1318.

Mahshie, S. N. (1995). *Educating deaf children bilingually.* Washington, DC: Gallaudet University Pre-College Programs.

Markides, A. (1970). The speech of deaf and partially hearing children with special reference to factors affecting intelligibility. *British Journal of Disordered Communication, 5,* 126–140.

Markides, A. (1988). Speech intelligibility: Auditory-oral approach versus total communication. *Journal of the British Association for Teachers of the Deaf, 12,* 136–141.

Marler, P. (1989). Learning by instinct: Birdsong. *Asha, 31,* 75–79.

Marmor, G., & Petitito, L. (1979). Simultaneous communication in the classroom: How well is English Grammar represented? In W. Tokoe (Ed.), *Sign language studies.* Silver Spring, MD: Linstok Press.

Massaro, D. W. (1987). *Speech perception by ear and eye: A paradigm for psychological inquiry.* Hillsdale, NJ: Lawrence Erlbaum Associates.

Mauze, E., & Frederick, E. (1995). *Communication-based aural rehabilitation class for hearing-impaired adults.* St. Louis, MO: Central Institute for the Deaf.

McFadden, K. (1982). *Tinnitus: Facts, theories, and treatments.* Washington, D.C.: National Academy Press.

McFall, R. M. (1970). Effects of selfmonitoring on normal smoking behavior. *Journal of Consulting and Clinical Psychology, 35,* 135–142.

McGarr, N. (1987). Communication skills of hearing-impaired children in schools for the deaf. In H. Levitt, N. McGarr, & D. Geffner (Eds.), Development of language and communication in hearing-impaired children. *ASHA Monographs, 26,* 91–107.

McGarr, N., & Lofqvist, A. (1982). Obstruent production in hearing-impaired speakers: Interarticulator timing and acoustics. *Journal of the Acoustical Society of America, 72,* 34–42.

McGurk, H., & MacDonald, J. (1976). Hearing lips and seeing voices. *Nature, 264,* 746–748.

Metz, D., Whitehead, R., & Whitehead, B. (1984). Mechanics of vocal fold vibration and laryngeal articulatory gestures produced by hearing-impaired speakers. *Journal of Speech and Hearing Research, 27,* 62–69.

Miller, G. A., & Nicely, P. E. (1955). An analysis of perceptual confusions among some English consonants. *Journal of the Acoustical Society of America, 27,* 338–352.

Monsen, R. (1976). The production of English stop consonants in the speech of deaf children. *Journal of Phonetics, 4,* 29–42.

Monsen, R. (1978). Toward measuring how well hearing-impaired children speak. *Journal of Speech and Hearing Research, 21,* 197–219.

Montgomery, A. A. (1994). WATCH: A practical approach to brief auditory rehabilitation. *The Hearing Journal, 10,* 10–55.

Montgomery, A., & Demorest, M. (1988). Issues and developments in the evaluation of speechreading. *Volta Review, 90,* 119–148.

Moog, J., Biedenstein, J., & Davidson, L. (1995). *The SPICE.* St. Louis, MO: Central Institute for the Deaf.

Moog, J. S., & Geers, A. E. (1975). *Scales of early communication skills for hearing impaired chidren.* St. Louis, MO: Central Institute for the Deaf.

Moog, J., & Geers, A. (1979). *Grammatical Analysis of Elicited Language: Simple Sentence Level.* St. Louis, MO: Central Institute for the Deaf.

Moog, J. S., Kozak, V. J., & Geers, A. (1983). *Grammatical Analysis of Elicited Language (GAEL-p).* St. Louis, MO: Central Institute for the Deaf.

Moores, D. F. (1992). An historical perspective on school placement. In T. N. Kluwin, D. F. Moores, & M. G. Gaustad (Eds.), *Toward effective public school programs for deaf students: Context, process, and outcomes.* New York, NY: Teachers College Press.

Moores, D. F. (1996). *Educating the deaf: Psychology, principles, and practices* (4th ed.). Boston, MA: Houghton Mifflin Co.

Mueller, H. G. (1994). CIC hearing aids: What is their impact on the occlusion effect? *The Hearing Journal, 47,* 29–30, 32–35.

Mueller, H., & Bender, D. (1988). Reasons for obtaining hearing aids: Do they relate to subsequent benefit? [Abstract]. *Corti's Organ, 11.*

Mueller, H., Bryant, M., Brown, W., & Budinger, A. (1991). Hearing aid selection for high-frequency hearing loss. In G. Studebaker, F. Bess, & L. Beck (Eds.), *The Vanderbilt Hearing-Aid Report II* (pp. 3551). Parkton, MD: York Press.

Mueller, H. G., & Grimes, A. (1987). Amplification systems for the hearing impaired. In J. G. Alpiner & P. A. McCarthy (Eds.), *Rehabilitative audiology: Children and adults* (pp. 116–162). Baltimore, MD: Williams and Williams.

Mulrow, C., Aguilar, C., & Endicott, J. (1990). Association between hearing impairment and the quality of life of elderly individuals. *Journal of the American Geriatric Society, 38,* 45–50.

Musselman, C., Wilson, A., & Lindsay, P. (1988). Effects of early intervention on hearing-impaired children. *Exceptional Children, 55,* 222–228.

National Center for Health Statistics. (1987). *Current estimates from the National Health Interview Survey: United States, 1987.* (Vital and Health Statistics. Series 10). Washington, DC: United States Government Printing Office.

Nevins, M. E., & Chute, P. M. (1996). *Children with cochlear implants in educational settings.* San Diego, CA: Singular Publishing Group.

Newby, H. A., & Popelka, G. R. (1992). *Audiology* (6th ed.). Englewood Cliffs, NJ: Prentice-Hall.

Nidday, K. J., & Elfenbein, J. L. (1991). The effects of visual barriers used during auditory training on sound transmission. *Journal of Speech and Hearing Research, 34,* 694–696.

Nix, G. W. (1983). How total is total communication? *Journal of British Association for Teachers of the Deaf, 7,* 177–181.

Nober, E. (1967). Articulation of the deaf. *Exceptional Children, 33,* 611–621.

Northcott, W. H. (1990). Mainstreaming: Roots and wings. In M. Ross (Ed.), *Hearing-impaired children in the mainstream* (pp. 1–26). Parkton, MD: York Press.

Northern, J., & Downs, M. P. (1991). *Hearing in children* (4th ed.). Baltimore, MD: Williams and Wilkins.

Nussbaum, J. F., Thompson, T., & Robinson, J. D. (1989). *Communication and aging.* New York, NY: Harper and Row.

Osberger, M. J., Robbins, A. M., Lybolt, J., Kent, R., & Peters, J. (1986). Speech evaluation. In M. J. Osberger (Ed.), *Language and learning skills of hearingimpaired students. ASHA Monographs, 23,* 24–31.

Osberger, M. J., Robbins, A. M., Todd, S. L., Riley, A. I., & Miyamoto, R. T. (1994). Speech production skills of children with multichannel cochlear implants. In I. J. Hochmair-Desoyer & E. S. Hochmair (Eds.), *Advances in cochlear implants* (pp. 503–508). Wien, Germany: Manz.

Parving, A. (1985). Hearing disorders in childhood: Some procedures for detection, idenification and diagnostic evaluation. *Pediatric Otorhinolaryngology, 9,* 31–57.

Pascoe, D. P. (1991). *Hearing aids: Who needs them?* St. Louis, MO: Big Bend Books.

Pascoe, D. P. (1995). Post-fitting and rehabilitative management of the adult hearing-aid user. In R. E. Sandlin (Ed.), *Handbook of hearing aid amplification* (Vol. 2, pp. 61–86). San Diego, CA: Singular Publishing Group.

Paul, P. V., & Jackson, D. W. (1993). *Toward a psychology of deafness.* Boston, MA: Allyn and Bacon.

Pederson, K. E., Rosenhall, U., & Moller, M. B. (1991). Longitudinal study of changes in speech perception between 70 and 81 years of age. *Audiology, 30,* 201–211.

Pichora-Fuller, M. K. (1997). Language comprehension in older listeners. *Journal of Speech-Language Pathology and Audiology, 21,* 125–142.

Pickett, J. M. (1980). *The sounds of speech communication: A primer of acoustic phonetics and speech perception.* Austin, TX: Pro-Ed.

Plath, P. (1991). Speech recognition in the elderly. *Acta Otolaryngology, 476*(Suppl.), 127–130.

Pollack, D. (1970). *Educational audiology for the limited hearing infant.* Springfield, IL: Charles C. Thomas.

Pratt, S. R., & Tye-Murray, N. (1997). Speech impairment secondary to hearing loss. In M. McNeil (Ed.), *The clinical management of sensorimotor speech disorders* (pp. 345–387). New York, NY: Thieme Medical Publishers, Inc.

Quigley, S. P., & Kretschmer, R. E. (1982). *The education of deaf children.* Austin, TX: Pro-Ed.

Quigley, S. P., Monranelli, D. S., & Wilbur, R. B. (1976). Some aspects of the verb system in the language of deaf students. *Journal of Speech and Hearing Research, 19,* 536–550.

Quigley, S. P., & Paul, P. V. (1984). *Language and deafness.* London, England: Croom Helm.

Quittner, A., & Steck, J. (1989, November). *Impact of hearing loss on child development and family adjustment.* Paper presented at the meeting of the American Speech-Language-Hearing Association, St. Louis, MO.

Reich, C., Hambleton, D., & Houldin, B. K. (1977). The integration of hearing-impaired children into regular classrooms. *American Annals of the Deaf, 122,* 534–543.

Reynell, J. K. (1977). *Reynell Development Language Scale.* Windsor, Ontario: NFER Publishing.

Ries, P.W. (1991). The demography of hearing loss. In H. Orlans (Ed.) *Adjustment to adult hearing loss* (2nd Edition), San Diego, CA: Singular Publishing Group, 3–22.

Robards-Armstrong, C., & Stone, H. E. (1994). Research in audiological rehabilitation: Current and future directions, the consumer's perspective. *Journal of the Academy of Rehabilitative Audiology 27*(Suppl.), 25–46.

Robb, M., & Pang-Ching, G. (1992). Relative timing characteristics of hearingimpaired speakers. *Journal of the Acoustical Society of America, 91,* 29542960.

Robinson, L. F., & Reis, H. T. (1989). The effects of interruption, gender, and status on interpersonal perceptions. *Journal of Nonverbal Behavior, 13,* 141–151.

Rosen, S. M., Fourcin, A. J., & Moore, B. C. J. (1981). Voice pitch as an aid to lipreading. *Nature, 291,* 150–152.

Ross, M. (1990). Definitions and descriptions. In J. Davis (Ed.), *Our forgotten children: Hard of hearing pupils in the schools.* Washington, DC: Self Help for Hard of Hearing People, Inc.

Ross, M., & Lerman, J. (1971). *Word Intelligibility by Picture Identification.* Pittsburgh, PA: Stanwix House, Inc.

Roush, J. (1994). Strengthening familyprofessional relations: Advice from parents. In J. Rousch & N. D. Matkin (Eds.), *Infants and toddlers with hearing loss* (pp. 337–350). Baltimore, MD: York Press, Inc.

Roush, J., & McWilliam, R. (1990). A new challenge for pediatric audiology: Public Law 99–457. *Journal of the American Academy of Audiology, 1,* 196–208.

Rubinstein, A., & Boothroyd, A. (1987). Effects of two approaches to auditory training on speech recognition by hearingimpaired adults. *Journal of Speech and Hearing Research, 30,* 153–160.

Sachs, J. S. (1967). Recognition memory for syntactic and semantic aspects of connected discourse. *Perception and Psychophysics, 12,* 437–442.

Samar, V., & Metz, D. (1988). Criterion validity of speech intelligibility ratingscale procedures for the hearing-impaired population. *Journal of Speech and Hearing Research, 31,* 307–316.

Samar, V. J., & Sims, D. G. (1983). Visual evoked response correlates of speechreading performance in normal–hearing adults: A replication and factor analytic extension. *Journal of Speech and Hearing Research, 26,* 2–9.

Scarborough, H. (1990). Index of productive syntax. *Applied Psycholinguistics, 11,* 122.

Scheetz, N. (1993). *Orientation to deafness,* Needham Heights, NJ: Allyn & Bacon.

Schegloff, E. A., & Sacks, J. S. (1973). Opening up closings. *Semiotica, 7,* 289327.

Schien, J., & Delk, M. (1974). *The deaf population of the United States.* Silver Spring, MD: National Association of the Deaf.

Schlesinger, H., & Acree, M. (1984). Antecedents to achievement and adjustment in deaf adolescents: A longitudinal study of deaf children. In G. B. Anderson & D. Watson (Eds.), *The habilitation and rehabilitation of deaf adolescents* (pp. 48–61). Washington, DC: The National Academy of Gallaudet College.

Schloss, P. J., & Smith, M. A. (1990). *Teaching social skills to hearingimpaired students.* Washington, DC: Alexander Graham Bell Association for the Deaf.

Schneider, B. (1997). Psychoacoustics and aging: Implications for everyday listening. *Journal of Speech-Language Pathology and Audiology, 21,* 111–124.

Schow, R., & Nerbonne, M. (1980). Hearing levels among elderly nursing home residents. *Journal of Speech and Hearing Disorders, 45,* 124–132.

Schulz, J. H. (1992). *The economics of aging* (5th ed.). New York, NY: Auburn.

Schum, L. K., & Tye-Murray, N. (1995). Alerting and assistive systems: Counseling implications for cochlear implant users. In R. S. Tyler & D. J. Schum (Eds.), *Assistive devices for persons with hearing impairment* (pp. 86122). Needham Heights, MD: Allyn and Bacon.

Schum, R. L. (1991). Communication and social growth: A developmental model of social behavior in deaf children. *Ear and Hearing, 12,* 320–327.

Schum, R., & Gfeller, K. (1994). Requisites for conversation: Engendering social skills. In N. Tye-Murray (Ed.), *Let's converse: A how-to-guide to develop and expand conversational skills of children and teenagers who are hearing impaired* (pp. 147–176). Washington, DC: Alexander Graham Bell Association for the Deaf.

Secord, W. (1981). *T-MAC: Test of Minimal Articulation Competence.* Columbus, OH: Charles E. Merrill.

Seyfried, D. N., & Kricos, P. B. (1996). Language and speech of the deaf and hard of hearing. In R. L. Schow & M. A. Nerbonne (Eds.), *Introduction to audiologic rehabilitation* (3rd ed. pp. 168228). Boston, MA: Allyn and Bacon.

Shatner, W. (1997). Sound of Silence. *People Magazine, 47,* 153–155.

Shepherd, D. (1982). Visual-neural correlates of speech-reading ability in normal-hearing adults: Reliability. *Journal of Speech and Hearing Research, 25,* 521–527.

Shepherd, D. C., de Lavergne, R. W., Fruneh, F. X., & Colbridge, C. (1977). Visualneural correlate of speech-reading abilities in normal-hearing adults. *Journal of Speech and Hearing Research, 20,* 752–765.

Shimon, D. A. (1992). *Coping with hearing loss and hearing aids.* San Diego, CA: Singular Publishing Group.

Shultz, D., & Mowry, R. B. (1995). Older adults in long-term care facilities. In P. B. Kricos & S. A. Lesner (Eds.), *Hearing care for the older adults: Audiologic rehabilitation* (pp. 167–179). Newton, MA: Butterworth-Heinemann.

Smith, C. (1975). Residual hearing and speech production in the deaf. *Journal of Speech and Hearing Research, 19,* 795–811.

Speaks, C. S., Jerger, J., & Trammell, J. (1970). Measurement of hearing handicap. *Journal of Speech and Hearing Research, 13,* 768–776.

Spencer, L. (1994). Some ways to nurture children's conversational and language skills.

In N. Tye-Murray (Ed.), *Let's converse: A how-to guide to develop and expand the conversational skills of children and teenagers who are hearing impaired* (pp. 51–84). Washington, DC: Alexander Graham Bell Association for the Deaf.

Sptizer, J. B. (1997). Cochlear implant and other options for persons with profound impairment. In H. T. Tobin (Ed.), *Practical hearing aid selection and fitting* (pp. 121–132). Washington, DC: Department of Veterans Affairs.

Staab, W. J. (1992). The peritympanic instrument: Fitting rationale and test results. *The Hearing Journal, 45,* 21–26.

Stach, B. A. (1997). *Comprehensive dictionary of audiology illustrated.* Baltimore, MD: Williams & Wilkins.

Stephens, D., & Hetu, R. (1991). Impairment, disability, and handicap in audiology: Towards a consensus. *Audiology, 30,* 185–200.

Stoel-Gammon, C. (1988). Prelinguistic vocalizations of hearing-impaired and normally hearing subjects: A comparison of consonantal inventories. *Journal of Speech and Hearing Disorders, 53,* 302315.

Stouffer, J.L. and Tyler, R.S. (1990). Characterization of tinnitus by tinnitus patients. *Journal of Speech and Hearing Disorders, 55,* 439–453.

Stout, G., & Windel, J. (1992). Developmental approach to successful listening II. Englewood, CO: Resource Point, Inc.

Strawbridge, W. J., Cohen, R. D., Shemna, S. J., & Kaplan, G. A. (1996). Successful aging: Predictors and associated activities. *American Journal of Epidemiology, 144,* 135–141.

Subtelny, J. D., Orlando, N. A., & Whitehead, R. L. (1981). *Speech and voice characteristics of the deaf.* Washington, DC: Alexander Graham Bell Association for the Deaf.

Summerfield, Q. (1989). Visual perception of phonetic gestures. In I. G. Mattingly (Ed.), *Modularity and the motor theory of speech perception* (pp. 117–137). Hillsdale, NJ: Laurence Erbaum Associates.

Summerfield, Q. (1992). Lipreading and audiovisual speech perception. *Phil. Royal Society of London,* 71–78.

Sutherland, G. (1995). Increasing consumer acceptance of assistive devices. In R. S. Tyler & D. J. Schum (Eds.), *Assistive devices for persons with hearing impairment* (pp. 251–266). Needham Heights, MD: Allyn and Bacon.

Teele, D., Klein, J., & Rosner, B. (1989). Epidemiology of otitis media during the first seven years of life in children in greater Boston. *Journal of Infectious Diseases, 160,* 83–94.

Thomas, A. and Herbst, K.G. (1980). Social and psychological implications of acquired deafness for adults of employment age. *British Journal of Audiology,* 14, 76–85.

Thorn, F., & Thorn, S. (1989). Speechreading with reduced vision: A problem of aging. *Journal of Optometry Society of America, 6,* 491–499.

Tillman, T. W., & Carhart, R. (1966). *An expanded test for speech discrimination utilizing CNC monosyllabic words: Northwestern University Auditory Test No. 6.* [Technical Report No. SAM-TR-6655. USAF School of Aerospace Medicine]. San Antonio, TX: Brooks Air Force Base.

Tobey, E., Geers, A. E., & Brenner, C. (1994). Speech production results: Speech feature acquisition. *Volta Review, 96,* 109–129.

Tong, Y. C., Busby, P. A., & Clark, G. M. (1988). Perceptual studies on cochlear implant patients with early onset of profound hearing impairment prior to normal development of auditory, speech, and language skills. *Journal of the Acoustical Society of America, 84,* 951–962.

Traynor, R. M. (1995). Financial and marketing considerations in the rehabilitation of older adults. In P. B. Kricos & S. A. Lesner (Eds.), *Hearing care for the older adults: Audiologic rehabilitation* (pp. 185–202). Newton, MA: BuHerworth-Heinemann.

Trybus, R. J., & Karchmer, M. A. (1977). School achievement scores of hearingimpaired children: National data on achievement status and growth patterns. *American Annals of the Deaf, 122,* 6269.

Trychin, S. (1987a). *Did I do that?* (manual). Washington DC: Gallaudet University Press.

Trychin, S. (1987b). *Did I do that?* [videotape]. Washington DC: Gallaudet University Press.

Trychin, S. (1994). Helping people cope with hearing loss. In J. G. Clark & F. N. Martin (Eds.), *Effective counseling in audiology: Perspectives and practice* (pp. 247277). Englewood Cliffs, NJ: Simon and Schuster Co.

Tullos, D. C. (1990). Strategies for assessing and training social skillsfacilitator behavior. In P. J. Schloss & M. A. Smith (Eds.), *Teaching social skills to hearing-impaired students* (pp. 45–57). Washington, DC: Alexander Graham Bell Association for the Deaf.

Tye-Murray, N. (1987). Effects of vowel context on the articulatory closure postures of deaf speakers. *Journal of Speech and Hearing Research, 30,* 90–104.

Tye-Murray, N. (1991). The establishment of open articulatory postures by deaf and hearing talkers. *Journal of Speech and Hearing Research, 34,* 453–459.

Tye-Murray, N. (1992a). Communication therapy. In N. Tye-Murray (Ed.), *Children with cochlear implants: A handbook for parents, teachers and speech and hearing professionals* (pp. 137–168). Washington, DC: Alexander Graham Bell Association for the Deaf.

Tye-Murray, N. (1992b). Auditory training. In N. Tye-Murray (Ed.), *Children with cochlear implants: A handbook for parents, teachers and speech and hearing professionals* (pp. 91–114). Washington, DC: Alexander Graham Bell Association for the Deaf.

Tye-Murray, N. (1992c). Speechreading training. In N. Tye-Murray (Ed.), *Children with cochlear implants: A handbook for parents, teachers and speech and hearing professionals* (pp. 115–136). Washington, DC: Alexander Graham Bell Association for the Deaf.

Tye-Murray, N. (1992d). Teaching speech perception skills: General guidelines. In N. Tye-Murray (Ed.), *Children with cochlear implants: A handbook for parents, teachers and speech and hearing professionals* (pp. 79–90). Washington, DC: Alexander Graham Bell Association for the Deaf.

Tye-Murray, N. (1993a). *Cochlear implants: Audiological foundations.* San Diego, CA: Singular Publishing.

Tye-Murray, N. (1993b). *Communication training for hearing-impaired children and teenagers: Speechreading, listening, and using repair strategies.* Austin, TX; Pro-Ed.

Tye-Murray, N. (1994a). Some conversation strategies for adults who interact with hard-of-hearing children. In N. TyeMurray (Ed.), *Let's converse! A how-to guide to develop and expand the conversational skills of children and teenagers who are hearing impaired* (pp. 11–50). Washington, DC: Alexander Graham Bell Association for the Deaf.

Tye-Murray, N. (1994b). Communication breakdowns in conversations: Adultinitiated repair strategies. In N. TyeMurray (Ed.), *Let's converse! A how-to guide to develop and expand the conversational skills of children and teenagers who are hearing impaired* (pp. 85–121). Washington, DC: Alexander Graham Bell Association.

Tye-Murray, N. (1994c). Communication therapy. In N. Tye-Murray (Ed.), *Let's converse! A how-to guide to develop and expand the conversational skills of children and teenagers who are hearing impaired* (pp. 137–168). Washington, DC: Alexander Graham Bell Association for the Deaf.

Tye-Murray, N. (1997). *Communication strategies training for older adults and teenagers.* Austin, TX: Pro-Ed.

Tye-Murray, N., & Folkins, J. (1990). Jaw and lip movements of deaf talkers producing utterances with known stress patterns. *Journal of the Acoustical Society of America, 87,* 2675–2683.

Tye-Murray, N., & Fryauf-Bertschy, H. (1992). Auditory training. In N. TyeMurray (Ed.), *Children with cochlear implants: A handbook for parents, teachers and speech and hearing professionals.* Washington, DC: Alexander Graham Bell Association for the Deaf.

Tye-Murray, N., & Geers, A. (1997). *The Children's Speechreading Enhancement Test (CHIVE).* St. Louis, MO: Central Institute for the Deaf.

Tye-Murray, N., Knutson, J. F., & Lemke, J. (1993). Assessment of communication strategies use: Questionnaires and daily diaries. *Seminars in Hearing, 14,* 338–353.

Tye-Murray, N., Purdy, S. C., & Woodworth, G. (1992). The reported use of communication strategies by members of SHHH and its relationship to client, talker, and situational variables. *Journal of Speech and Hearing Research, 35,* 708–717.

Tye-Murray, N., Purdy, S. C., Woodworth, G., & Tyler, R. S. (1990). Effects of repair strategies on visual identification of sentences. *Journal of Speech and Hearing Disorders, 55,* 621–627.

Tye-Murray, N., Spencer, L., Witt, S., & Bedia, E. G. (1997). *Cochlear implant rehabilitation* (pp. 65–82). Basel, Switzerland: Karger Publishing Co.

Tye-Murray, N., Spencer, L., & Woodworth, G. (1995). Acquisition of speech by children who have prolonged cochlear implant experience. *Journal of Speech and Hearing Research, 38,* 327–337.

Tye-Murray, N., Tomblin, B., & Spencer, L., November (1997). Speech and language acquisition over time in children with cochlear implants. Paper presented at the American Speech-Language Hearing Convention. Boston, MA.

Tye-Murray, N., & Tyler, R. (1988). A critique of continuous discourse tracking as a test procedure. *Journal of Speech and Hearing Disorders, 53,* 226–231.

Tye-Murray, N., Tyler, R., Bong, B., & Nares, T. (1988). Using laser videodisc technology to train speechreading and assertive listening skills. *Journal of the Academy of Rehabilitative Audiology, 21,* 143–152.

Tye-Murray, N., Tyler, R., Woodworth, G., & Gantz, B. J. (1992). Performance over time with a multichannel cochlear implant. *Ear and Hearing, 13,* 200–209.

Tye-Murray, N., & Witt, S. (1996). Conversational moves and conversational styles of adult cochlear-implant users. *Journal of the Academy of Rehabilitative Audiology, 29,* 11–25.

Tye-Murray, N., Witt, S., & Castelloe, J. (1996). Initial evaluation of an interactive test of sentence gist recognition. *Journal of the American Academy of Audiology, 7,* 396–405.

Tye-Murray, N., Witt, S., & Schum, L. (1995). Effects of talker familiarity on communication breakdown in conversation with adult cochlear-implant users. *Ear and Hearing, 16,* 459–469.

Tye-Murray, N., Witt, S., Schum, L., & Sobaski, C. (1995). Communication breakdowns: Partner contingencies and partner reactions. *Journal of the Academy of Rehabilitative Audiology, 25,* 1–27.

Tye-Murray, N., Zimmermann, G., & Folkins, J. (1987). Movement timing in deaf and hearing speakers: Comparison of phonetically heterogeneous syllable strings. *Journal of Speech and Hearing Research, 30,* 411–417.

Tyler, R. (1993). Speech perception by children. In R. Tyler (Ed.), *Cochlear implants: Audiological foundations* (pp. 191–256). San Diego, CA: Singular Publishing Group.

Tyler, R., Fryauf-Bertschy, H., & Kelsay, D. (1991). *Audiovisual Feature Test for Young Children.* Iowa City: The University of Iowa Hospitals and Clinics.

Tyler, R., Preece, J., & Tye-Murray, N. (1986). *The Iowa phoneme and sentence tests.* Iowa City: The University of Iowa Hospitals and Clinics.

Tyler, R.S. and Baker, L.J. (1983). Difficulties experienced by tinnitus sufferers. *Journal of Speech and Hearing Disorders, 48,* 150–154.

U.S. Department of Commerce Bureau of the Census. (1986). *Statistical abstract of the U.S.* (106th ed.). Washington, DC: Government Printing Office.

U.S. Department of Labor CFR 29, 1910.95. (1983). Occupational noise exposure standard. *Code of Federal Regulations,* Title 29, Chapter XVII part 1910, Subpart G, 48FR9776, March 8,1983.

U.S. Public Health Service. (1990). *Healthy People 2000.* Washington, DC: Government Printing Office.

Van Hecke, M. (1994). Emotional responses to hearing loss. In J.G. Clark and F.N. Martin (Eds.) *Effective Counseling in Audiology: Perspectives and practice.* Englewood Cliffs, N.J.: Prentice-Hall Inc., 92–115.

van Uden, A. (1988). Interrelating reception and expression in speechreading training. *Volta Review, 90,* 261–272.

Ventry, I., & Weinstein, B. (1982). The Hearing Inventory for the Elderly: A new tool. *Ear and Hearing, 3,*128.

Ventry, I., & Weinstein, B. (1983). Identification of elderly people with hearing problems. *Asha, 25,* 37–47.

Vergara, K. C., & Miskiel, L. W. (1994). CHATS: *The Miami cochlear implant, auditory and tactile skills curriculum.* Miami, FL: Intelligent Hearing Systems.

Vinding, T. (1989). Age-related macular degeneration. Macular changes, prevalence, and sex ratio. *Acta Ophthalmology, 67,* 609–616.

Voeks, S., Gallagher, C., Langer, E., & Drinka, P. (1990). Hearing loss in the nursing home: An institutional issue. *Journal of the American Geriatrics Society, 38,* 141–145.

Voelker, C. (1938). An experimental study of the comparative rate of utterances of deaf and normal-hearing speakers. *American Annals of the Deaf, 83,* 274284.

Wagner, D. and Abrahamson, J. (1996). Learning to hear again: An audiological rehabilitation curriculum guide. Austin, TX: Hear Again.

Walden, B. E., Erdman, S. A., Montgomery, A. A., Schwartz, D. M., & Prosek, R. A. (1981). Effects of training on the visual recognition of consonants. *Journal of Speech and Hearing Research, 20,* 130145.

Walden, B. E., Prosek, R. A., Montgomery, A. A., Scherr, C. K., & Jones, C. J. (1977). Effects of training on the visual recognition of concepts. *Journal of Speech and Hearing Research, 20,* 130145.

Waltzman, S., Cohen, N., Gomolin, R., Green, J., Shapiro, W., Brackett, D., & Zara, C. (1997). Perception and production results in children implanted between 2 and 5 years of age. *Advances in OtoRhino-Laryngology, 52,* 177–180.

Wardhaugh, R. (1985). *How conversation works.* New York, NY: Blackwell.

Wayner, D. S., & Abrahamson, J. E. (1996). *Learning to hear again.* Austin, TX: Hear Again.

Weinstein, B. E. (1991). The quantification of hearing aid benefit in the elderly: The role of self-assessment measures. *Acta Otolaryngology, 476*(Suppl.), 257–261.

Weinstein, B. E., & Ventry, I. M. (1983). Audiometric correlates of the Hearing Handicap Inventory for the Elderly. *Journal of Speech and Hearing Disorders, 48,* 379–384.

White, S. (1984). *Antecedents of language functioning in the deaf: Implicationsfor early intervention. Project summary* (EDD0001). Washington, DC: U.S. Department of Education.

White, S., & White, R. (1987). The effects of hearing status of the family and age of intervention on reception and expressive oral language skills in hearing-impaired infants. In H. Levitt, N. S. McGarr, & D. Geffner (Eds.), *Development of language and communication skills in hearingimpaired children.* Washington, DC: ASHA.

Whitehead, R., & Barefoot, S. (1980). Some aerodynamic characteristics of plosive consonants produced by hearing-impaired speakers. *American Annals of the Deaf, 125,* 366–373.

Williams-Scott, B., & Kipila, E. (1987). Cued speech: A professional point of view. In S. Schwartz (Ed.), *Choices in deafness: A parent's guide.* Washington, DC: Woodbine House.

Williamson, J. D., & Fired, M. D. (1996). Characterization of older adults who attribute functional decrements to "old age." *Journal of the American Geriatrics Society, 44,* 1429–1434.

Willott, J. F. (1996). Anatomic and physiologic aging: A behavioral neuroscience perspective. *Journal of the American Academy of Audiology, 7,* 141151.

Witt, S. (1997). *Effectiveness of an intensive aural rehabilitation program for adult cochlear implant users: A demonstration project.* Unpublished master's thesis. University of Iowa, Iowa City.

Wolff, A. B., & Harkins, J. E. (1986). Multihandicapped students. In A. N. Schildroth & M. A. Karchmer (Eds.), *Deaf children in America* (pp. 55–82). San Diego, CA: College-Hill Press.

Wood, D., Wood, H., Griffiths, A., & Howarth, I. (1986). *Teaching and talking with deaf children.* New York, NY: John Wiley and Sons.

Woodward, M. F., & Barber, C. G. (1960). Phoneme perception in lipreading. *Journal of Speech and Hearing Research, 17,* 212–222.

World Health Organization. (1980). *International classification of impairments, disabilities, and handicaps: A manual of classification relating to the consequences of disease.* Geneva, Switzerland: World Health Organization.

Wylde, M. A. (1982). The remediation process: Psychologic and counseling aspects. In J. G. Alpiner (Ed.), *Handbook of adult rehabilitation audiology* (2nd ed.). Baltimore, MD: Williams and Wilkins.

Yoshinaga-Itano, C. (1988). Speechreading instruction for children. *Volta Review, 90,* 241–260.

Yoshinaga-Itano, C., & Downey, D. M. (1996). Development of school-aged deaf, hard-of-hearing and normally hearing students' written language. *Volta Review, 98,* 3–7.

Yoshinaga-Itano, C., & Ruberry, J. (1992). The Colorado individual performance profile for hearing-impaired students: A data driven approach to decision making. *Volta Review, 95,* 159–187.

Yoshinaga-Itano, C., Snyder, L. S., & Mayberry, R. (1996). How deaf and normally hearing students convey meaning within and between written sentences. *Volta Review, 98,* 9–38.

Zones, J., Estes, C., & Binney, E. (1987). Gender, public policy and the oldest old. *Aging Society, 7,* 275–302.

Index